NEONATOLOGY AND LA
MEDICINE

Anne Green PhD, FRSC, FRCPath, FIBiol, FRCPCH
Consultant Paediatric Clinical Biochemist, Birmingham Children's Hospital, Birmingham, UK

Imogen Morgan FRCPCH, FRCP(Lond), FRCP(Glasg), DCH
Consultant Neonatologist, Birmingham Women's Hospital, Birmingham, UK

Jim Gray MB ChB, MRCP(UK), FRCPath
Consultant Medical Microbiologist, Birmingham Children's Hospital, Birmingham, UK

Editors:
Beverley Harris BSc, MSc, DipRCPath
Principal Biochemist, Royal United Hospital, Bath, UK

William Marshall, FRCP, FRCPath, FRCPEdin, FIBiol
Reader in Clinical Biochemistry, King's College Hospital, London, UK

ACB VENTURE PUBLICATIONS
with generous support from HemoCue

ACB VENTURE PUBLICATIONS
Chairman - Roy Sherwood

British Library Cataloguing in Publication Data

A catalogue record for the book is available from the British Library

ISBN 0 902429 41 8 ACB Venture Publications

Cover design by Alan Sherwood of burntcanvasdesign, Kent,
www.burntcanvasdesign.btinternet.co.uk

Layout and typesetting by Roy Sherwood in Palatino.

Printed by KSC Printers, Tunbridge Wells, Kent

Preface

The purpose of this monograph is to bring together those aspects of laboratory medicine that are particularly relevant to the investigation and management of the neonate. The book has been expanded from the first edition, which previously only considered clinical biochemistry. We have aimed to provide the reader with a series of clinical situations covering the fetal and neonatal period, and guide the use of laboratory tests in this context. We thank Venture Publications for providing this platform and are indebted to Beverley Harris and William Marshall, our editors, for their help, support and editorial skill.

This book is intended to be a basic handbook for junior doctors, laboratory scientists and neonatal nurses, who require background information and a practical approach to the management of common problems in neonates.

We are extremely grateful to our many clinical colleagues, and staff in the Paediatric Laboratory Medicine and Neonatal Departments at both Birmingham Children's Hospital and Birmingham Women's Hospital respectively, especially Dr Daisy Obeid, Consultant Haematologist, and Mrs Susan Standing, Consultant Biochemist, for help with some of the detail. We also thank Dr John Puntis, Senior Lecturer in Paediatrics and Child Health, Neonatal Unit, Leeds General Infirmary, for help and advice with the chapter on parenteral nutrition. Finally, our thanks go to Mary Dowling for her excellent secretarial skills, which have supported us throughout the writing phase.

Anne Green, Imogen Morgan and Jim Gray
April 2003

ACKNOWLEDGEMENTS

The authors are grateful to the following for permission to reproduce or adapt material for certain figures used in this publication:

Annals of Clinical Biochemistry 1988; 25: 199-209 (Fig 10.7)

Churchill Livingstone, Paediatric Haematology 1977, Michael L N Willoughby

Dr Mario Werner and John Wiley and Sons, Microtechniques for the Clinical Laboratory; Concepts and Applications 1976, (Fig 10.2)

Hodder and Stoughton Ltd, Paediatric Vade Mecum, 12th edition, Editor Jack Insley, 1990 (Figs 6.2 and 7.3)

Mark Allen Publishing Ltd, Brit J Hosp Med 1989, 41: 426-34 (Figs 10.5 and 10.9)

The Lancet Ltd, Blumenfield TA, Turi GK, Blanc WA, Lancet 1979, Feb 3 230-33 (Fig A.1)

Elsevier, Haematology of Infancy and Childhood 3rd edition 1987, Nathan DG, Oski FA (Haematology reference ranges)

Elsevier, Care of the High Risk Neonate 5th edition 2001, Klaus MH, Fanaroff AA (Haematology reference ranges)

The authors are grateful to colleagues at Birmingham Children's Hospital and Birmingham Women's Hospital who contributed to the production of the reference range data.

Contents

Chapter 1

Neonatology for the non-specialist

Of the nearly 700,000 babies born annually in the UK, about 5% will require admission to a neonatal unit. Many admissions are brief. The commonest reason for prolonged admission is prematurity. Other reasons include poor condition at birth, congenital abnormality, postnatal problems, or anticipated postnatal difficulties such as known Rhesus incompatibility.

Neonatal units are categorised (1, 2, 3, 4) according to the complexity of care they offer (see later). The obstetric services offered on the same site will be appropriately provided to take account of this categorisation. For instance, a small district general hospital with a Category 1 neonatal service will not be able to undertake prolonged intensive care of newborns, nor is it likely to have the consultant expertise to deal with complex obstetric cases. Women booking with such a service might have their care transferred during pregnancy if there were an abnormality, or if preterm delivery were anticipated. A sick baby born at such a location would usually be resuscitated and stabilised on site, then collected by a transport team and taken to a tertiary service with appropriate and available facilities.

All units where babies are delivered, therefore, must have laboratory facilities for immediate analysis for blood gases, basic biochemistry (glucose, bilirubin, electrolytes); coagulation (fibrinogen, prothrombin time (PT), activated partial thromboplastin time (APTT)) and full blood count; microscopy of urine or CSF, and standard microbiology facilities to culture neonatal blood and urine specimens.

Although a 'neonate' is a baby in the first four weeks of life, neonatal care covers a much wider age range than this. Very ill or preterm babies – from a minimum of 23-24 weeks gestation – may require intensive care for several weeks, followed by high dependency care, then specialised support care, then pre-home preparation. In all, their stay in the neonatal unit may be 3-4 months.

After discharge, the baby may still be receiving treatment at home, such as medication or oxygen (for the management of chronic lung disease).

Community follow-up by neonatal nurses and the primary care team is accompanied by outpatient follow-up for months or years. These provisions are mainly required for babies who weighed less than one kilogram at birth.

POSTNATAL WARD AND COMMUNITY CARE

About one third of babies will develop visible jaundice (equivalent to a plasma bilirubin of approximately 80 μmol/L). This usually appears on the second day or later and has resolved by day 10, though later than this in breast-fed babies. In a well infant, in the first 14 days, no investigation is indicated. If the baby is unwell, or the jaundice is severe, or if the baby is clinically jaundiced on day 1 or after day 14, then clinical examination is required, plasma bilirubin (total and conjugated) should be measured, and other investigations will be indicated (*see Chapter 6*).

Hypoglycaemia may develop postnatally, particularly in certain subgroups of babies (*see Chapter 7*). Asymptomatic hypoglycaemia has not been proven to be harmful when other fuels are available and can be utilised by the baby's brain. Symptomatic hypoglycaemia is an emergency, requiring prompt treatment.

Surveillance monitoring of whole blood glucose in at-risk babies from birth is used to detect low concentrations (less than 2 mmol/L) so that management can be initiated – for instance early or frequent feeding – to prevent development of a very low glucose concentration (less than 1.4 mmol/L) requiring immediate correction, or the appearance of symptoms.

Three hourly monitoring of whole blood glucose before feeds, by stix testing, should be provided for the following groups:

- birth weight below 10th centile
- preterm < 37 weeks
- low Apgar score (0-3) at 1 minute
- hypothermia
- infants of diabetic mothers.

Other at-risk babies are likely to be already on the neonatal unit and, therefore, undergoing glucose monitoring.

Most babies born at term require no routine haematological or microbiological testing, and the only blood sample that will be required is for neonatal screening tests, which are, in the UK, taken by heelprick, usually in the community, at around six days (*see Chapter 9*).

If there has been prolonged rupture of the membranes and the baby is delivered before 36 weeks, surface swabs and a gastric aspirate are taken for microbial culture.

NEONATAL UNITS

Babies with particular nursing or medical requirements in the newborn period are brought together in specialised wards. In the UK, these are always on the same site as a maternity unit but this is not the case worldwide. In the USA, for instance, babies are often transported from the unit of delivery to a different hospital if they require intensive care.

Nurses on neonatal units have specialised training in the disorders of the newborn. Medical staff are paediatricians. A Category 2 or 3 unit will have 24 hour cover by a neonatal specialist. Many large neonatal units share services, and sometimes staffing, with a neonatal surgical service, so that the medical aspects of care – for instance, parenteral nutrition – can be shared.

Reasons for admission – either from the delivery room or from the postnatal ward – are listed below. Most units have strict criteria for readmitting babies from home because of the risk of introducing viral infection. Such readmissions are always to an isolation area within the unit.

Babies requiring admission to a neonatal unit may have any of the following conditions:

- severe birth asphyxia (still depressed at 5 minutes)
- obvious congenital abnormality requiring early surgery
- weight < 1.7 kg or gestation < 34 weeks
- illness requiring investigation or treatment
- tachypnoea > 60 per minute
- cyanosis
- persistent or symptomatic hypoglycaemia
- at-risk because of maternal illness or behaviour, e.g. addiction
- requirement for parenteral nutrition
- dying, if ward or home facility not available.

Babies not usually requiring admission to a neonatal unit include:

- well, operatively delivered babies
- babies with Down's syndrome who are well
- babies with cleft lip or palate who can feed

- babies with transiently low Apgar scores who have recovered
- well infants of diabetic mothers.

LEVELS OF CARE

Neonatal units are specially staffed and equipped according to their ability to provide different levels of care. Category 1 units provide short term (stabilising) intensive care only, in addition to high dependency and special care. Category 2 units provide full intensive care for babies born on site. Category 3 units transport babies in from elsewhere for intensive care and may include a neonatal surgical service. Category 4 is used in USA classifications and refers to units with ECMO (extracorporeal membrane oxygenation) and NO (inhaled nitric oxide treatment) on site in addition to the above. The British Association of Perinatal Medicine has recently (2001) redefined appropriate care levels.

Intensive care is required for:

- intubated babies and for 24 hours after extubation
- all babies < 1000 g receiving nasal continuous positive airways pressure (CPAP) and for 24 hours after
- babies receiving nasal CPAP who fulfil other categories
- babies with respiratory distress requiring > 60% O_2, age < 48 hours
- babies of gestation < 29 weeks, age < 48 hours
- babies requiring inotrope, pulmonary vasodilator, or prostaglandin infusion, and for 24 hours after treatment
- pre-operative babies and for 48 hours post-operatively (emergency surgery)
- babies on the day of death
- babies being transported by a medical and nursing team
- babies undergoing peritoneal dialysis
- babies undergoing exchange transfusion.

High dependency care is required for:

- babies receiving nasal CPAP who do not fulfil the categories above
- babies less than 1000 g who do not fulfil the categories above
- babies receiving parenteral nutrition
- babies with convulsions

- babies being transported by a trained nurse
- babies with an arterial catheter or a chest drain
- babies with respiratory disease requiring 40-60% O_2
- babies with apnoeas requiring any resuscitation
- babies more than 48 hours post-operatively and requiring complex nursing
- babies with a tracheostomy (first 2 weeks)
- babies receiving a partial exchange transfusion
- babies receiving treatment for neonatal abstinence syndrome.

Special care is required for:

- babies requiring continuous monitoring of heart rate or respiration
- babies receiving added oxygen
- babies with a tracheostomy after first 2 weeks
- babies receiving intravenous treatment with glucose or electrolyte solutions
- babies being fed via nasogastric tube
- babies < 24 hours after minor surgery
- barrier nursing
- babies requiring phototherapy (sometimes administered on the postnatal ward using a light-emitting mattress or blanket)
- special monitoring, e.g. frequent glucose or bilirubin estimation
- babies receiving antibiotic treatment.

SURVIVAL

Figure 1.1 shows typical figures for survival to discharge of babies admitted to a tertiary UK neonatal service (Birmingham Women's Hospital's Neonatal Unit, 2000).

Most deaths are in the first week of life, with an excess on the first day. The commonest cause of death in premature babies remains respiratory distress syndrome and its complications, despite the use of prenatal steroids and postnatal exogenous surfactant.

Survival to discharge

Birth weight band (g)	Number of babies	% Survivors
<750	28	72
750-999	29	86
1000-1499	85	93
1500-1999	104	99
2000-2499	113	100
>2500	262	98
Total	621	96
Gestation band (weeks)	**Number of babies**	**% Survivors**
<25	13	62
25-26	13	84
27-28	37	79
29-30	48	95
31-32	73	98
33-34	117	99
35-36	98*	100
>36	222*	98
Total	621	96

*most babies >34 weeks are cared for on a transitional care ward beside their mothers, or at 36 weeks and beyond, on the postnatal ward, until discharge

Figure 1.1 Survival to discharge, babies admitted to Birmingham Women's Hospital's Neonatal Unit, 2000

ETHICS AND CONSENT

In the UK, explicit consent from parents for intensive neonatal care treatment is not routinely requested or required, unless the baby is to undergo a surgical procedure. It is, however, vital that parents are kept informed about all aspects of their baby's care. An explanatory booklet given on admission is the usual way in which parents can be helped to understand the equipment and treatments their baby will require.

Documentation in the records of discussions with parents is extremely important, and information may have to be repeated several times. When parents can understand the basis on which decisions are made, they are much more likely to accept these as being in their baby's interests.

Specific situations arise in which the welfare of the baby must take precedence over parents' expressed wishes, such as in a lifesaving emergency situation or, for instance, when parents' beliefs preclude blood transfusion and this treatment is felt to be very important. Where possible these can be anticipated and discussed in advance. At least two senior clinicians should document the need for a particular treatment if parents are not in accord, and Social Services may need to be involved in child protection issues.

In some cases, initiation of, or continuation of, neonatal intensive care is not in the baby's best interests. This decision should be made by the clinical team, on the basis of good evidence. This situation may arise, for instance, with the delivery of an extremely premature baby – 23 weeks gestation or below – whose chances of intact survival are very poor, and for whom even active resuscitation at birth may not be appropriate. Such situations, where they can be anticipated, are best managed by discussion between the parents and a senior paediatrician in advance.

BIOCHEMICAL CHANGES IN THE PERINATAL PERIOD

The birth process and the adjustment of the newborn to independent life have a major effect on the production, metabolism and excretion of many metabolites, hormones and enzymes. Rapid growth and maturation, particularly of the liver and kidney, further modify these parameters over ensuing weeks.

Consequently, reference ranges for biochemical analytes in neonates not only differ from those in infants and older children, but many of them change significantly during the first four weeks of life. Differences in solute intake, e.g. breast or bottle feeding, make an additional contribution to reference range variability. It is particularly important to appreciate these changes when interpreting the results of biochemical tests in the neonate.

Available data on reference ranges are limited for ethical and logistical reasons: they often relate either to cord blood, or to blood collected at around six days (in the UK) as part of the neonatal screening programme. Changes in instrument technology or methodology may invalidate historical data. Reference data provided in this book are intended to be a guide only and are no substitute for good data provided by the local laboratory.

BIRTH PROCESS

The stress of birth provides the stimulus required by the baby to begin the process of adaptation to survival outside the womb. This stress response brings about marked changes in hormone secretion: plasma concentrations of TSH, thyroxine and cortisol are markedly increased in the first twenty four hours of life compared with those found in older babies.

In response to these processes, the term baby mobilises fuel and regulates its metabolism appropriately to maintain homeostasis. By contrast, the preterm or poorly grown baby has a much poorer ability to regulate metabolic processes for energy production.

The process of vaginal delivery causes release of enzymes from muscle. There is a rapid, marked rise in plasma creatine kinase activity immediately after birth, followed by a decline over the first week. Awareness of this is important when investigating for Duchenne muscular dystrophy.

MATERNAL CONTRIBUTIONS

At birth, the biochemistry of the baby's plasma resembles the mother's in many respects, with modifications due to placental function. Any secondary abnormality, for instance, elevated bilirubin or creatinine secondary to maternal disease, may take several days to revert to normal owing to low neonatal glomerular filtration rates.

Plasma concentrations of hormones, metabolites and proteins that are maternal in origin fall sharply after birth. 17-hydroxyprogesterone and cortisol fall over the first 24-48 hours. Therefore, use of these parameters for diagnosis of congenital adrenal hyperplasia, for example, is therefore difficult in the first few days of life.

As the infant begins to increase its own protein synthesis (e.g. of immunoglobulins, caeruloplasmin) the concentrations of these gradually increase over ensuing weeks or months.

The placenta actively transports calcium to the fetus via placental vitamin D, (the fetus acquires about 3.7 mmoL (150 mg)/kg/24h throughout the 3rd trimester) and, therefore, plasma concentrations before and at birth will be slightly higher than maternal, decreasing in the subsequent 24 to 48 hours. Total alkaline phosphatase activity is elevated at birth owing to the presence of placental enzyme, and, therefore, is only of value as a marker of nutritional assessment after the first week.

Plasma proteins, which are not freely diffusable across the placenta, have very variable concentrations at birth. They can be affected by fetal nutrition and well-being. The only protein measured routinely in neonatal units is albumin, which can serve as an indicator of inadequate intake of protein and energy. Plasma values can vary at birth from 20 g/L in a growth-restricted, preterm baby, to 40 g/L in a well grown term infant. Lower concentrations in preterm infants are thought to reflect rapid turnover of a small plasma pool rather than decreased synthesis.

FEEDING REGIMEN

Plasma urea is higher in formula-fed than in breast-fed infants, and some amino acid concentrations differ depending on whether the milk is predominantly a curd based or a whey based formula, reflecting the protein content. Plasma and urinary osmolality vary according to the overall solute load. Historical reference values may relate to babies fed with higher protein formulae than those used now.

MATURATION OF ORGAN FUNCTION

Changes in kidney function have a marked effect on plasma creatinine concentration. This, therefore, depends on gestational age as well as actual age. Renal tubular function matures over the first six months, resulting in markedly different ranges for urinary amino acid and phosphate excretion during this period.

Some proteins (e.g. α-fetoprotein) and enzymes are specific to the fetus and are not produced by the baby. Deficiency of the fetal isoenzyme of cytochrome C oxidase may cause a transient lactic acidosis in infancy. The same phenomenon may account for other transient 'abnormalities' that resolve spontaneously as the infant matures. Relative immaturity of tissue enzyme systems will cause a different profile of metabolites at different ages. For example, a stressed preterm baby will have increased concentrations of cortisol precursors, but not of cortisol, owing to immaturity of the steroid synthesis pathway.

SPECIAL CHARACTERISTICS OF NEONATAL LABORATORY SAMPLES

NEONATAL BLOOD

The blood volume of a term neonate is about 275 mL, while a premature baby weighing 1 kg will have a blood volume of only 80 mL.

At birth, neonates have a relatively high haemoglobin and haematocrit, which rise further in the first 12 hours owing to redistribution of extracellular fluid from plasma to interstitial spaces. Normal haemoglobin values for cord blood at term average 16.8 g/dL, rising to 18.4 g/dL after 24 hours. Equivalent haematocrits average 53% for cord blood, 58% after 24 hours (Figure 1.2). Plasma volume in a well baby remains constant at about 50 mL/kg. This high neonatal haematocrit means that the plasma yield (for testing) from a given blood volume is up to 30% lower for a neonate than for an older child or adult.

The volume of extracellular fluid, about 40% of body weight at birth in the full term infant, falls to 35% over the first 5 days of life, contributing to normal post-natal weight loss. These values have implications for the number and size of blood samples that can safely be taken, particularly from a very low birth weight (<1500 g) baby (Figure 1.3).

In babies requiring intensive care, the volumes of blood taken should be monitored, and blood replaced by transfusion if the haemoglobin falls below 11 g/dL or if more than 10% of the circulating volume has been removed.

Sufficient blood volumes for most routine tests can be collected by capillary puncture of the heel. Usually, 600 μL of blood can be collected by this route (*see Appendix A*), which is sufficient for most commonly requested analyses, e.g. total and conjugated bilirubin, creatinine, sodium, potassium, albumin, and calcium. After collection, blood should be suitably protected from light if bilirubin analysis is required.

SPECIMEN COLLECTION

Capillary puncture and blood collection is a skilled process (*see Appendix A*). Squeezing of the heel and scraping the tube over the skin is painful to a baby and is likely to produce a grossly haemolysed sample, possibly contaminated with tissue fluid. Results from such specimens may have elevated potassium and magnesium concentration, from release of red cell electrolytes, falsely low sodium and albumin, from tissue fluid contamination, or elevated ammonia or amino acids, from sweat.

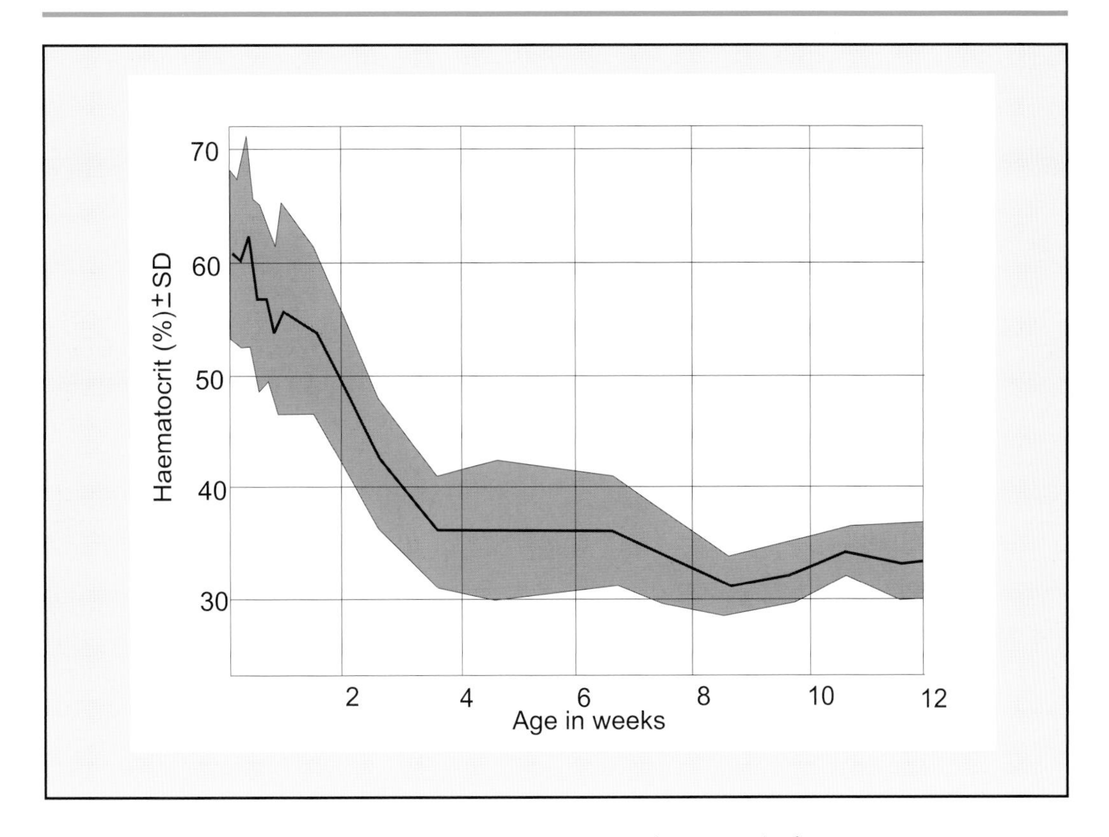

Figure 1.2 Haematocrit in the term neonate and young infant

Plasma potassium will be on average 1-1.5 mmol/L higher than in arterial blood, even without visible haemolysis.

Trained laboratory based phlebotomy staff are often the best people to collect capillary specimens, as they can become expert and appreciate the technical difficulties involved.

When small blood volumes are collected from an arterial line, particular care is needed to aspirate infusion fluid, then flush the line with sufficient blood volume, otherwise erroneous results can occur owing to dilution with the infusate.

NEONATAL PAIN PERCEPTION AND THE NEED FOR ANALGESIA

Neonates in a neonatal unit undergo a vast number of uncomfortable or frankly painful procedures and treatments, for example having an endotracheal tube sucked out, having an intravenous cannula inserted or undergoing heelpricks for blood tests.

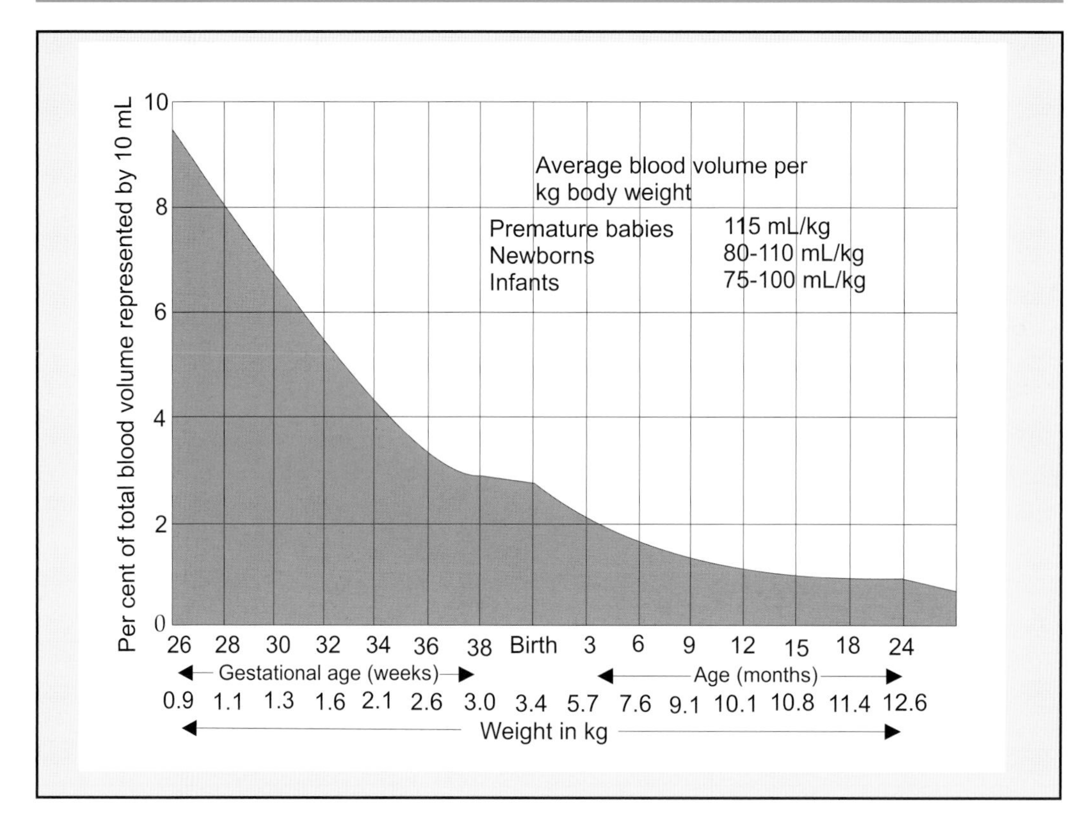

Figure 1.3 Relationship of a 10 mL blood sample to total blood volume

Studies have shown that a baby of less than 30 weeks gestation may have up to 2000 painful procedures during its care. Adverse effects of pain include well documented physiological changes – apnoeas, crying that may interfere with ventilation, increased blood pressure, increased risk of intracranial haemorrhage and increased pulmonary pressures leading to right-left circulatory shunting. Repeated experience of pain can lead to sensitisation, so that simple touch in future can lead to a 'pain' response. Anatomical studies have confirmed the presence of pain pathways to cortical and subcortical levels even in the most immature babies cared for on neonatal units.

These adverse effects can be minimised by considering the following:

- is the specimen necessary? Will the result potentially change the baby's care?
- is there an indwelling arterial line that can be used for some or all of the blood samples instead of a venepuncture or heelprick?
- is the procedure being performed optimally by a trained person – no

squeezing with a heelprick, few or no 'second shots' at procedures?

- grouping potentially painful handling and procedures together in time, so the baby can then have a rest period
- giving comfort from sucking a dummy, or comfort touch, e.g. from a parent; these reduce a baby's physiological reactions to pain
- giving sucrose gel or 25% solution orally. This can act as an analgesic and is beginning to be widely employed in neonatal units
- local anaesthesia, if this will not make the procedure more difficult (and hence prolong it).

FURTHER READING

Levene MI, Thearle MJ, Tudehope DI. Essentials of Neonatal Medicine. Oxford: Blackwell Science, 2000.

Roberton NRC. A Manual of Normal Neonatal Care. London: Arnold, 1996.

Roberton NRC, Rennie J. A Manual of Neonatal Intensive Care. London: Arnold, 2001.

Chapter 2

Laboratory services

In the UK, most neonatal units (NNUs) are served by the hospital's main laboratories, which usually provide a comprehensive test repertoire onsite. Although neonatal work represents only a small part of the workload of such laboratories, provided that there is adequate provision to meet the needs of the NNU on a 24 hour basis, this model generally works well. However, reconfiguration of laboratory services, often involving an element of rationalisation and centralisation, is not uncommonly considered by hospital managers seeking to achieve cost savings. Such changes must be planned with the full involvement of laboratory staff and the clinical users, to ensure that there is no detrimental effect on service delivery. A clearly defined service specification, which recognises the special needs of the NNU, is a prerequisite for this process. The service specification must include consideration of all elements of the laboratory service, which extend well beyond the analytical part of the service.

ELEMENTS OF A LABORATORY SERVICE

LOCATION OF THE LABORATORIES

NNU patients, especially those requiring intensive or high dependency care, are often in a very unstable condition, and require close laboratory monitoring. The amount of neonatal work, together with the urgency of a large proportion of the requests, provides strong operational and economic justification for provision of at least core laboratory services on the same site as the NNU. Ensuring adequate turnaround times for results is a key determinant of where laboratory tests are performed: at the very least, it is recommended that, where results may be required within one hour, investigations should be undertaken on the same hospital site as the NNU. Suggested acceptable turnaround times for commonly requested, or important, routine and urgent requests are shown in Figure 2.1.

The local laboratory should be responsible for selecting and monitoring the quality of other laboratories to which work is referred. This will include consideration of many of the topics discussed in detail below, including the ability to handle small sample volumes, turnaround times, the provision of interpretation as well as results, and evidence of continuing accreditation.

Suggested turnaround times for routine and urgent requests

Analysis	Recommended maximum turnaround times for requests that are: Routine	Urgent
Clinical biochemistry		
Acyl carnitine species	5 working days	1 working day
Albumin	4 hours	Rarely required
Amino acids	5 working days	1 working day
Ammonia	All requests are urgent	Analysed immediately
Bilirubin	1-2 hours	<1 hour
Blood gases	All requests are urgent	Analysed immediately
Calcium	4 hours	30 minutes
Creatinine, urea	4 hours	<1 hour
Glucose	1-2 hours	30 minutes
Lactate	All requests are urgent	1-2 hours
Liver enzymes	1 working day	Rarely required
Magnesium	4 hours	<1 hour
Organic acids (urine)	5 working days	1 working day
Phosphate	1 working day	Rarely required
Sodium, potassium	1-2 hours	30 minutes
17OH-progesterone	1 working day	Same working day
Haematology		
Full blood count	1-2 hours	30 minutes
PT & APTT	1-2 hours	30 minutes
Cross-match	4 hours	1 hour
Microbiology		
Antibiotic assays	Same day	<1 hour
CSF microscopy	All requests are urgent	<1 hour
Endotracheal tube aspirate microscopy	<4 hours	<1 hour
Urine microscopy	<4 hours	<1 hour
HIV antibodies	1-2 working days	<4 hours
Hepatitis screen	1-2 working days	1 working day
Bacterial & fungal culture	Set up in <4 hours	Set up at same time as microscopy
Direct immunofluorescence: respiratory secretions	Same day	<2 hours
Direct immunofluorescence: skin samples	Same day	<2 hours
Rotavirus screen	Same day	<2 hours

Figure 2.1 Suggested specification for turnaround times for routine and urgent requests

SPECIMEN COLLECTION AND TRANSPORT

The quality of results is dependent on the quality of the specimen, which must be collected correctly and transported to the laboratory in a timely manner. Specimens from neonates are particularly precious because of the difficulties in collection, and the morbidity caused to the baby during sampling: in particular, repeated venepuncture can quickly lead to anaemia. Therefore, it is important to ensure both that specimens are collected and handled correctly, and that unnecessary sampling is avoided. In most cases, capillary samples from a warmed heel will suffice for monitoring investigations. Venous samples are essential for reliable measurement of certain analytes (e.g. potassium, calcium, ammonia), and for blood cultures (*see Appendix A*).

Functions of the laboratory include:

- ordering and maintaining stocks of specimen containers and specimen collection systems suitable for neonatal samples
- provision of a phlebotomy service. Collection of blood samples, especially capillary sampling, from neonates is a skilled procedure to ensure a quality specimen, and in particular to minimise haemolysis. This is best performed by trained laboratory-based personnel
- development of standard operating procedures for specimen collection, and guidelines for requesting appropriate tests
- management of specimen delivery services, including air tube systems, specimen porters, and inter-hospital specimen transport.

SAMPLE ANALYSIS

Although a large number of laboratory tests required for neonates are similar to those used for older age groups, there are some important differences in sample processing and analysis for neonatal patients. For all laboratory specialties, both analysers and manual methodologies must be compatible with small sample volumes, including minimising sample evaporation. They must also be sufficiently sensitive to measure accurately those neonatal values that are normally lower than in other age groups, e.g. creatinine. In clinical biochemistry, it is important that methods are evaluated for potential interference from haemoglobin or bilirubin, to ensure that true results can be obtained from haemolysed and/or jaundiced samples. Clinical biochemistry and haematology services must be able to facilitate same day diagnosis of serious conditions that may present in the neonatal period, including inherited metabolic disorders, clotting problems and haemolytic disease of the newborn (*see Chapters 10 & 11*). Where these services are not provided onsite, close liaison with the appropriate specialist laboratories is vital. In particular, it is important to ensure that the correct specimens (sample type, type of anticoagulant for blood samples) are taken, relevant clinical details (e.g. feeding regimen, drug therapy) are provided and that rapid transport is arranged.

Microbiology standard operating procedures should recognise that microorganisms usually dismissed as contaminants in other age groups may be important neonatal pathogens (e.g. coagulase-negative staphylococci isolated from endotracheal tube aspirates). Specialist culture techniques are necessary for detection of mycoplasmas, which may be important neonatal pathogens (especially *Ureaplasma urealyticum*). A commercial blood culture system, using paediatric bottles formulated to enhance the growth of neonatal and childhood pathogens from small volumes of blood, is recommended. The choice of antibiotics for susceptibility testing should reflect the NNU antimicrobial prescribing policy.

REPORTING OF RESULTS

Clinically acceptable turnaround times for results must be achieved (see Figure 2.1). This depends on timely delivery of the specimen to the laboratory, and on there being a robust system in the laboratory for prioritisation of urgent work. Where applicable, results should be reported with appropriate reference ranges, which are often different from those for other age groups. Electronic transmission of results to the NNU is desirable, because it gives clinicians immediate access to authorised results. There should be agreed protocols for liaison over potentially serious abnormal results; examples of results that justify immediate verbal communication are shown in Figures 2.2 to 2.4. Appropriately experienced and interested senior staff should provide clinical advice and liaison.

Clinical biochemistry results for immediate notification

Test	Value	Possible symptoms/complications
Ammonia	> 100 μmol/L	Seizures, coma
Bilirubin	> 400 μmol/L	Kernicterus
Calcium	< 1.5 mmol/L	Seizures
Glucose	< 2.0 mmol/L	Seizures
Magnesium	< 0.5 mmol/L	Seizures
Phosphate	< 0.3 mmol/L	Myocardial dysfunction, respiratory failure, muscle weakness, seizures, death
Potassium	> 7.5 mmol/L	Cardiac dysrhythmias, sudden death
Sodium	< 130 mmol/L	Seizures, cerebral oedema
	> 150 mmol/L	Seizures

Figure 2.2 Clinical biochemistry laboratory test results that should be notified immediately to the responsible clinician

Haematology results for immediate notification		
Test	**Value**	**Possible symptoms/complications**
Fibrinogen	Elevated concentrations	Suggestive of infection
Haemoglobin	< 8 g/dL	Anaemia, cardiac failure
Neutrophils	< 1.0×10^9/L	Risk of bacterial or fungal infection
Platelets	< 50×10^9/L	Baby requires close monitoring for evidence of bleeding
PT/APTT	Prolonged	Risk of bleeding

Figure 2.3 Haematology laboratory test results that should be notified immediately to the responsible clinician

Microbiology results for immediate notification		
Test	**Results**	**Rationale**
Antibiotic assays	All results > 20% outside target range	Low levels sub-therapeutic High levels toxic
Antibiotic susceptibility tests	Unexpected antibiotic resistances, e.g. MRSA, gentamicin-resistant Gram-negative bacteria	To optimise therapy and implement infection control precautions, where indicated
Blood cultures	All positive results	To optimise therapy
CSF microscopy & culture	All microscopy results All positive culture results	To optimise therapy
Detection of microorganisms that may cause outbreaks of infection (*see also Chapter 12*)	All positive results	To implement infection control precautions
Detection of *N.gonorrhoeae* or *C.trachomatis*	All positive results	To optimise therapy of infant and parents
Microbial serology/PCR	All results consistent with recent infection	To expedite patient management
Urine microscopy & culture	All microscopy results All positive culture results	To optimise therapy

Figure 2.4 Microbiology laboratory test results that should be notified immediately to the responsible clinician

QUALITY ASSURANCE AND ACCREDITATION

Quality is paramount in all aspects of laboratory work. Laboratories should have a comprehensive internal quality control programme and should be able to provide evidence of satisfactory performance in all relevant external quality assurance schemes, such as those organised by NEQAS in the UK. There should be a programme of departmental audit, and also a willingness to participate with users in multidisciplinary audits. Accreditation by a relevant professional body is a good indication that quality standards are adequate; all laboratories should be accredited or at least actively working towards obtaining accreditation. In the UK, Clinical Pathology Accreditation (CPA(UK)Ltd.) is the main accreditation body.

MANAGEMENT OF POINT OF CARE TESTING

The main reason for moving analytical procedures to the bedside is to expedite rapid adjustments to patients' management. A wide range of biochemical, haematological and microbiological assays can be undertaken at the point of care. However, at the present time, point of care testing (POCT) should be seen as augmenting, and not replacing, local laboratory services. Determining which bedside tests are appropriate for a NNU entails consideration of several factors, including:

- the urgency with which results are required
- availability of resources to ensure that clinical staff have sufficient time and training to operate point of care testing equipment safely and reliably
- the proximity of the laboratory, which is an important determinant of result turnaround times
- availability of space on the NNU to accommodate POCT equipment
- the reliability and accuracy of results obtained with the equipment available
- the cost of equipment and consumables necessary to perform the test
- the demand for the test.

POCT is most well-established in clinical biochemistry. Blood glucose and arterial blood gas measurement are the most common point of care tests, the demand for these investigations in most NNUs easily justifying the cost of any equipment. Equipment is also readily available for other tests, including sodium, potassium, lactate, ionised and total calcium concentrations, and C-reactive protein. Bilirubin meters are used in some NNUs; however, in the authors' experience these are potential sources of serious errors, and we do not recommend their use. If they are used, it is essential that regular checks are made to ensure accurate standardisation and good correlation with the laboratory methods.

POCT is used less for haematology, although equipment is available for a range of blood count and coagulation measurements. However, these tests do not provide an adequate substitute for full haematological profiles available from the laboratory, and many have also been found to be unreliable in practice. Likewise, although various microbiological tests are transferable to the bedside (usually based on detection of microbial antigens by latex agglutination), their relatively poor sensitivity and specificity, together with the low level of demand in NNUs, rarely justifies their use in neonatology.

POCT must be under the control of the laboratory, and performed to the same standard as laboratory-based tests. Functions of the laboratory include:

- evaluation and procurement of suitable equipment
- ensuring that equipment is appropriately and safely sited
- production of policies and protocols relating to the use of the equipment
- training, certification, and revalidation of operators
- equipment maintenance and troubleshooting
- quality assurance monitoring
- provision of backup testing in the event of equipment failure, and to confirm unexpectedly high or low results.

OUT OF HOURS SERVICE

NNUs have a significant requirement for laboratory support outside the traditional working hours of 09:00 to 17:00, with most of the urgent work being requested before midnight. Many laboratories, especially in larger hospitals, now operate an extended working day, sometimes even a 24 hour shift system. Other laboratories continue to deal with out of hours work on an on-call basis. Whatever the system, it is important that clinical users are clear about their laboratories' arrangements to ensure that urgent work is processed appropriately.

If a local onsite (satellite) laboratory provides daytime services, but another laboratory provides the out of hours on-call service, it is essential that the laboratories use methods that give comparable results. This is especially important when following trends in measurements such as sodium, bilirubin or haematological parameters. Not all specimens collected out of hours require immediate processing. Most specimens that are not sent directly to the laboratory should be stored in a refrigerator designated for specimen storage. The exception is blood cultures; these should be incubated immediately to obtain the greatest and most rapid yield of positive results.

BLOOD PRODUCT SERVICE

The haematology department must ensure the supply and identification of blood products, and provide guidance on, and audit, their use. In the UK, hospitals are required to have a Blood Transfusion Committee to oversee these functions.

INFECTION CONTROL

The Infection Control Team has an important role in the prevention and control of infection (*see also Chapter 13*), including:

- production of policies and procedures relating to the prevention and management of infection
- infection surveillance and audit
- training and education
- management of outbreaks of infection.

COMMUNICABLE DISEASE EPIDEMIOLOGY

Microbiology departments play an important role in the collation of national statistics on infection. In the UK, a range of important infections, including bacteraemia, meningitis and viral infections, are reported to the Public Health Laboratory Service Communicable Disease Surveillance Centre. There is also cooperation with other national organisations, such as the British Paediatric Surveillance Unit. Liaison with Consultants for Communicable Disease Control is important to ensure that statutorily notifiable diseases and important hospital-acquired infections are reported locally.

TEACHING AND RESEARCH

Laboratory personnel have an important role in training users on all aspects of use of the laboratories. Especially in larger centres, laboratories should be able to support clinical research projects, as well as initiating laboratory-based research.

ETHICAL ISSUES FOR LABORATORY TESTING

Ideally, informed consent should be obtained for any procedure, including blood sampling. In practice, consent for 'routine' investigations is often assumed. In an emergency, it is certainly acceptable to collect and test specimens without consent, where the results will have a direct and immediate impact on the care of the patient. It is normally the responsibility of the doctor treating the patient to obtain consent for testing for diagnostic purposes, and laboratories may assume that consent has been given for the tests that are requested. Examination of specimens collected from the patient immediately after death may help to determine the cause of sudden unexplained death. Only a coroner (or equivalent) has the authority to consent to such investigations, which are best undertaken under the aegis of an agreed routine protocol (*see Appendix C*). Laboratories should not initiate tests that have not been requested, unless they are closely related to the original request, and in the direct interest of the patient.

Important samples from patients may be stored for possible further use. This should be explained to parents at the time of sampling. Subsequent testing on stored samples for clinical reasons, for example in inherited conditions where technological advances allow new genetic information to be ascertained, should not be undertaken unless consent has been obtained. For any research using clinical material, approval must be obtained from a Research Ethics Committee, and specific consent obtained from the parents of each infant. This is the case even if specimens are to be processed anonymously.

Sometimes it may be in the best interests of the child to undertake an investigation that has been refused by the parents. This may be because of concerns about the implications of a diagnosis such as HIV infection, or because of an attempt to conceal a diagnosis of Munchausen's syndrome. Laws relating to sample collection and testing vary from country to country, even within the UK. However, anyone collecting or testing samples in such circumstances should feel able to justify their decision in the courts or to their professional body. Prior discussion with experienced colleagues, hospital managers and/or legal advisors is advisable, and where a suitable sample that has been collected previously is available, it is preferable to test this, rather than collecting a further sample under duress.

When a health care worker suffers an occupational exposure to blood or body fluids, it is usual to seek consent to test the source patient for evidence of hepatitis B or HIV infection, to determine whether post-exposure prophylaxis is indicated. Testing against the parent's wishes in this circumstance is justified only in exceptional circumstances.

FUTURE TRENDS

Whatever changes occur in the organisation of laboratory services, there will continue to be a need for onsite provision of core laboratory support for NNUs. However, there is likely to be greater centralisation of more specialised tests, both to achieve economy of scale and to ensure that there is adequate expertise in performing and interpreting the results of such tests. Significant developments in neonatal screening in the UK are already being planned, and the use of molecular biological techniques to investigate inherited metabolic and haematological disorders will increase. Molecular biology in microbiology is currently less well developed, but has considerable potential, especially for improved diagnosis of viral infections and rapid detection of antibiotic resistance.

FURTHER READING

Clinical Pathology Accreditation (UK) Ltd. Standards for the Medical Laboratory. Sheffield: CPA(UK)Ltd, 2001.

Joint Working Group on Quality Assurance. Guidelines on the control of near-patient tests (NPT) and procedures performed on patients by non-pathology staff. Birmingham: UKNEQAS, 1999.

Management of in vitro diagnostic medical devices. MDA DB2002(02). London: Medical Devices Agency, 2002.

Management and use of IVD point of care test devices. MDA DB2002(03). London: Medical Devices Agency, 2002.

Reference guide of consent for examination or treatment. Department of Health: London, 2001.

Seeking patients' consent: the ethical considerations. London: General Medical Council, 1998.

Chapter 3

Pregnancy and delivery

THE UNCOMPLICATED PREGNANCY

The unborn baby can be at risk from genetic, maternal, environmental or social disadvantages. Most pregnancies, however, are uncomplicated, and antenatal care in the UK is now organised so as to tailor care appropriately to those who require it. The majority of pregnant women are cared for in the community by family doctors and midwives, in liaison with an appropriate obstetric unit.

Delivery is still mainly hospital based, with only 2% of deliveries in the UK occurring in the mother's home. Currently, 19% of labours in the UK are 'induced'. Intervention during delivery occurs with increasing frequency, the incidence increasing when continuous fetal monitoring in labour (by fetal heart monitoring supplemented by fetal scalp blood sampling when indicated) is used.

Up to 20% of babies in the UK are now delivered by caesarean section, of which 40% are performed as an emergency. A further 11% of babies are delivered with the aid of ventouse suction cup or forceps.

In a pre-pregnancy clinic, potential medical and obstetric problems can be anticipated. Women will be advised of the risks of smoking (reduced fetal weight, increased sudden infant death, increased childhood respiratory problems), screening tests will be performed, and diet and folic acid supplementation discussed. It is currently recommended that all women planning pregnancy be advised to take 400 µg of folic acid daily because of its proven role in reducing the incidence of neural tube defects. If there has been a previously affected pregnancy, 5 mg daily is recommended.

Maternal age is less of an additional risk factor than previously thought: indeed, the average age of women in their first pregnancy is rising steadily owing to social factors, and in the UK is currently about 28 years.

At the first booking appointment with an antenatal clinic, the expected date of delivery is established from the date of the last menstrual period (LMP) (Naegele's rule: expected date of delivery = (LMP date + 7 days) – 3 months + 12 months), adjusted for cycle length. Many units confirm this date by a first trimester ultrasound scan: this will also confirm a singleton, intrauterine pregnancy.

Potential problems in the pregnancy can be identified at this initial appointment, e.g. maternal health or social problems, past medical or obstetric complications, or family history of a potentially recurrent condition. In the UK, 'low risk' women will then be cared for predominantly in the community, while 'higher risk' women will have a plan for hospital attendance and supervision by a consultant obstetrician.

In the low risk population, the aim of antenatal care is to screen for problems that may develop without risk markers, e.g. a proportion of growth retardation, hypertension, and pre-eclampsia. Blood pressure is checked regularly, and urinalysis performed for protein and glucose. A haemoglobin check is performed – often by a slide method, e.g. HemoCue – and iron supplements prescribed as necessary.

Medical problems managed through hospital clinics will include diabetes, whose control may be difficult, and which is ideally managed by a combined obstetrician/diabetologist team. Drug management of epilepsy may need to be altered either before pregnancy, to reduce teratogenicity as far as possible, or during pregnancy, owing to altered drug pharmacokinetics, as blood volume, glomerular filtration rate, protein binding and gut absorption all alter during pregnancy. The treatment of hypertension may also need to be modified.

Fetal health in low risk pregnancies is monitored by listening to the fetal heart, assessing uterine size using symphyseal-fundal height measurement by tape measure, and maternal monitoring of fetal movements either informally or using a chart. Fundal height measurements are not sensitive detectors of poor fetal growth; probably only just over half of babies with weight below the 5th centile are detected in this way. Where there is doubt, confirmatory ultrasound scanning is indicated.

An example of an antenatal schedule for a low risk pregnancy in the UK is shown in Figure 3.1.

SCREENING TESTS IN PREGNANCY

In the UK, all women are offered a routine surveillance screening programme. Since 2000, this now includes counselling regarding HIV screening and performance of this serology screen on request. This change results from compelling evidence that intrapartum treatment of the affected mother, plus neonatal drug therapy, can substantially reduce vertical transmission of HIV.

Antenatal schedule for a low risk pregnancy		
Gestation	**Event**	**Aims**
6-12 weeks	Dating scan	Dating, viability, multiplicity
	Booking	Pregnancy plan, fix expected date of delivery
	Bloods	Routine screening and special investigations
16 weeks	AFP/HCG	Neural tube defect/Down's risk
20 weeks	Mid trimester scan	Structural anomaly scan
24 weeks	Community	Review of results
28-30 weeks	Community	Blood pressure, urinalysis, fundal height, presentation
34 weeks	Community/ hospital	As above plus blood group antibody screen
36 and 40 weeks	Community	As above
41 weeks	Hospital visit	Assessment to determine possible date for induction

Figure 3.1 Antenatal schedule for a low risk pregnancy

Minimum routine surveillance screening comprises:

- general medical examination, weight, blood pressure, urinalysis, mid-stream urine (for culture)
- abdominal examination
- full blood count, blood group and antibody screen, syphilis screen, hepatitis B screen, rubella serology, HIV serology
- anomaly detection screening (after counselling) – ultrasound and blood tests.

Note that positive rubella serology does not exclude a rubella infection earlier in the pregnancy: the usefulness of this test is that a negative result indicates the need for immunisation postpartum. In some areas, the following additional tests are also offered as part of surveillance screening:

- haemoglobinopathy screen: sickle cell and thalassaemia (*see Chapter 11*). In high prevalence areas of the UK, these tests will be offered routinely from 2004
- toxoplasmosis (routine screen in France and some other European countries)
- phenylketonuria (urine Phenistix test at booking)
- cytomegalovirus.

Anomaly detection screening comprises a combination of blood tests and ultrasound screening. It should be undertaken only after full explanation to the mother of the purpose of the screening and the nature of the tests involved. Unwillingness to consider termination of pregnancy in any circumstance is not necessarily a reason for an informed woman not to have anomaly screening; some families have derived great benefit from being able to plan for the birth of a baby with problems.

The first antenatal screening test performed on pregnant women was the measurement of α-fetoprotein (AFP) in maternal serum, to identify those pregnancies most at risk of an open neural tube defect (NTD). The optimum time for this screening is between 16 and 18 weeks gestation. Results are expressed as 'multiples of the median' (MOMs) and values above 2.5 MOMs should trigger further investigation. The presence of such a defect can be confirmed by measurement of AFP and electrophoresis of acetylcholinesterase isoenzymes in amniotic fluid and/or ultrasound examination. Other causes of raised AFP are impending or actual fetal death, congenital nephrosis or other open defect, e.g. of the abdominal wall. In addition, multiple pregnancy or incorrect gestational age can cause the AFP to appear abnormally high.

Screening for Down's syndrome using maternal blood evolved from NTD screening, and the observation that Down's syndrome affected pregnancies are associated with lower than usual concentrations of AFP in maternal serum. It was later discovered that a number of other biochemical substances are present in higher or lower concentrations in maternal blood in a Down's affected pregnancy. Maternal age has long been known to be a risk factor (term incidence approximately 1 in 1400 at maternal age 25 years and 1 in 30 at age 45). Currently, most screening for Down's syndrome takes place in the second trimester in conjunction with NTD screening. The age-related risk is refined by taking into account the concentrations of several of these biochemical substances. Much effort has gone into using a combination of these factors to provide a 'level of risk' for an affected fetus in a given pregnancy, in order to reduce as far as possible false negative and false positive results, while minimising the number of women having the diagnostic test, i.e. fetal blood sampling or amniocentesis for fetal chromosome analysis. Most widely used are combinations of maternal serum AFP and chorionic gonadotrophin (HCG), with or without unconjugated estriol as a third analyte (double or triple test). Women with a predicted risk of around 1 in 250 or worse are offered karyotyping or other DNA studies on amniotic fluid to achieve a definitive diagnosis. This strategy achieves a detection rate up to about 70% with around 5% of all pregnant women being selected for the diagnostic test.

Increasingly, women are being offered testing for Down's syndrome earlier in pregnancy (10-14 weeks). This is based on the age-related risk and an ultrasound measurement of the thickness of a specific area of the fetal neck (nuchal translucency). Ultrasound assessment of nuchal translucency is not yet available in all centres but, in combination with biochemical markers, can achieve slightly better detection rates, with fewer women having to undergo amniocentesis.

Ultrasound examination to screen for abnormality is usually performed after the 20th week of gestation. Some structural abnormalities, such as defects of the anterior abdominal wall or major spinal abnormalities, are readily detected: others, such as some potentially major heart defects, are much harder to see and detection rates are lower. An apparently normal scan does not totally exclude the possibility of a pathological condition.

THE HIGH RISK PREGNANCY

INVASIVE PRENATAL DIAGNOSIS

CHORIONIC VILLUS SAMPLING OR PLACENTAL BIOPSY.

This early test, usually carried out trans-cervically at 11 weeks of pregnancy or shortly after, provides trophoblastic cells, which are a source of fetal DNA. This can be used for chromosomal or genetic investigations in women with a fetus at high risk of chromosomal abnormality or with a family history of selected genetic diseases (*see Chapter 10*). Results from direct genetic analysis are usually available within a week, so that if termination of pregnancy is required, it can be carried out within the first trimester. If cell culture is required prior to analysis, results will not be available for at least 3 to 4 weeks. The risk of miscarriage after the procedure is about 2%, twice that for amniocentesis

AMNIOCENTESIS

Amniocentesis is a simpler procedure, involving removal of liquor from the amniotic sac under ultrasound guidance. The earliest time at which the test is usually done is the 14th week of pregnancy; the risk of miscarriage is between 0.5 to 1%.

Fetal cells (amniocytes) can be used for chromosomal DNA analysis, fetal sexing and enzyme assay in cultured cells. Cultures take at least 2-3 weeks but sometimes may fail completely. The fluid can also be analysed for bilirubin concentrations in blood group isoimmunisation, AFP, or for acetylcholinesterase (elevated in neural tube defects), as well as lecithin/sphingomyelin ratio (mature ratio > 2.5:1). The latter test is not available routinely, but can be used to evaluate fetal lung maturity before planned preterm delivery.

FETAL BLOOD SAMPLING

Cordocentesis, or fetal blood sampling, provides rapidly available, direct fetal information including:

- karyotyping
- fetal haemoglobin in isoimmunisation or hydrops
- infection investigations in a very small baby or one with intracranial abnormality (CMV, toxoplasma, parvovirus, rubella)
- fetal blood group
- DNA analysis for specific genetic conditions
- fetal blood gases and biochemistry
- diagnosis of haemoglobinopathy
- diagnosis of some inborn errors of metabolism.

This procedure is done in larger centres with appropriate technical expertise and laboratory support. There is a risk of sudden fetal compromise or death during the procedure if there is bleeding into the cord.

ASSESSMENT OF THE FETUS

In the low risk pregnancy, this consists of clinical evaluation of fetal growth, and maternal attention to fetal kicking movements in the second half of the pregnancy. In a pregnancy perceived as higher risk, whether because of maternal disease, relevant past obstetric history, or a detected problem such as poor growth or developing maternal hypertension, more formal assessment is done.

Fetal growth can be followed ultrasonically (fetal biometry) if the uterine size is small or there are other reasons for concern about fetal growth. Measurements made include the length of the femur, (useful in dating a pregnancy from 12 weeks on), biparietal diameter (the distance across the widest diameter of the fetal skull – used in the second trimester), and fetal head circumference and abdominal circumference – used in the late second and early third trimester. In a fetus whose growth is faltering, a discrepancy may develop between these two measures, thought to be due to shrinkage of the fetal liver.

The liquor volume around the fetus is also important, as it reflects fetal renal function and placental function. When placental function is reduced, the fetus grows poorly and there is a reduction in the proportion of the fetal blood supply going to the viscera, leading to reduced fetal urine production and reduced liquor volume. This is assessed by measuring the maximum depth in centimetres of pools of liquor in the four uterine quadrants – the 'amniotic fluid index'.

Combined assessment of fetal movements, fetal tone or posture, fetal breathing, amniotic fluid volume and fetal heart reactivity on CTG (cardiotocograph) comprise the 'biophysical profile'. Each element scores 0 or 2 for a total score out of 10.

Doppler assessment of the diastolic flow velocity in the umbilical cord – affected by changes in the resistance of placental blood vessels – is increasingly used as a risk predictor in the small fetus for whom early delivery may be the best option. Absent or reversed end-diastolic flow is associated with 40% perinatal mortality and high perinatal morbidity without intervention.

MATERNAL DISORDERS AFFECTING THE BABY

MATERNAL DIABETES

The achievement of good diabetic control usually becomes more difficult in pregnancy owing to effects on carbohydrate metabolism, and glucose tolerance can become abnormal for the first time during pregnancy. Optimisation of maternal blood glucose control can reduce the incidence of fetal malformations, particularly congenital heart disease, and the risk of sudden fetal death in late pregnancy. Maternal hyperglycaemia causes the fetus to receive an increased glucose load and become hyperinsulinaemic. This predisposes to macrosomia, the severity of which is related to the adequacy of third trimester maternal glycaemic control.

Polyhydramnios can lead to preterm delivery; macrosomia can lead to intrapartum hypoxia or birth trauma, particularly shoulder dystocia, with its associated risks of fractured clavicle and brachial plexus nerve injury (Erb's palsy, phrenic nerve palsy).

The neonate is at risk of early hypoglycaemia, particularly if macrosomic. An early feed should be offered and blood glucose should be measured every three hours prior to feeds for 48 hours. Hypoglycaemia despite feeds will require neonatal unit admission and intravenous dextrose infusion as a feed complement for up to three days (*see Chapter 7*).

EPILEPSY

All anticonvulsants cross the placenta and all the established therapies are associated with a variably increased risk of fetal abnormality. There is no 'neonatal withdrawal' from their effects and breast feeding is not contraindicated.

HAEMOGLOBINOPATHIES AND SICKLE CELL DISEASE

All women of Afro-Caribbean, Asian or Eastern Mediterranean origin should be tested for sickle cell disease, thalassaemia and other clinically important haemoglobinopathies at their initial booking with an antenatal clinic. If the woman is heterozygous, her partner should be screened. If both parents are heterozygous, counselling regarding invasive diagnostic prenatal testing should be offered.

THALASSAEMIAS

An affected fetus with alpha thalassaemia major will develop lethal hydrops. Heterozygous beta thalassaemia produces only mild microcytic anaemia, but the homozygous form is a life-limiting condition requiring transfusions and chelation therapy. These conditions are discussed in more detail in Chapter 11.

THROMBOCYTOPENIA

Maternal thrombocytopenia (platelets $<100{,}000 \times 10^9/L$) can be due to ITP (idiopathic thrombocytopenic purpura), benign idiopathic thrombocytopenia of pregnancy, systemic lupus erythematosus, hypertensive disease, maternal viral infections, or be a side effect of heparin or non-steroidal drugs. In the vast majority of such cases, the baby is unaffected or has only mild thrombocytopenia at birth. There is no correlation between maternal and neonatal platelet counts. Treatment of the baby is with group-compatible platelet infusion or intravenous immunoglobulin if there is active bleeding or if the platelet count is less than $20{,}000 \times 10^9/L$.

Allo-immune thrombocytopenia is a rare and potentially serious condition, in which the mother's platelet count is normal but she has IgG anti-platelet antibodies that may cross the placenta and produce fetal intracerebral bleeding or death. The usual antibody is directed against PLA1 antigen, and the presence/absence of this antibody in the mother's blood should be investigated if a thrombocytopenic baby is delivered. First pregnancies can be affected. Where the diagnosis is known in pregnancy, fetal platelet transfusions and early delivery are indicated.

BLOOD GROUP ISOIMMUNISATION

This is discussed in Chapter 11.

FETAL COMPLICATIONS

HYDROPS FETALIS

This condition is characterised by soft tissue oedema plus fluid within at least one body cavity, such as pleural or pericardial effusions or abdominal ascites (*see Appendix D*). Diagnosis is by ultrasound examination. Hydrops fetalis can be divided into two types according to aetiology. The immune type is due to haematological causes, mainly Rhesus isoimmunisation. The non-immune type has many causes and an overall worse prognosis. Appropriate fetal and maternal investigations, which should be performed in a specialised centre, are shown in Figure 3.2.

Investigations required for hydrops fetalis

Test	Possible causes of fetal hydrops
Maternal haematological antibody screen	Isoimmunisation
Maternal haemoglobinopathy screen	Fetal homozygosity
Detailed ultrasound scan	Heart or lung defect
Fetal karyotyping (cordocentesis)	Trisomy
Screen for toxoplasmosis IgM, rubella IgM, CMV IgM, parvovirus	Fetal infection
Kleihauer test	Fetomaternal bleed
Maternal G6PD deficiency screen	Fetal anaemia

Figure 3.2 Investigations required for hydrops fetalis

When the affected baby is delivered, at least two experienced resuscitators should be present. Intubation and ventilation are always required. Frequent suction is needed to clear lung fluid. Ascites or pleural effusions should be immediately drained if they are embarrassing respiration. High pressure ventilation may be needed because of poor compliance of the oedematous chest wall.

Samples for investigation should be collected before any transfusion to exclude the following:

- fetal anaemia: isoimmunisation, haemoglobinopathy, bleeding, parvovirus
- congenital infection: syphilis, CMV, toxoplasma, parvovirus
- cardiac failure: structural defect or tachyarrhythmia
- hypoproteinaemia: congenital nephrotic syndrome, hepatitis
- twin-twin transfusion syndrome (hypervolaemic twin)
- trisomy (especially trisomy 21) with pulmonary lymphatic abnormality
- chylothorax, which carries a relatively good prognosis, presenting with left sided pleural effusion (oedema, confirmed by cytology of pleural fluid containing lymphocytes)
- inherited metabolic disease: a rare possibility (*see Chapter 10*).

Ongoing treatment of the baby will be supportive, depending on the underlying diagnosis. The outlook in non-immune hydrops is generally poor, with only about 10% neonatal survival. Better outcomes are obtained where there is fetal tachyarrhythmia, which can be treated prenatally via medication to the mother, and fetal isolated chylothorax, which can sometimes be drained prenatally.

PRETERM DELIVERY

Preterm labour is often secondary to underlying pathology that can affect the outcome. Such processes include systemic or local genital infection, abruption, fetal or uterine abnormalities, multiple pregnancy, polyhydramnios or ruptured membranes. Prior to 32 weeks, tocolytics are sometimes used to prolong pregnancy, to allow administration of steroids. If delivery is anticipated between 24 and 36 weeks gestation, antenatal steroids given within seven days of delivery improve neonatal survival. Betamethasone may be less likely than dexamethasone to produce undesirable neurological effects in the fetus.

Many preterm births are elective, induced either to protect the wellbeing of the mother – for instance, with hypertension slipping out of control – or the baby – for instance, a fetus with poor growth, oligohydramnios, and absent end diastolic flow on umbilical artery Doppler monitoring.

The care of the preterm baby is complex, involving close monitoring and attention to temperature, fluid balance, energy supply, and circulatory stability, as well as management of the specific problems of prematurity. The interested reader should consult a specialised text (see Further Reading). The major medical problems of preterm babies are summarised in Figure 3.3.

Major medical problems in preterm babies

Condition	Origin	Management
Anaemia	Repeated venepunctures Marrow unresponsive Increased blood volume with growth Iron deficiency	Replace losses by transfusion (taking care to minimise number of donors)
Chronic lung disease	Volutrauma and oxygen toxicity in the extreme preterm with respiratory distress syndrome	Prolonged oxygen requirement Supportive monitoring, nutritional and pulmonary care
Dehydration	Transdermal water losses in the extreme preterm Polyuria in recovering tubular necrosis	Humidified environment Monitor urinary losses Adequate water intake
Hyperglycaemia	Diabetogenic effect of steroid ± parenteral nutrition	May require insulin infusion
Hypernatraemia	Dehydration	Adequate fluid intake
Hypocalcaemia	Immature parathyroid regulation Low albumin	Replace in i.v. fluids 1 mmol/kg/24h as calcium gluconate
Hypoglycaemia	Inadequate intake Low glycogen stores	i.v. dextrose according to local protocol
Hyponatraemia	Renal tubular immaturity	Adequate replacement of urinary losses

continued...

Major medical problems in preterm babies (continued)

Condition	Origin	Management
Hypothermia	Large surface area Poor insulation Immature skin structure Nursed naked	Clothing Warm environment Consider added humidity
Infection	Invasive management Low immunoglobulins Ineffective localisation of infections	High index of suspicion Early parenteral antibiotics
Irregular respiration/ apnoea	Immature respiratory centre	Monitor respiration Caffeine Seek pathological cause e.g. infection, oesophageal reflux
Jaundice	Hepatic immaturity Bruising Delayed feeding	Phototherapy Exchange transfusion
Malnutrition	Low energy stores Inadequate nutrition Energy expenditure can be large	Minimal enteral feeding as soon as tolerated Parenteral nutrition Fortified milks
Metabolic acidosis	Renal immaturity (in presence of protein load)	May need to reduce protein intake Sodium bicarbonate infusion
Necrotising enterocolitis	Inadequate perfusion of sections of gut in response to food	Supportive Surgical resection of infarcted tissue may be required
Nephrocalcinosis	Oliguria, poor acidification, hypercalciuria Use of frusemide	Avoid prolonged use of loop diuretics
Osteopenia of prematurity	Demineralisation of bones if nutrition inadequate	Adequate mineral content of feeds

continued...

Major medical problems in preterm babies (continued)		
Condition	**Origin**	**Management**
Periventricular haemorrhage	Immaturity Cerebrovascular instability	Supportive care Rarely progresses to hydrocephalus
Periventricular leucomalacia	Cerebral white matter infarction after ischaemic insult	Supportive care Minimise hypocapnia Avoid hypoperfusion
Persistent patent ductus arteriosus	Immaturity Hypoxia Acidosis	Indomethacin or ibuprofen Diuretics and fluid restriction
Respiratory distress syndrome	Surfactant deficiency	Exogenous surfactant intra-tracheally Monitor blood gases, heart rate, respiration rate, SaO_2 CPAP, IPPV IV fluids/nutrition
Retinopathy of prematurity	Local oxygen toxicity affects retinal vasculature	Ophthalmic screening of at-risk babies (< 31 weeks) Laser treatment
Unable to suck	Immature suck/swallow coordination	Nasogastric tube feeds if well

Figure 3.3 Major medical problems in preterm babies

Mortality and morbidity increase as gestation and size at birth decrease. Knowledge of local survival figures at given gestations and birthweights is useful in counselling parents, both before and after delivery.

In the UK, prematurity is the leading cause for 55% of deaths in the first week of life, other causes being congenital abnormalities (26%), intrapartum events (9%), and other specific events (11%).

LABOUR AND DELIVERY

MONITORING IN LABOUR

Where delivery of the baby is planned at home or in a low technology setting, then monitoring of fetal wellbeing during labour will be only by direct auscultation of the fetal heart rate using a Pinard or equivalent stethoscope. In hospitals generally, intrapartum cardiotocography is the mainstay of fetal monitoring in labour.

In the low risk pregnancy, continuous monitoring has not been shown to have any benefit over intermittent, and is likely to increase the intervention rate. For high risk cases, including presence of meconium, breech presentation, preterm, post-term, diabetes, intrauterine growth retardation, antepartum haemorrhage, previous caesarean section, poor obstetric history and multiple pregnancy, continuous monitoring is usually employed.

Cardiotocographs (CTGs) are evaluated in terms of baseline rate, short term variability, accelerations and decelerations. The underlying heart rate reflects interactions between intrinsic heart control mechanisms, parasympathetic and sympathetic influences, and CNS control.

If fetal distress is suspected, fetal condition is first optimised (mother placed in left lateral position and given facial oxygen, hypotension corrected and oxytocics discontinued) before a fetal blood sample is obtained from the fetal scalp. Situations requiring this investigation include abnormal CTG at artificial rupture of membranes, fresh thick meconium, fetal tachycardia, rising baseline heart rate, unreactive trace, or variable or late decelerations.

The main focus of interest in fetal scalp blood sample analysis is the hydrogen ion concentration, as lactate accumulation and developing acidosis may reflect fetal compromise. The action required in response to the fetal hydrogen ion concentration on scalp sampling will vary according to the severity of the problem (Figure 3.4).

CORD GASES AT DELIVERY

Cord gases will give an assessment of the acid-base status of the baby *at the moment of birth*. This may be very useful in attributing possible diagnoses to a baby who has respiratory depression at birth or behaves abnormally afterwards. Paired samples from one of the umbilical arteries and from the umbilical vein should be taken, as soon as practical after delivery, from a section of cord that has been clamped at both ends (double clamping). In all deliveries, the person carrying out the delivery should double clamp a section of cord so that gases can be checked if needed. In all complex deliveries – instrumental or operative deliveries, breech or twin deliveries, after fetal distress in labour, when there is concern about fetal growth or if the 1 minute Apgar score for the baby is 3 or less – cord gases should be measured and the results recorded.

These requirements mean that a blood gas analyser should be constantly available in, or directly adjacent to, the delivery suite.

Acidosis at birth is only a reflection of the situation at that time, and the duration or severity of any problem cannot be deduced from this measure alone. Umbilical arterial hydrogen ion concentration of more than 100 nmol/L (pH < 7.00) correlates with a need for active resuscitation of the baby at birth. High cord hydrogen ion concentration is neither a sensitive nor a specific indicator of poor neonatal outcome unless combined with other factors such as prolonged depression of neonatal Apgar score (<6 at 5 minutes).

Most babies with severe acidosis at birth do not go on to develop cerebral palsy, and the vast majority of children with cerebral palsy had normal cord gases and were in good condition at birth.

Monitoring of fetal hydrogen ion concentration

$[H^+]$ (nmol/L)	pH	Base deficit	Interpretation	Action
< 56	> 7.25	< -6	Normal	Manage as usual
56-63	7.20-7.25	-6 to -10	Borderline	Repeat in 30 minutes if no deterioration
> 63	< 7.20	> -10	Hypoxia/acidosis	Deliver

Figure 3.4 Monitoring of fetal hydrogen ion concentration

INFECTION CONTROL IN THE DELIVERY SUITE

The delivery presents significant risks of infection for the mother, her baby, and birth attendants. Both general infection control precautions and specific interventions can greatly reduce these risks. This section focuses on aspects of infection control at the time of delivery that relate to the paediatrician.

PREVENTION OF INFECTION IN THE MOTHER

Puerperal sepsis is a life threatening condition where *Streptococcus pyogenes* (group A streptococci) invades local tissues around the time of delivery, leading to endometritis and septicaemia. The organism may originate from the throat of the mother, or from other personnel in the delivery room. Although the majority of sore throats are viral in aetiology, it is recommended that healthcare workers with a sore throat persisting for more than 48 hours should have a throat swab examined.

PREVENTION OF INFECTION IN THE NEONATE

During delivery, the neonate may acquire infection with microorganisms present in the maternal genital tract (Figure 3.5). Important pathogens in all neonates include microorganisms that are regarded as normal inhabitants (commensals) of the maternal genital tract (especially group B streptococci), as well as others that are unequivocal maternal pathogens (e.g. *Neisseria gonorrhoeae*, herpes simplex virus). A number of factors predispose to serious neonatal sepsis not only with group B streptococci, but also with many other maternal genital tract commensals. These include low birth weight (less than 1000 g), prematurity, prolonged rupture of membranes and maternal chorioamnionitis. Vaginal delivery is also the time when most cases of vertically transmitted infections with blood-borne viruses (most importantly hepatitis B and HIV) are acquired.

Where a mother is infected with a blood-borne virus, a number of simple precautions during the immediate care of the neonate can reduce the risk of infection. Special care should be taken to minimise trauma to the baby, especially during resuscitation. The neonate's skin should be cleaned as soon as possible to remove maternal blood and body fluids, taking care to wipe away from mucous membranes. Vitamin K injections should not be given, nor blood samples taken, until the baby has been cleaned.

Specific preventative measures, e.g. antimicrobial prophylaxis and immunisation, are effective in protecting the infant from certain infections. For infections that are potentially serious, and where such measures are either not available or have limited efficacy, delivery by caesarean section can protect the neonate from infection.

Measures to prevent intrapartum infection from mother to infant	
Indication	**Preventative measure(s)**
Risk factors for neonatal group B streptococcal (GBS) disease Maternal GBS colonisation documented at any time during pregnancy GBS infection in a previous baby	Penicillin given to mother from onset of labour
Risk factors for serious neonatal sepsis Low birth weight (< 1000 g) Prematurity Prolonged rupture of membranes Maternal chorioamnionitis	Broad spectrum antibiotics given to neonate (e.g. penicillin and gentamicin) for at least 48 hours
Maternal HIV infection	Anti-retroviral prophylaxis given to mother and neonate Delivery by caesarean section
Maternal hepatitis B carriage	Immunisation of neonate (vaccination ± administration of immunoglobulin)
Primary genital herpes at time of delivery	Delivery by caesarean section

Figure 3.5 Measures that are widely used to prevent intrapartum transmission of infections from mother to infant

PREVENTION OF INFECTION IN THE PAEDIATRICIAN

The main risk to staff attending a delivery is exposure to blood-borne viruses. High standards (Universal Precautions) should always be observed, to ensure protection from patients who are unexpectedly infected with blood-borne viruses (Figure 3.6). Additional precautions are required where there is a risk of contact with blood or body fluids from patients who are either known or suspected to have these infections (Figure 3.7).

Universal Precautions against exposure to blood-borne viruses
Good basic hygiene practices with regular hand washing
Appropriate protective clothing
Water-repellent gown
Surgical gloves
Mask and protective eyewear or full face visor, especially if risk of aerosols (e.g. during suction)
Avoid sharps usage wherever possible
Handle and dispose of sharps safely
Clear up spillages of blood promptly and disinfect surfaces
Dispose of contaminated waste safely

Figure 3.6 Universal Precautions to protect against exposure to blood-borne viruses

Additional infection control precautions for high risk patients
Full protective clothing when handling the baby before it is cleaned
Full length long-sleeved waterproof gowns worn over a full length plastic apron
Wellington boots
Mask and protective eyewear or full face visor, especially if risk of aerosols (e.g. during suction)
Double surgical gloves
Avoid cord blood sampling where possible. If essential:
use a needle and syringe (do not bleed the cord directly into a tube)
use forceps to isolate and steady the cord, rather than holding it between the thumb and finger

Figure 3.7 Additional infection control precautions where a patient is known to have, or to be at high risk of having, an infection with a blood-borne virus

FURTHER READING

Campbell S, Lees C (Eds). Obstetrics by Ten Teachers. London: Arnold, 2000.

Drew D, Jevon P, Raby M. Resuscitation of the Newborn, a Practical Approach. London: Butterworth Heinemann, 2000.

Henderson C, Jones K. Essential Midwifery. London: Mosby, 1997.

Smith NC. Obstetric Ultrasound Made Easy. Edinburgh: Churchill Livingstone, 2001.

Wald N, Leck J. Antenatal and Neonatal Screening, 2nd edn. Oxford: Oxford University Press, 2000.

Chapter 4

Water, sodium and potassium

INTRODUCTION

THE NEONATAL ENVIRONMENT

At birth, the baby is transferred suddenly from a temperature-controlled aqueous environment into a gaseous environment of variable temperature and humidity. It becomes dependent for maintenance of body temperature and hydration on its carers and its own homeostatic mechanisms.

TEMPERATURE REGULATION AND WATER BALANCE

Maintenance of the thermal environment of the newborn baby is an important aspect of care. Thermal stress has been linked to increased morbidity and mortality; the newborn baby is vulnerable to temperature instability because of various anatomical and physiological factors, summarised in Figure 4.1. Temperature regulation is relevant to water homeostasis as cutaneous loss of water is a significant source of heat loss. In neonatal care, the aim is to maintain a core temperature between 36°C and 37°C at all times. The most critical period is immediately following delivery.

HEAT PRODUCTION AND HEAT LOSS

To maintain a normal body temperature, heat production must balance heat lost to the environment. Heat production uses energy that might otherwise contribute to growth. Clinical care aims to nurse a baby in a neutral thermal environment, that is, one in which the energy expenditure required for heat exchange is minimised. Heat loss occurs by conduction, convection, radiation and evaporation. The relative contribution of each of these factors will vary depending on the gestation and postnatal age of the baby, the temperature, air flow and humidity of the environment, the proportion of the body exposed to air and the presence of clothing. For a term infant after the immediate postnatal period, neutral environmental temperature represents a minimum dry heat loss equivalent to about 6 cal/sec/m^2.

For a baby in a steady state, the major route of heat loss (46%) is by radiation if the baby is nursed naked in a single walled incubator, whereas the same baby nursed under a radiant warmer would have net radiant heat gain. Heat loss by evaporation, however, increases from about 30% in an incubator to about 75%

under a radiant warmer, and can be much greater in a very immature newborn infant.

Heat production depends on the body's resting metabolic rate. This increases from about 35-40 kcal/kg/24h on day 1 to 40-60 kcal/kg/24h after the first week. Heat production increases with activity, with feeding, and with cold stress.

Conservation of body heat when exposed to cold stress is achieved by peripheral vasoconstriction (measured clinically as an increased toe:core temperature difference) – although this response takes 2 to 3 days after birth to develop in very low birth weight infants – and by increasing heat production by non-shivering thermogenesis in brown adipose tissue, triggered when the mean skin temperature falls below about 35°C. Conversely, vasodilatation occurs at a rectal temperature above 37°C and sweating above about 37.2°C.

Factors increasing neonatal vulnerability to cooling
Change in environmental temperature at birth (from 0.5°C above maternal core)
Large surface area relative to body mass (this ratio in a small preterm baby is five times that of an adult)
Moist naked skin at delivery – temperature may fall by 2-3°C in the first 30 minutes
Thin skin of preterm babies allows easy water transudation and increased evaporative water losses
Thermal insulation by body fat is low (0.05°C/m^2/h/kcal cf. 0.13 for an adult) – but addition of clothing can improve this
Ability to modify skin blood flow is reduced
Ability to adjust position is limited
Ability to shiver is reduced
Immature or absent thermoregulatory mechanisms, especially in premature babies

Figure 4.1 Factors increasing neonatal vulnerability to cooling

EFFECTS ON WATER BALANCE

Evaporative insensible water loss, if not reduced by modification of the baby's environment, can be significant. Average losses of 2.4 g/kg/h have been described in low birth weight babies under radiant warmers, increasing to 3.5 g/kg/h if phototherapy is added.

If these losses are unrecognised, the very preterm baby is at risk of developing hypovolaemic circulatory failure with electrolyte imbalance (hypernatraemia, hyperkalaemia), prerenal uraemia, oliguria and excessive weight loss. Prompt resuscitation with crystalloid will then be necessary, using either 5% dextrose or 4% dextrose with 0.18% saline.

The use of plastic blankets under radiant warmers, humidification of incubator air to 80-90% relative humidity, use of 'air mode' rather than 'servo mode' regulation of air temperature, use of clothing (particularly head covering) and blankets, and minimisation of door opening and air flow disturbance, can all be helpful. The adequate humidification of inspired warmed gases in headboxes, CPAP (continuous positive airways pressure) and ventilator circuits is also important.

WATER

DISTRIBUTION

At term, about 75% of body weight is represented by water (30% intracellular and 45% extracellular). In premature babies, a greater proportion of body weight is due to water, although the intracellular amount remains approximately constant. A 32 week baby comprises about 85% water at birth.

Body water falls – mainly as a reduction in extracellular fluid – in all babies after birth, being responsible for the frequently observed 5-10% weight loss that occurs in the first week of life. The mechanism is a diuresis related to altered renal perfusion and increasing glomerular filtration rate. This fluid loss represents isotonic contraction of body fluids, that is, loss of water and electrolytes together. A high fluid intake during this period can overcome this loss, but is thought to be disadvantageous, and is associated with increased frequency of both necrotising enterocolitis and symptomatic patent ductus arteriosus.

HOMEOSTASIS

Body water is regulated through several feedback systems. These result in control of both the amount of water in the body and the osmolality of plasma, that is, the concentration of solute particles in plasma, which is maintained at 275-295 mmol/kg. Body water gain, derived from intake and from oxidation of protein, fat and carbohydrate, must balance losses from the kidneys, lungs, skin and gastrointestinal tract. Intake in the suckling infant is regulated by thirst, a sensation governed by the hypothalamus. Physiologically, the main stimulus of thirst is an increase in plasma osmolality, detected by osmoreceptors in the hypothalamus. In addition, thirst is stimulated by hypovolaemia, through the activation of baroreceptors in the cardiac atria and blood vessels, and an increase in the secretion of renin; the latter causes increased production of angiotensin II, which acts on the hypothalamus to stimulate thirst.

Activation of osmoreceptors also causes release of vasopressin (antidiuretic hormone, ADH), which is synthesised in the supraoptic nuclei and released from the posterior pituitary into the bloodstream to act on the renal collecting ducts by increasing their permeability to water. Parallel to the dual control of thirst by osmolality and hypovolaemia, vasopressin secretion is also stimulated by hypovolaemia, through mechanisms involving the secretion of angiotensin II and the stimulation of low- and high-pressure baroreceptors in the cardiac atria and great veins, and carotid sinuses and aortic arch, respectively. Vasopressin secretion increases linearly with increasing plasma osmolality. Hypovolaemia causes an exponential increase in vasopressin secretion and shifts the osmotic response curve to the left, that is, it reduces the osmotic threshold for the secretion of vasopressin. Thus, in severe hypovolaemia, plasma volume is defended at the expense of a fall in osmolality.

Obligatory water losses, equivalent to the minimum necessary daily fluid intake to maintain fluid balance, include insensible losses from lungs and skin, urinary excretion and stool water (5-10 mL/kg/24h). In the term neonate, these total a minimum 50 mL/kg/24h in the first week and 60-80 mL/kg/24h by the end of the second week of life. In addition, a net 20-25 mL/kg/24h is needed to account for growth. Pulmonary insensible loss is increased in tachypnoea and if inhaled air is dry. Evaporative water loss from the skin depends on temperature and environment. Losses by both of these routes occur independently of body water content. Some urinary water excretion is obligatory to excrete the solute load; the remainder reflects the regulation of the volume and composition of the extracellular fluid.

The kidneys in the newborn have limited capacity to adjust to a fluid load, in part due to the poorly developed response of receptors in the collecting ducts to vasopressin. Even a healthy term infant can concentrate urine only up to an osmolality of 800 mmol/kg – half that of an adult – and can maximally dilute urine to 50 mmol/kg. Newborn babies are at risk of dehydration or fluid overload if there is any error in calculating fluid requirements. In sick neonates, excess vasopressin may be secreted as part of a stress response, resulting in water retention and hyponatraemia. This is seen in ventilated, asphyxiated, or septic babies as well as those with brain trauma or intraventricular haemorrhage. Diagnosis is by clinical suspicion (at-risk baby, excess weight gain, hyponatraemia and low plasma creatinine concentration) confirmed by simultaneous measurement of plasma osmolality (low) and urine osmolality (greater than 100 mmol/kg). Restriction of fluid intake to 60 mL/kg or less is indicated.

REQUIREMENTS

The fluid volumes normally offered to bottle-fed infants are indicated in Figure 4.2. Requirements during the first week are calculated based on birth weight; thereafter, actual weight or birth weight (whichever is greater) should be used. These volumes are also appropriate for a standard parenteral nutrition regimen, provided that there is neither fluid deficit nor ongoing increased loss. An additional 30 mL/kg should be given to babies under a radiant warmer. The figure also indicates the amounts of major minerals appropriate for a standard parenteral nutrition regimen.

Fluid and mineral requirements for healthy neonates

Day	Water (as 5 or 10% dextrose)	Sodium (as 30% NaCl = 5 mmol/mL)	Potassium (as 15% KCl = 2 mmol/mL)	Calcium (as 10% Ca gluconate)
1	60 mL/kg	0	0	0
2	90 mL/kg[1]	2-3 mmol/kg[2]	2-3 mmol/kg[3]	1 mmol/kg
3	120 mL/kg	3-4 mmol/kg	2-3 mmol/kg	1 mmol/kg
4	150 mL/kg	3-4 mmol/kg	2-3 mmol/kg	1 mmol/kg
5	180 mL/kg	3-4 mmol/kg	2-3 mmol/kg	1 mmol/kg

[1] Restrict to 60 in babies with respiratory distress, asphyxia or infection

[2] In babies below 30 weeks requirements are sometimes higher: check plasma sodium concentration daily

[3] Start potassium only after urine output of at least 1 mL/kg/h is established

Figure 4.2 Fluid and mineral requirements for healthy neonates

Low birth weight babies have a high incidence of requiring parenteral fluids, very variable requirements for the composition of these, very limited renal capacity to cope with fluid imbalance, and extreme vulnerability to complications arising from imbalances.

DEFICIT AND EXCESS

Water losses are often not directly measurable. They may be estimated by taking into account clinical hydration status (skin turgor, peripheral perfusion, oedema), possible excessive losses (e.g. due to skin immaturity or damage, radiant heaters, diarrhoea and necrotising enterocolitis with hidden fluid loss into the abdomen), urine output and plasma sodium concentration (though bearing in mind that concentration reflects the amounts of both solvent and solute in the solution). Accurate daily weighing using electronic scales is possible in almost every infant, however sick.

After the first week, a daily weight gain of 25 to 30 g/kg should be expected. Abnormal losses should be replaced according to their volume and electrolyte composition (see Figure 4.3).

Water overload can occur if fluids are administered too rapidly. It should be apparent from clinical examination (oedema, or the reopening of the ductus arteriosus in a preterm baby) and from the concomitant excessive gain in weight. Hyponatraemia may be present, but not if the excess fluid is isotonic with respect to plasma.

Approximate electrolyte content of body fluids

Fluid source/type	Na^+ (mmol/L)	K^+ (mmol/L)	Cl^- (mmol/L)
Stomach	20-80	5-20	100-150
Small intestine	100-140	5-15	90-120
Bile	120-140	5-15	90-120
Ileostomy	45-135	3-15	20-120
Diarrhoea	10-90	10-80	10-110

Figure 4.3 Approximate electrolyte content of body fluids

SODIUM

DISTRIBUTION

Sodium is the main cation in extracellular fluid, 40% of total body sodium residing in plasma and interstitial fluid. Intracellular sodium concentration is generally low (about 10 mmol/L), while extracellular concentration is maintained at around 140 mmol/L. Sodium ions are the major osmotically active species in the extracellular fluid, and because of the primacy of the control of osmolality through the mechanisms described above, body sodium content is the major determinant of extracellular fluid volume.

SODIUM HOMEOSTASIS

Sodium homeostasis depends on the maintenance of a balance between input, sodium retained as the extracellular fluid volume expands with growth, and output. In healthy infants, relatively little sodium loss occurs through the skin and gut. The kidneys provide the major route for controlled excretion.

Renal regulation of sodium excretion relies on the reabsorption of over 99% of filtered sodium by the renal tubules. This is a two stage process: reabsorption of a constant proportion of the filtered load in the proximal tubules (about 67%) and loops of Henle (about 20%), then reabsorption in the distal tubules (7%) and collecting ducts (5%), in part regulated by aldosterone. The secretion of aldosterone itself varies according to production of renin and angiotensin, and with potassium balance. Renin, a proteolytic enzyme, is released from the juxtaglomerular apparatus, a cluster of specialised cells in the afferent arterioles, in response to hypovolaemia, hypotension or increased sympathetic nervous system activity. Renin releases angiotensin I from its inactive precursor, the plasma protein angiotensinogen, and angiotensin I is converted to angiotensin II by angiotensin converting enzyme. Angiotensin II stimulates aldosterone production by the adrenal cortex; aldosterone acts on the distal convoluted tubules and proximal collecting ducts to promote sodium reabsorption. Natriuretic peptides, produced by cardiac muscle, are released in response to increased circulating volume and act to increase both renal sodium and water excretion.

SODIUM DEFICIT AND EXCESS

Where an infant has become sodium depleted, it is possible to calculate the deficit of solute, assuming an expected total body water of 0.7 L/kg. The aim should be to replace this over 24-48 hours.

Sodium deficit (mmol) = (135 - plasma [Na^+]) x 0.7 x body weight (kg)

Breast milk supplied at 150 mL/kg/24h will provide only 1 mmol/kg/24h each of sodium and chloride. Renal conservation of sodium is impaired in the immediate post-delivery period, in immature infants, in sick infants and when loop diuretics have been used. Obligatory renal loss can be estimated by calculating fractional sodium excretion, the value varying from less than 1% to over 15% in a sick, very preterm baby.

$$\text{Fractional sodium excretion} = \frac{\text{Urine } [Na^+]}{\text{Urine [creatinine]}} \times \frac{\text{Plasma [creatinine]} \times 100}{\text{Plasma } [Na^+]}$$

Enteral salt intake can be increased by use of a preterm formula milk, a proprietary breast milk fortifier, or by adding salt to breast milk, e.g. 0.5 mL of 1 mmol/mL NaCl added to 25 mL of breast milk for all babies less than the equivalent of 34 weeks gestation (e.g. a 32 week gestation baby up to two weeks old). Adequacy of supplementation in well, preterm, orally fed babies can be monitored by weekly checks of urinary $[Na^+]/[K^+]$ molar ratio on a spot sample. The value should be greater than unity.

Sodium excess is invariably iatrogenic. Plasma sodium concentration will be normal if excessive isotonic fluid has been given and there may be physical signs of fluid overload. Hypernatraemia is more frequently a feature of water deficit than salt overload, but may reflect the inappropriate replacement of hypotonic fluid with isotonic saline.

POTASSIUM

DISTRIBUTION AND REGULATION

Potassium is the main intracellular cation, only 0.4% of total body potassium being in the plasma and interstitial fluid. The intracellular concentration of potassium is about 150 mmol/L while the extracellular concentration averages 4 mmol/L. The difference is maintained by action of the cell membrane enzyme, Na^+, K^+-ATPase.

Potassium intake in a healthy baby is approximately 1-2 mmol/kg/24h. Regulation maintains the intracellular concentration and matches intake by adjusting renal excretion, normally 10 to 15% of the filtered load.

Potassium is freely filtered by the renal glomeruli and reabsorbed in the proximal convoluted tubules proportionately with water. Both the distal convoluted tubules and the collecting ducts can secrete and reabsorb potassium. Secretion of potassium in the distal convoluted tubule varies with plasma potassium concentration, and is promoted by aldosterone (secretion of which is directly increased in hyperkalaemia). Atrial natriuretic peptide and low plasma potassium concentration inhibit aldosterone secretion. Acid-base status also has an effect: alkalosis increases potassium secretion and acidosis reduces it. Obligatory potassium excretion increases in proportion to the flow rate of fluid through the tubules. Most diuretics increase potassium losses by increasing tubular flow rate and sodium concentration.

Potassium depletion is usually associated with hypokalaemia, and potassium excess with hyperkalaemia, but because the major fraction of the body's potassium is intracellular, hypokalaemia can occur in the absence of potassium depletion, and hyperkalaemia without potassium excess. Accompanying metabolic alkalosis suggests that hypokalaemia is due to depletion of potassium.

DISTURBANCES OF SODIUM AND POTASSIUM CONCENTRATION

HYPONATRAEMIA

Hyponatraemia, (plasma sodium concentration of less than 133 mmol/L), is caused by decreased extracellular sodium content, an increase in body water, or a combination of these. It is common in the low birthweight infants in the first week of life. The aetiology, clinical features, management and causes are listed in Figure 4.4. Severe hyponatraemia can lead to seizures, possibly because of effects on membrane depolarisation in the central nervous system. Hyponatraemia present at birth is a reflection of maternal plasma sodium concentration.

In immature infants, the most frequent cause of hyponatraemia is excess renal loss of sodium due to immature tubular function and consequently reduced ability to conserve sodium. For this reason, salt supplementation of human milk feeds is recommended for babies of less than 33 weeks gestation (*see p.52*). Babies receiving parenteral fluids should be provided with at least 3 mmol sodium/kg/24h.

In some preterm babies, even this will be insufficient. The urine Na:K ratio will fall below one, indicating greater than average soidum losses. In these individuals, supplementation should be increased until the urine Na:K ratio is above unity. This may occasionally require short-term sodum intakes of 10 mmol/kg/24h or more.

Causes and management of hyponatraemia

Aetiology	Condition	Presenting feature	Management
Maternal water excess	Reflects maternal sodium at delivery: - large fluid volume during labour - maternal diuretics or laxatives	Low sodium concentration for 48 hours	Recovers spontaneously
Iatrogenic water excess	Prolonged parenteral administration of dextrose	Hyponatraemia	Add NaCl to fluids but restrict volume
Excess ADH secretion ('pure' water retention)	Birth injury Systemic sepsis Intraventricular haemorrhage Positive pressure ventilation Surgery	Weight gain/oedema Poor urine output Plasma osmolality reduced	Fluid restriction to 40-60 mL/kg/24h
Retention of water and sodium	Acute (oliguric) or chronic renal failure Cardiac failure	Water retention exceeds sodium retention	Fluid restriction
Renal loss of sodium and chloride	Immaturity Recovery phase of acute tubular necrosis Congenital renal diseases Loop diuretics Osmotic diuresis (hyperglycaemia)	Hyponatraemia	Tolerate values of 130-135 mmol/L if actively treating e.g. heart failure Otherwise replace deficit in full Treat underlying problem
	Congenital adrenal hyperplasia	Glucocorticoid deficiency Mineralocorticoid deficiency Males pigmented scrotum Females virilisation (variable)	Add NaCl to feeds Diagnose and treat underlying condition

continued...

Causes and management of hyponatraemia (continued)			
Aetiology	**Condition**	**Presenting feature**	**Management**
Renal loss of sodium and bicarbonate	Proximal renal acidosis	Acidosis Plasma potassium low or normal High bicarbonate requirement	Confirm diagnosis Treat with sodium bicarbonate and potassium citrate

Figure 4.4 Causes and management of hyponatraemia

HYPERNATRAEMIA

Hypernatraemia (plasma sodium concentration greater than 145 mmol/L) is caused either by an excessive sodium intake (usually iatrogenic), or a loss of body water, or a combination of these. The aetiology, clinical features and management of hypernatraemia are summarised in Figure 4.5.

Causes and management of hypernatraemia			
Aetiology	**Condition**	**Presenting feature**	**Management**
Sodium excess	Administration of sodium bicarbonate Excess sodium chloride	Oedema Excess weight gain	Reduce sodium intake
Inadequate fluid intake	Starvation – failed breast feeding Iatrogenic	Dehydration Hypotension	Gradual volume re-expansion with 4% dextrose/0.18% saline (avoid rapid change in plasma [Na^+])
Water loss			
• Cutaneous	Prematurity, skin damage or disease, evaporative losses (including very preterm infant under overhead heater)	Dehydration Hypotension	Humidified environment Volume re-expansion (see above)

continued...

Causes and management of hypernatraemia (continued)			
Aetiology	**Condition**	**Presenting feature**	**Management**
• Gastrointestinal	Necrotising enterocolitis – third space losses Vomiting, diarrhoea	Dehydration Hypotension Gastrointestinal disease	Volume re-expansion (see above) Measure electrolytes in liquid stool
• Renal	Diabetes mellitus – especially preterm baby on parenteral nutrition or systemic steroid treatment	Polyuria, dehydration Glycosuria Hyperglycaemia	Reduce glucose intake or use insulin infusion Rehydrate
	Diabetes insipidus (DI) – central or nephrogenic (X-linked recessive)	Polyuria, dehydration Low urinary osmolality with high plasma osmolality	Diagnosis – brain imaging, test pituitary function DDAVP for cranial DI, thiazide for nephrogenic DI
	Congenital hyperaldosteronism	Hypokalaemia, hypertension	Spironolactone

Figure 4.5 Causes and management of hypernatraemia

HYPOKALAEMIA

Both hypo- and hyperkalaemia are potentially harmful, largely because of the effects of potassium on the excitability of nerve and muscle cell membranes. Hypokalaemia (plasma potassium concentration less than 3.0 mmol/L) may be asymptomatic or lead to muscle weakness (increased apnoeas in a baby) or ileus with abdominal distension and vomiting. Hypokalaemia can be caused by inadequate intake, excessive loss, redistribution (from extra- to intracellular fluid) or dilution. The causes, clinical features and management of hypokalaemia are summarised in Figure 4.6. Treatment should be aimed at correcting the underlying cause, and replacement of potassium if necessary. In giving parenteral potassium, care must be taken both with regard to the concentration and rate of infusion in order to avoid hyperkalaemia.

Causes and management of hypokalaemia			
Aetiology	**Condition**	**Presenting feature**	**Management**
Dilutional, due to excess ADH	Birth asphyxia Intracranial trauma or disease Some lung conditions	Hyponatraemia Hypokalaemia Water retention Reduced plasma osmolality without urinary dilution	Fluid restriction to 40-60 mL/kg/24h
Gastrointestinal losses		Diarrhoea Vomiting Aspiration of gastric fluid	Replace lost fluid
Increased renal excretion			
• Excretion of K^+ in place of H^+ in systemic alkalosis	Pyloric stenosis with loss of HCl Administration of alkali	Recurrent vomiting Laboratory test results	Replace lost fluid with saline Correct alkalosis
• Excretion of K^+ in place of H^+ in renal tubular acidosis	Renal tubular acidosis	Acidosis	Give bicarbonate
• Diuretic administration	Use of any loop diuretic	Laboratory test results	Give potassium-sparing diuretics or oral KCl
• Hyperaldo-steronism	Primary or secondary hyperaldosteronism	Hypernatraemia Hypokalaemia	Spironolactone, treat underlying cause

Figure 4.6 Causes and management of hypokalaemia

HYPERKALAEMIA

Hyperkalaemia (potassium concentration in a venous blood sample > 5.5 mmol/L) produces neuromuscular effects to which the heart is especially sensitive. ECG changes with peaking of T waves, lengthening of the P-R interval, then widening of the QRS complex, may herald the onset of ventricular arrhythmias and fibrillation. These abnormalities may develop rapidly. Babies deemed to be at risk of hyperkalaemia should have ECG monitoring.

Neonates appear to be more resistant to these effects than children or adults, so in practice potassium concentrations up to 7.0 mmol/L are generally well tolerated. Potassium concentrations of 7.0 mmol/L or more must be telephoned to a clinician and responded to urgently. The causes, clinical features and management of hyperkalaemia are summarised in Figure 4.7.

Spurious (or artefactual) hyperkalaemia, due to loss of red cell potassium into the plasma during capillary blood sampling, is a particular problem in neonatal practice. Scrupulous attention to phlebotomy procedure is essential to avoid this. A reported high potassium concentration should lead the clinician to request an immediate repeat venous sample.

TREATMENT OF HYPERKALAEMIA

Asymptomatic hyperkalaemia can be well tolerated in a neonate in the short-term, but arrhythmias can develop without warning, potentiated by any hypocalcaemia or hypomagnesaemia. This risk increases with increasing concentration.

Management involves correcting any dehydration, withdrawing any supplementary potassium from administered fluids in affected or at-risk babies and correction of any hypocalcaemia with intravenous 10% calcium gluconate (1 ml/kg) with ECG monitoring. Any metabolic acidosis should be corrected with intravenous sodium bicarbonate (amount in mmol = 0.3 x body weight in kg x base deficit). Rectal calcium resonium resin (1 g/kg/24h), made into a suppository with a little water, will allow removal of moderate amounts of potassium (gastric resonium produces abdominal distension and is not recommended).

In an emergency, with an arrhythmia, either intravenous salbutamol 4 µg/kg stat or an infusion of glucose and insulin (soluble insulin 0.1 units/kg with 10 mL/kg of 10% dextrose over 30 to 60 minutes) will lower the potassium concentration temporarily by stimulating its intracellular uptake. If there is anuria or severe oliguria due to renal failure, renal replacement treatment (peritoneal dialysis) may be needed.

Causes and management of hyperkalaemia

Aetiology	Condition	Presenting feature	Management*
Artefact	Poorly taken sample with haemolysis	Unexplained laboratory test result	Repeat sample – venous or arterial
Cell membrane failure	Asphyxia Hypothermia Sepsis	Sick infant Laboratory test result	Treat underlying condition
Excessive intake			
• Intravenous fluid	Parenteral fluids, including nutrition	Laboratory test result	Reduce intake
• Blood transfusion	Administration of large volumes of stored blood	History of exchange transfusion or use of blood > 5 days old	Increase fluid input
Red cell or tissue catabolism	Trauma Bruising Haemorrhage Swallowed blood	Laboratory test result	Increase fluid input
Water loss	Excess insensible or third space losses in a preterm baby	Signs of dehydration or circulatory collapse	Increase fluid input
Decreased renal excretion			
• Acute renal failure	Oliguria	Laboratory test results	Renal replacement treatment
• Adrenocortical disease	Mineralocorticoid deficiency	Shock with hypoglycaemia May have family history Pigmented genitalia or female virilisation	Give gluco- and mineralocorticoids and NaCl

***Hyperkalaemia may require rapid correction: see text for details**

Figure 4.7 Causes and management of hyperkalaemia

SPECIFIC CONDITIONS ASSOCIATED WITH SODIUM OR POTASSIUM DISTURBANCES

RENAL TUBULAR ACIDOSES

In these disorders, systemic acidosis results either from deficient secretion of hydrogen ions or deficient reabsorption of bicarbonate by renal tubular cells. Proximal (type 2) RTA can be inherited or acquired, but when it presents in the neonatal period it is usually inherited, as an autosomal recessive disorder. The defect is impaired reabsorption of bicarbonate in the proximal tubules, leading to massive loss of bicarbonate. However, the urine can be acidified because the distal acidification mechanism is normal; because the bicarbonate loss leads to a fall in plasma concentration, the amount filtered falls to a level at which total reabsorption is possible. Presentation in infancy is with failure to thrive and metabolic acidosis. This defect can be part of a generalised tubular defect (primary or secondary), e.g. the Fanconi syndrome, Lowe's syndrome, cystinosis or tyrosinaemia. Treatment is with sodium bicarbonate or citrate supplementation (10-25 mmol/kg/24h).

Distal RTA (type 1) is an autosomal dominantly inherited condition. The renal tubular cells are unable to generate the high hydrogen ion gradient needed to adequately acidify the urine and, as a result, urinary pH cannot be reduced below 6.2. Presentation is with failure to thrive, with hypokalaemia and metabolic acidosis, and treatment is with sodium and potassium citrate (1-3 mmol/kg/24h).

Renal tubular acidosis type 4 refers to disorders in which hydrogen ion secretion is impaired because of either impaired secretion of, or decreased sensitivity to, aldosterone.

CONGENITAL ADRENAL HYPERPLASIA (CAH)

This term refers to a group of inherited (autosomal recessive) disorders of adrenal steroid hormone biosynthesis. They can result in a deficiency of cortisol or aldosterone or both. Cortisol deficiency leads to stimulation of the hypothalamo-pituitary axis, adrenocortical hyperplasia, and overproduction of precursors and androgens. Depending on which enzymatic step is deficient, and whether the genetic mutation is severe or mild, there may be:

- mineralocorticoid deficiency (leading to renal sodium loss and hyponatraemia, with or without signs of extracellular fluid volume depletion)
- mineralocorticoid excess (leading to renal sodium retention and hypertension)
- incomplete virilisation of an affected male (ambiguous genitalia)

- premature androgenisation of an affected male
- virilisation of an affected female (ambiguous genitalia)
- sexual infantilism presenting during later childhood in an affected female
- excessive pigmentation of the genitalia at birth
- neonatal hypoglycaemia, secondary to cortisol deficiency.

21-HYDROXYLASE DEFICIENCY

Ninety per cent of patients with CAH have deficiency of 21-hydroxylase, an enzyme that hydroxylates progesterone and 17-hydroxyprogesterone to yield 11-deoxycorticosterone (DOC) and 11-deoxycortisol. These are precursors in the formation of aldosterone and cortisol, respectively. The genetic defect usually results from point mutations or deletions of the CYP21 A2 gene. The incidence of these conditions is estimated to be about 1 in 10,000 to 15,000 in Europe and North America.

Clinical presentation

Presentation is classically, in females, with virilisation and salt wasting (75%) or virilisation alone (25%). The clitoris is enlarged and the labia may be fused. Internal genital organs are those of a normal female. Without treatment, masculinisation progresses. Males often appear normal at birth, although there may be excess genital pigmentation. In patients with a salt losing variant, there is immediate failure to thrive, then weight loss, vomiting, poor appetite and progressive dehydration. Hypoglycaemia may be present. Clinical presentation may be at any time in the first month. Those without salt loss develop signs of premature sexual development during infancy or early childhood, with advanced bone age and tall stature.

Laboratory findings

Plasma concentrations of sodium and chloride will be low in salt losing disease, while plasma potassium, urea and creatinine may be elevated. Plasma renin activity is increased and plasma aldosterone concentration is inappropriately low for the renin activity.

Plasma 17-hydroxyprogesterone concentration is markedly elevated in 21-hydroxylase deficiency, and is a useful diagnostic test. The sample must be taken after the age of 48 hours, as concentrations are normally somewhat elevated after birth particularly in preterm or stressed babies.

Cortisol concentrations are low in salt-wasting disease, and normal (but inappropriately low) for the concentration of ACTH in simple virilising disease.

11β-HYDROXYLASE DEFICIENCY

Five to eight percent of patients with CAH have this defect. The enzyme converts 11-deoxycortisol to cortisol and 11-deoxycorticosterone to corticosterone. Salt wasting does not occur because 11-deoxycorticosterone is a mineralocorticoid. Female virilisation at birth and male premature sexual development are seen, but without salt wasting. Hypertension occurs in childhood. Plasma concentrations of 11-deoxycortisol and 11-deoxycorticosterone are both elevated. Plasma renin activity is suppressed.

OTHER FORMS OF CONGENITAL ADRENAL HYPERPLASIA

Other rarer defects include 3β-hydroxysteroid dehydrogenase, defects of aldosterone synthesis and 17-hydroxylase deficiencies (Figure 4.8). Urinary steroid profiles by gas chromatography/mass spectrometry are required to make a definitive diagnosis and are advisable in all cases of CAH. 17-hydroxylase deficiency can be a cause of ambigous genitalia in genetic males, but usually presents later.

NEPHROGENIC DIABETES INSIPIDUS

When this condition occurs in infancy, it is invariably as a sex-linked recessive inherited disorder. It is caused by a defect in vasopressin receptors in the collecting tubules. The onset is neonatal or in early infancy. There is vomiting, constipation, failure to thrive, recurrent fever, and recurrent episodes of dehydration. Polyuria and polydipsia may not be obvious features. The glomerular filtration rate is usually normal. During episodes of dehydration there is hypernatraemia and hyperchloraemia. Lack of response to exogenous vasopressin differentiates this condition from pituitary diabetes insipidus. There may be massive urinary tract dilation (hydronephrosis and hydroureter).

Diagnosis is on the basis of the clinical findings, hypernatraemia and lack of response to vasopressin. Treatment consists of maintenance of adequate water intake and the use of thiazide diuretics.

Inherited disorders of adrenal steroid synthesis

Enzyme deficiency	Biochemical abnormalities Plasma	Urine*
21-hydroxylase	↑17-hydroxyprogesterone	↑pregnanetriol ↑11-oxopregnanetriol
11β-hydroxylase	↑11-deoxycortisol ↑11-deoxycorticosterone	↑tetrahydro-11-deoxy cortisol
3β-hydroxysteroid dehydrogenase	↑dehydroepiandrosterone ↑17-hydroxypregnenolone	↑pregnenetriol
17α-hydroxylase	↓testosterone ↓cortisol ↑progesterone	↑corticosterone metabolites ↓cortisol metabolites ↓androgen metabolites
18-hydroxylase (corticosterone methyl oxidase Type 1)	↑renin ↓aldosterone	↓aldosterone ↓18-hydroxycorticosterone
18-hydroxylase (corticosterone methyl oxidase Type 2)	↑renin ↓aldosterone	↓aldosterone ↑18-hydroxycorticosterone

*Urine steroid profiles by GC-MS are required to make a definitive diagnosis. Samples should be collected before treatment with steroids or correction of electrolyte imbalances.

Figure 4.8 Inherited disorders of adrenal steroid synthesis

GASTROINTESTINAL DISORDERS

Some 'surgical' disorders such as pyloric stenosis, gut atresia and necrotising enterocolitis can lead to large losses of fluid and electrolytes, either externally as vomitus or into an unavailable 'third space' such as the gut lumen or peritoneal cavity. Dehydration with peripheral circulatory failure and electrolyte abnormalities may occur. These must be corrected prior to surgery. In some situations, such as established pyloric stenosis with loss of gastric hydrochloric acid leading to a hypochloraemic, hypokalaemic alkalosis, this may take 24 to 48 hours of treatment with saline and potassium supplements prior to surgical repair.

A suitable regimen in pyloric stenosis is infusion of 0.9% or 0.45% saline with added potassium chloride sufficient to replace the chloride deficit, calculated from the following formula:

$[Cl^-]$ deficit (mmol) = (100-measured plasma $[Cl^-]$ (mmol/L)) x body weight (kg).

Plasma chloride measurement obviates the need for bicarbonate measurement.

During surgery for any neonatal gastrointestinal disorder, calculated fluid and electrolyte requirements should be given in addition to replacement of losses of blood or fluids as they occur. All such losses must be recorded as accurately as possible. Immediately post-operatively, urine output will be reduced secondarily to the stress-mediated increased vasopressin secretion. Insensible water loss is also likely to be reduced due to decreased skin perfusion. Parenteral fluid intake should therefore be reduced to 40 mL/kg/24h, with careful monitoring of fluid balance, measurement of plasma and urinary sodium and potassium, and regular assessment of clinical hydration status, body weight and urine output.

CYSTIC FIBROSIS (CF)

Ten per cent of infants with cystic fibrosis present with meconium ileus, the features of which are abdominal distension and failure to pass meconium within 48 hours of birth. A family history of CF or neonatal bowel obstruction are suggestive of the diagnosis. All babies with meconium ileus should be investigated for CF by DNA testing followed by a sweat test at four weeks, as DNA testing currently does not detect all mutations causing cystic fibrosis.

More rarely, CF presents as persistent conjugated hyperbilirubinaemia with raised plasma aspartate and alanine aminotransferase activities. The baby may be completely well, and the jaundice may resolve. Failure to thrive and pancreatic insufficiency then present later in infancy. CF testing, as described above, should be performed in all babies with unexplained conjugated hyperbilirubinaemia. In some places, there are neonatal screening programmes. Hyponatraemia due to excessive sweat loss is an even rarer presentation of CF.

RENAL DYSFUNCTION

In the fetus, most of the functions of the kidney are performed by the placenta. Presentation of renal dysfunction in the neonate is therefore different from presentation at later ages. Major abnormalities, such as absent or non-functioning kidneys, may present acutely in the first week after delivery in a baby whose plasma electrolyte composition is normal at birth.

Additionally, there is a background of immature and changing renal function. Glomerular filtration rate averages 1 mL/kg/min at birth. Three weeks later, it has doubled. This postnatal increase is thought to be due to increased renal plasma flow with increased blood pressure and redistribution of flow to the renal cortex. In the neonate, renal reserve capacity to cope with adverse environmental stresses is small. There is limited ability to excrete excessive sodium, probably due to the initial high plasma aldosterone concentrations and consequently high distal tubular sodium reabsorption.

The ability to cope with dehydration is limited by the restricted renal concentrating ability in the newborn, i.e. up to a maximum osmolality of 800 mmol/kg. Furthermore, the ability to excrete free water is limited in situations where vasopressin secretion is increased such as in acute respiratory distress syndrome and post-operatively.

In the preterm neonate, the low glomerular filtration rate, together with renal tubular immaturity, leads to a number of practical problems in clinical management. Many renally excreted drugs have an extremely prolonged half-life, leading to requirements for dosage interval adjustment and monitoring of plasma drug concentrations.

Renal dysfunction can be caused by a structural congenital abnormality such as posterior urethral valves, by perinatal problems such as hypoxia-ischaemia or blood loss, or by postnatal events, such as use of nephrotoxic drugs, septicaemia, shock, dehydration, renal vein thrombosis or major heart surgery.

Diagnosis

The diagnosis of renal failure depends on demonstration of a rising plasma creatinine concentration, with or without oliguria. This is defined as a urinary flow rate of <0.5 mL/kg/h after the first 24 hours of life. Plasma creatinine concentration is similar to the mother's at birth. By the second week, average plasma creatinine concentration is 35 μmol/L. In acute renal failure, plasma creatinine rises consistently by more than 20 μmol/L/24h.

Urine sodium concentration is of limited use in defining the causes of renal failure, particularly because of the immaturity of renal tubular sodium handling. Proteinuria, haematuria, and red cells or granular casts on microscopy of urinary sediment are all useful pointers to renal damage or disease.

Differentiation of established renal failure from prerenal failure owing to hypovolaemia is often clarified clinically rather than biochemically. Fractional excretion of sodium more than three in a term infant suggests renal disease with tubular involvement.

Management

The ultimate management option for severe, progressive renal disease is dialysis, usually peritoneal dialysis, although standard dialysis solutions present difficulties because of large glucose loads and slow metabolism of the lactate in the solutions. Another option is continuous renal replacement therapy by haemofiltration, utilising arteriovenous or venovenous access and an extracorporeal circuit with a highly permeable haemofilter.

Indications for dialysis (in an infant with a potentially reversible renal problem) are:

- hyperkalaemia
- severe acidosis
- volume overload
- progressively rising plasma creatinine concentration.

Early diagnosis of a renal problem, with meticulous attention to fluid and electrolyte balance, will frequently avert the need for dialysis in the baby with peri- or postnatally induced renal failure. Abdominal ultrasound and urinary catheterisation should be performed early. The baby's response to a fluid challenge of 10-15 mL/kg of 0.9% saline over one hour should indicate whether there is a prerenal component. Repeated intravenous frusemide, at doses of 1 mg/kg, should be given. If prerenal factors are excluded, fluid restriction to a level of 50 mL/kg/day plus urine and gastrointestinal losses is then appropriate.

Potassium-free intravenous fluids should be given on suspicion of dysfunction and in the acute phase, and ECG monitoring for arrhythmias performed. Acidosis with a base deficit of more than 10 mmol/L is usually treated using sodium bicarbonate to half correct it according to the formula:

$NaHCO_3$ to be infused (mmol) = (base deficit x 0.5) x (0.3 x body weight (kg)).

The infusion is usually administered as 4.2% sodium bicarbonate over 1-2 hours. In persisting renal failure, there is a danger of hypoglycaemia and malnutrition, and parenteral nutrition may be required. Plasma calcium and magnesium concentrations should be maintained because of the increased arrhythmogenicity of hyperkalaemia in the presence of hypocalcaemia or hypomagnesaemia. Drugs that are renally excreted will require adjustment of dose and/or dose interval, and monitoring of plasma concentrations. Potentially nephrotoxic drugs should, wherever possible, be discontinued.

The prognosis reflects the underlying cause and the extent to which other body organs, particularly the brain, have been affected by an ischaemic process. This may influence the extent to which aggressive management of the renal problem is continued. Up to 40% of survivors may have persisting decreased creatinine clearance, residual concentrating defects, or renal tubular acidosis.

FURTHER READING

Cartilidge P. The epidermal barrier. Semin Neonatol 2000; **5:** 273-80.

Modi N. Hyponatraemia in the newborn. (Annotation). Acta Dis Child Fetal Neonatl Ed. 1998; **78:** F81-4.

Modi N. Disorders of the kidney and urinary tract; Renal function, fluid and electrolyte balance and neonatal renal disease. In: Textbook of Neonatology 3rd edn. Rennie JM, Robertson NRC (Eds). London: Chruchill Livingstone, 1999, pp 1009-37.

Rutter N. Clinical consequences of an immature barrier. Semin Neonatol 2000; **5:** 281-7.

Chapter 5

Acid-base disorders

ADAPTATION TO INDEPENDENT LIFE

The perinatal period is one of major change for a baby. Before the onset of labour, the fetal environment, compared with that outside the womb, is relatively hypoxic. During labour, some tissue hypoxia and placental insufficiency occur, resulting in a mixed respiratory and metabolic acidosis. With the first breath, the lungs become inflated and the respiratory system rapidly adapts to take on respiratory gas exchange. The cardiovascular system also undergoes a dramatic change; difficulties in cardiorespiratory adaptation are frequent and can have serious consequences. Perinatal asphyxia occurs when there is inadequate gas exchange to meet the needs for oxygen consumption and carbon dioxide removal. Lactic acid, the product of anaerobic metabolism, and carbon dioxide accumulate. pH can be assessed in labour by fetal scalp blood sampling, and delivery expedited if necessary.

NEONATAL ACID-BASE HOMEOSTASIS

Normal extracellular hydrogen ion concentration in healthy newborn infants ranges from 38-48 nmol/L (pH 7.32 to 7.43). Normal metabolism and growth are dependent on maintaining a normal acid-base status. In a preterm baby, acidosis may prolong patency of the ductus arteriosus, allowing a left-to-right shunt, and may make the baby more susceptible to cerebral insults. Severe acidosis itself causes reduced peripheral perfusion and can produce or prolong pulmonary hypertension and left-to-right intracardiac shunting of blood through the patent foramen ovale and the ductus arteriosus. Maintenance of acid-base homeostasis in neonates is dependent upon maintaining adequate respiration and perfusion, and intact renal and hepatic function.

Neonates are particularly vulnerable to disturbance of acid-base balance because of the relative immaturity of their organ systems. This vulnerability is exacerbated in premature infants and/or if there is superimposed organ dysfunction, e.g. intrinsic renal disease or dysfunction secondary to poor perfusion or infection.

The maintenance of normal hydrogen ion concentration depends on a balance between acid production, consumption by metabolism and excretion. Short-term imbalances are absorbed through buffering.

The major buffer system in the extracellular fluid is carbonic acid (H_2CO_3)/bicarbonate (HCO_3^-):

$$H^+ + HCO_3^- \rightleftarrows H_2CO_3 \rightleftarrows H_2O + CO_2$$

The efficiency of this buffer system is increased by the fact that carbonic acid can be formed by the hydration of carbon dioxide or disposed of by the reverse process, and by carbon dioxide excretion in the expired breath. Buffering also occurs in the intracellular environment, with hydrogen ions crossing cell membranes in exchange for potassium, and bicarbonate in exchange for chloride; acute acidosis may, therefore, result in hyperkalaemia, whereas alkalosis can lower extracellular potassium concentration.

Long-term maintenance of hydrogen ion concentration depends on the balance between production and excretion of hydrogen ions. The kidney has a key role in acid-base homeostasis through the reabsorption of filtered bicarbonate in the proximal convoluted tubule, and excretion of acid in the distal convoluted tubule. The balance between carbon dioxide production and its excretion by the respiratory system, and bicarbonate utilisation in buffering and its reabsorption and regeneration in acid excretion, determines the extracellular fluid (ECF) hydrogen ion concentration or pH (Figure 5.1).

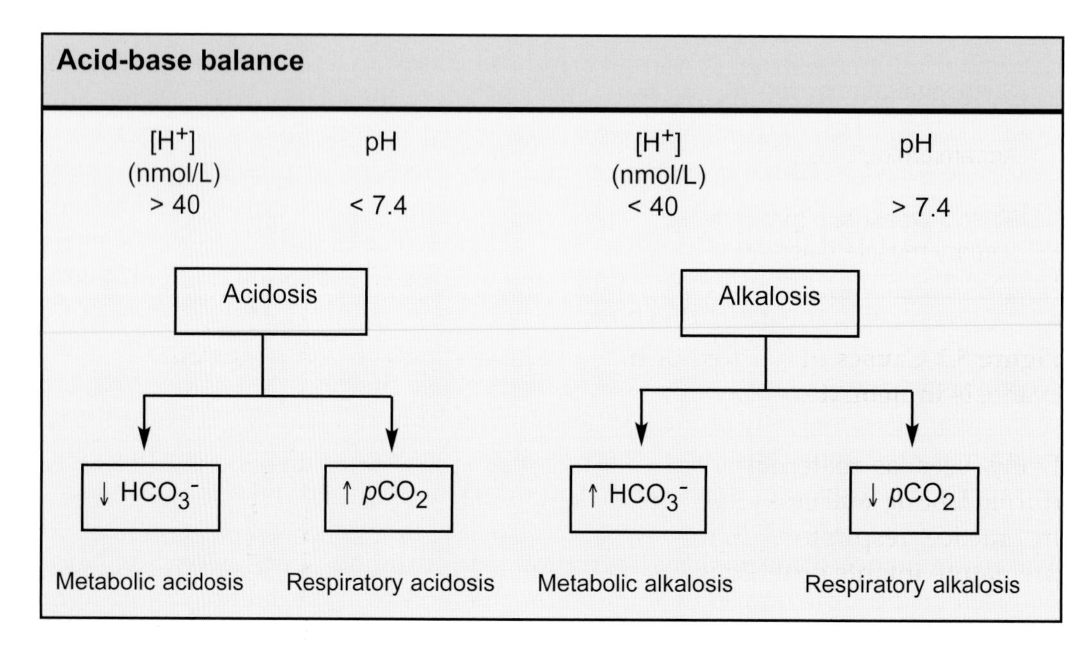

Figure 5.1 Acid-base balance

RESPIRATORY CAUSES OF ACID-BASE DISTURBANCE

RESPIRATORY DEPRESSION AT BIRTH

Urgent management of respiratory failure in newborn infants is of paramount importance. Hypoxia, and its consequences, is the commonest cause of perinatally acquired brain damage in term babies, although only a minority of cases of hypoxia-induced ischaemic damage arise during labour. In 70% of newborns requiring resuscitation, the cause is complications arising during labour. In the remainder, however, there is an apparently normal labour, with no evidence of fetal compromise. The baby may fail to establish adequate respiration (Figure 5.2) or, more rarely, may breathe regularly but fail to become centrally pink.

Causes of delayed or inadequate respiration and persistent cyanosis

Causes of delayed respiration	Causes of persistent cyanosis
Intrapartum asphyxia	Persistent pulmonary hypertension
Drugs (causing CNS depression)	Cyanotic congenital heart defect
Prematurity	Underexpansion of lungs (surfactant deficiency)
Trauma to CNS	Pneumothorax
Congenital abnormalities	Diaphragmatic hernia
Anaemia/blood loss	Anatomical abnormality of airways
Muscle weakness (prematurity or primary muscle disease)	

Figure 5.2 Causes of delayed or inadequate respiration and persistent cyanosis in neonates

Drugs used as maternal analgesics or sedatives, or general anaesthetics given during labour, will cross the placenta and can depress the fetal respiratory centre. In practice, respiratory depression from drugs is likely to be important only in premature infants or those whose respiratory drive is already compromised.

PREMATURE INFANTS

Premature infants often require active resuscitation. The mechanism of respiratory failure in this group is multifactorial, including hypoxia-ischaemia, drugs and the difficulty of establishing respiration with stiff, surfactant-deficient lungs. Avoidance of perinatal hypoxia is particularly important because of the association of hypoxia with more severe surfactant deficiency, persistent pulmonary hypertension, and with intraventricular haemorrhage and periventricular leucomalacia. Infants with established surfactant deficiency usually have a respiratory acidosis initially, because of carbon dioxide retention. Underventilation may be due to inadequate respiratory effort, irregular respiration, or muscle weakness. When hypoxia ensues, and if respiratory management is inadequate, the acidosis is compounded by a metabolic component due to increased lactic acid production from anaerobic metabolism. It is important that these disturbances are minimised by providing appropriate ventilatory support for the baby and maintaining adequate oxygenation.

APNOEA

Apnoeas, or pauses in respiration, are common in neonates. Their duration and severity are less in mature than in premature infants. Neonates, especially if preterm, often exhibit periodic breathing, with increasing and decreasing amplitude of breath; an apnoea represents a pause during the 'shallow breathing' phase. Maturation of the respiratory centre leads to the abolition of this pattern. Prolonged apnoea leads to hypoxaemia, carbon dioxide retention, acidosis and bradycardia. These episodes are usually self-limiting, but sometimes the hypoxaemia can itself lead to hypoventilation, or there is a mechanical obstructive element to the apnoea, which then becomes prolonged.

Monitoring on NNUs includes continuous oxygen saturation (SaO_2) and heart rate monitoring in at-risk babies, or, in more stable babies, the use of a pressure-sensitive external thoracic 'apnoea alarm' set to a 20 second time delay. Apnoeas usually respond to external stimulation, or can be reduced in frequency by administration of a respiratory stimulant (caffeine, theophylline) to preterm babies.

METABOLIC CAUSES OF ACID-BASE DISTURBANCES

RENAL DYSFUNCTION

Primary renal dysfunction, e.g. renal tubular acidosis (*see p.60*) may lead to an inability to excrete an acid load and hence the development of a metabolic acidosis. If there is significant acidosis, the baby will attempt to compensate by hyperventilation and pCO_2 will fall. Secondary, or transient, renal dysfunction, for instance following birth asphyxia, may also lead to metabolic acidosis, but this does not usually cause a problem in clinical management. Preterm babies may develop a chronic and mild metabolic acidosis due to renal immaturity and an inability to excrete the physiologically generated acid load. This may be exacerbated by the use of parenteral nutrition, and nitrogen intake may have to be reduced temporarily in this situation.

HYPOPERFUSION

The commonest cause of acidosis in newborn babies is lactic acidosis secondary to poor perfusion. There are numerous causes, including structural abnormalities, e.g. hypoplastic left heart, as well as sepsis, necrotising enterocolitis and loss of blood (*see p.82*).

OVERPRODUCTION OF ACID

Severe metabolic acidosis, usually with compensatory respiratory alkalosis, can occur in babies with a whole range of inherited defects of organic acid metabolism (*see Chapter 10*). In these situations, acidosis is not present at birth but will usually occur within 24-72 hours, often presenting as tachypnoea (respiratory rate > 60/min) in a previously well baby. Blood hydrogen ion concentration may be normal owing to the presence of a compensatory respiratory alkalosis.

MEASUREMENT OF BLOOD GASES AND ACID-BASE ASSESSMENT

All sick babies, particularly if there is clinical evidence of poor perfusion, respiratory insufficiency, dehydration or infection, should have their acid-base status assessed. A combination of blood gas measurements and complementary, non-invasive monitoring (transcutaneous gas analysis) allows the clinician to assess the patient and make therapeutic decisions. Non-invasive monitoring includes a combination of transcutaneous pO_2, pCO_2 and oxygen saturation monitoring (*see p.75*). Invasive arterial monitoring (umbilical artery or peripheral arterial line) is indicated if the baby is unstable, requires > 30% oxygen in the inspired gas or is on any respiratory support.

Particular challenges in assessment are the rapidly changing physiology of neonates, difficult access to arterial sampling and small blood volume.

COLLECTION AND TRANSPORT OF BLOOD

It is extremely important to pay attention to the quality of specimen obtained for acid-base monitoring. Capillary blood is not suitable in seriously ill patients, e.g. those with shock, hypotension or poor perfusion. The best specimens for measuring pO_2 are those collected with minimal disturbance through an indwelling catheter sited in the umbilical artery or a peripheral artery. Haemodilution can be a potential problem associated with peripheral arterial catheters if care is not taken to flush out the heparinised saline. Repeated sampling may itself change the pO_2 as the infant responds to pain by crying, leading to misleadingly low results. In many cases, capillary blood is used. In such situations, it is essential that the person collecting the blood has been properly trained to collect these specimens (*see p.285*). The blood must be free flowing, from a well perfused limb and collected into the special heparinised capillary tubes designed for blood gas analysis. Great care must be taken to ensure that air bubbles are not trapped in the tube, and, if the blood gas analyser is at a remote site, that the blood is maintained at 4°C during transit. Capillary values for hydrogen ion concentration and pCO_2 are usually close to arterial values ($[H^+]$ ± 5 nmol/L, pCO_2 + 1kPa). However, capillary pO_2 underestimates the arterial value. Transcutaneous pO_2 and pulse oximetry have now replaced capillary pO_2 measurement and capillary blood is *not* considered suitable for this purpose.

BLOOD GAS ANALYSIS

There are several blood gas analysers that are suitable to use for analysing samples from neonates. Small sample size and ease of use with capillary tubes or syringes are obviously key factors when choosing an instrument.

In units that have their own blood gas analyser, where non-laboratory clinical staff are trained to use the instruments, it is imperative that there is an appropriate quality assurance programme, maintenance programme, support for training and troubleshooting, all provided from the laboratory. This must include provision of a designated 'back up' instrument, which may be most appropriately located in the main laboratory.

NON-INVASIVE BLOOD GAS MONITORING

Pulse oximetry and transcutaneous oxygen monitoring are useful non-invasive techniques to estimate oxygenation and complement blood gas analysis. However, neither technique can replace arterial blood gas monitoring in critically ill infants.

TRANSCUTANEOUS GAS ANALYSIS

Blood gas analysis of arterial specimens gives measurements of pO_2, $[H^+]$ and pCO_2 at a particular time. In sick neonates, however, pO_2 in particular may be extremely variable, with profound falls after handling procedures, such as physiotherapy or suction, or respiratory irregularity. A fall in pO_2 may also provide early warning of significant clinical problems – for instance, pneumothorax, or air leak, in a baby with respiratory distress syndrome – before this could be detected by observing changes in colour, heart rate or respiration. Because of these factors, some form of continuous pO_2 monitoring or, alternatively, oxygen saturation monitoring, is usually employed in the care of babies receiving oxygen. This can reveal trends and facilitate rapid intervention when necessary.

For these reasons, electrodes for the transcutaneous measurement of oxygen tension ($TcpO_2$) are widely used in neonatal units. While these electrodes are extremely useful in monitoring arterial pO_2 non-invasively, there are problems associated with the technique. The operating temperature of the electrode is 43°C and this may cause first or second degree burning of the skin, especially in poorly perfused or very immature babies. The $TcpO_2$ probe should be crosschecked for accuracy by comparing its reading with four-hourly, or more frequent, arterial pO_2 measurements taken from an indwelling catheter. This is because, on occasions, unexpected discrepancies can arise between transcutaneous and arterial pO_2, necessitating correlation with direct arterial samples at frequent intervals. Over a period of hours, 'electrode drift' will occur, necessitating re-zeroing and recalibration of the electrodes. In some units, $TcpO_2$ is relied on alone, without any correlation with arterial values of pO_2; this is bad clinical practice and should be discouraged.

If a baby is shocked and poorly perfused, it may be impossible to obtain a $TcpO_2$ reading. In older babies, particularly those with chronic lung disease who have received steroids, the skin and subcutaneous tissue characteristics are altered and it is not possible to obtain accurate or consistent $TcpO_2$ measurements.

Oxygen saturation monitoring (pulse oximetry)

Oxygen is present in the blood in two physical forms:

- freely dissolved in plasma water
- bound reversibly to haemoglobin within red cells.

The first of these is directly related to the partial pressure of oxygen in blood (pO_2). This accounts for about 2% of total blood oxygen content. The other 98% is the oxygen bound to haemoglobin. This is also related to pO_2, although it cannot be increased by increasing the pO_2 above normal, as haemoglobin is fully saturated with oxygen at normal pO_2. This relationship is defined by the oxygen-haemoglobin affinity curve. This can be graphically represented as a comparison between the percentage of haemoglobin fully saturated with oxygen ($[HbO_2]$ $\times 100/[Hb]+[HbO_2]$) and blood pO_2. In neonates, this curve will tend to be shifted to the left because of the characteristics of neonatal red cells (Figure 5.3).

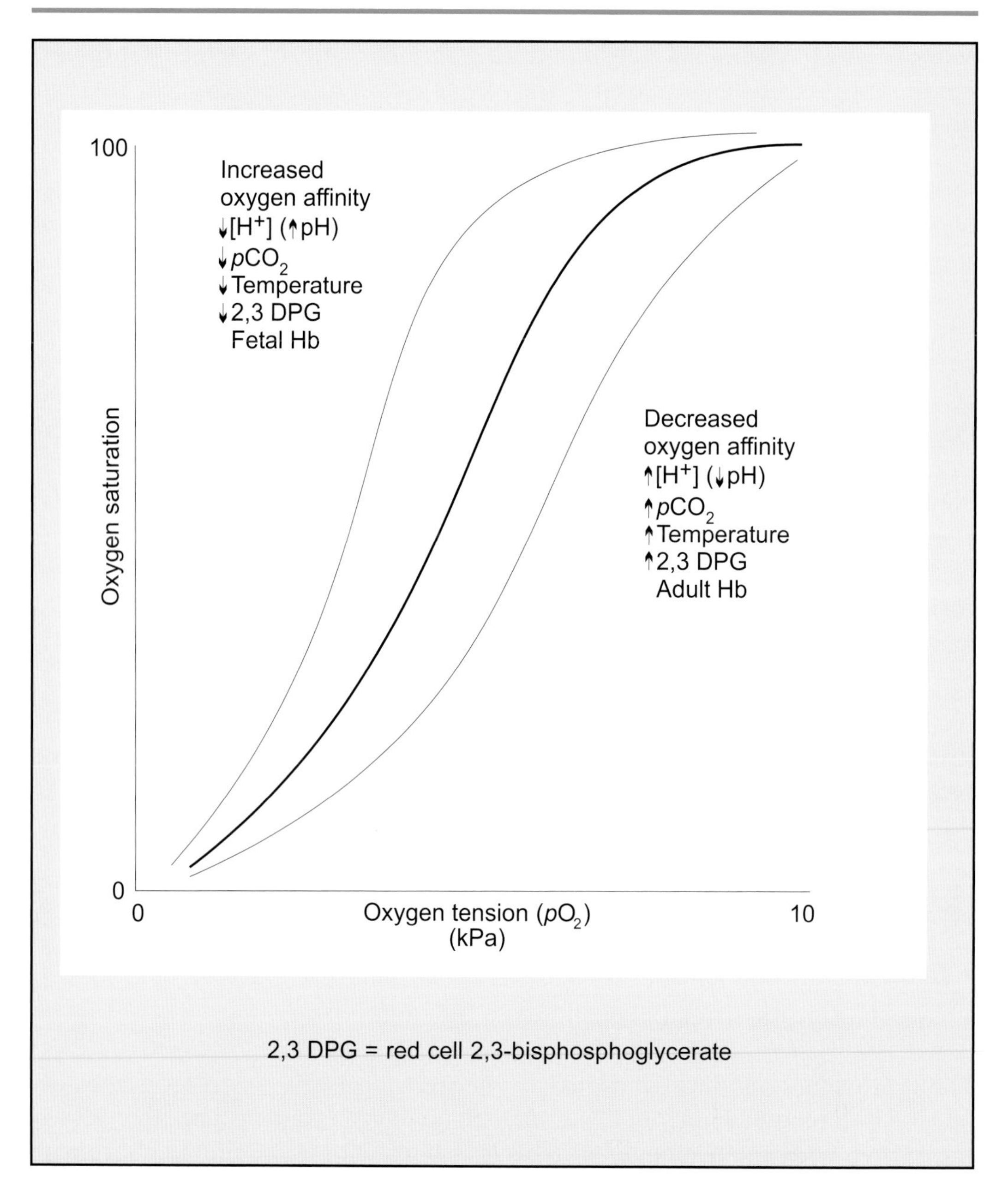

Figure 5.3 Factors affecting oxygen-haemoglobin affinity in neonates

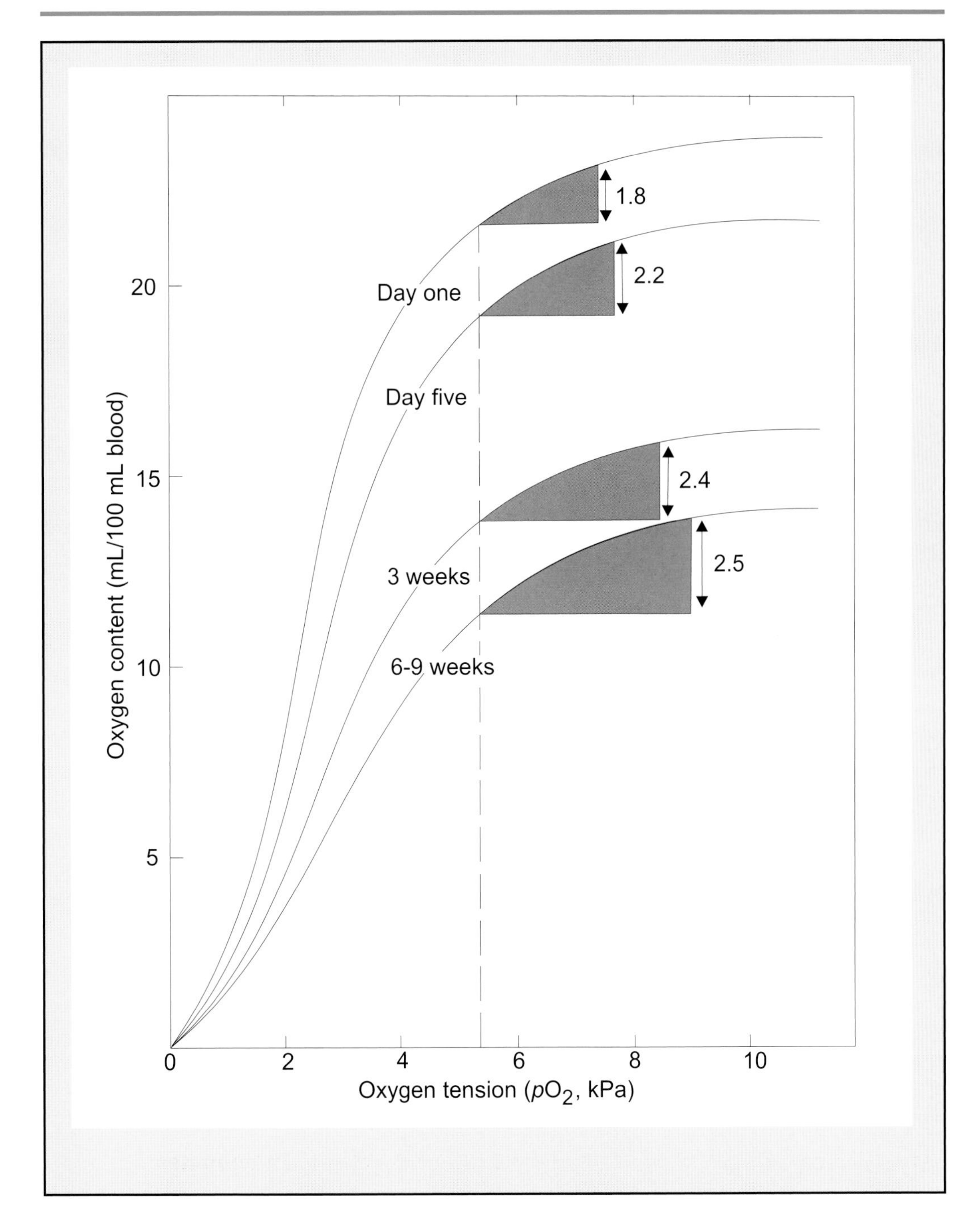

Figure 5.4 Relationship between blood oxygen content and pO_2 at different ages in normal term infants

Total oxygen carrying capacity thus depends on the haemoglobin concentration, which falls in the first weeks of postnatal life. During this period, however, the proportion of fetal haemoglobin also falls, and the oxygen released to tissues increases. The hatched areas shown in Figure 5.4 represent the volume of oxygen released as the pO_2 falls from a point at which haemoglobin is 95% saturated to an approximate tissue pO_2 of 5.3 kPa.

Direct measurement of the percentage of haemoglobin saturated with oxygen may be of theoretical as well as practical value. It provides an indication of the adequacy of tissue oxygen supply. This will be compromised if oxygen saturation (SaO_2) is less than 80%.

Pulse oximetry uses a light-emitting probe attached to a hand or foot, and computes oxygen saturation from the light absorption characteristics of the pulsatile flow (containing both oxygenated and deoxygenated haemoglobin) as it passes beneath the probe. The results correlate closely with validated arterial saturation measurements in some oximeters (e.g. Nellcor) but there is variability between results obtained with some other instruments. Rapidly responding saturation results can be obtained without initial calibration. They are obtainable in poorly perfused babies and in older babies with chronic oxygen dependency. No recalibration of probes is required during use. However, since the normal values of SaO_2 in the neonate are 95-98%, hyperoxaemia may go undetected unless the pO_2 is also known. This is because only small changes in SaO_2 occur, even with large alterations in partial pressure of oxygen at this upper end of the dissociation curve. A false estimate can occur if the probe is applied incorrectly or if there is movement of the patient or probe. The aim is to keep SaO_2 in the 88-92% range. Pulse oximetry must be supplemented with intermittent arterial blood gas measurements, particularly in high risk premature infants.

Pulmonary circulation, ductus arteriosus diameter, and cellular and tissue injury from oxygen free radical production all relate to pO_2 rather than to oxygen content. Knowledge of pO_2 is therefore vital when oxygen saturation monitoring is being used in acutely ill neonates.

ARTERIAL pCO_2

Arterial pCO_2 provides an assessment of adequacy of alveolar ventilation. The pCO_2 reflects the balance between the metabolic production of carbon dioxide and its excretion by ventilation. Reduction in pCO_2 can be achieved by reducing the metabolic rate or by increasing ventilation. Transcutaneous pCO_2 monitoring correlates well with directly measured pCO_2 and provides a good means of following trends. Unlike pO_2 monitors, pCO_2 monitors do not cause skin burns. *In vivo* calibration against arterial or capillary gases is required.

INTRAVASCULAR *p*O2 ELECTRODES

Umbilical artery catheters are available that have an intrinsic pO_2 electrode at their tip. They can provide continuous pO_2 data for as long as the umbilical catheter remains *in situ*. Regular recalibration of the system against directly measured arterial pO_2 remains essential.

INTERPRETATION OF ACID-BASE STATUS

Normal values for arterial blood $[H^+]$, pCO_2 and pO_2, are dependent on postnatal age. After birth, as pulmonary gas exchange is established, pCO_2, $[H^+]$ and pO_2 move towards adult values. There are dramatic changes in the first 30 minutes after birth ($pO_2\uparrow$, $pCO_2\downarrow$, $[H^+]\downarrow$, $pH\uparrow$). The changes continue over the first two hours (see Figure 5.5).

Interpretation of acid-base measurements must take into account the type of specimen (capillary/arterial), the clinical state of the baby and the results of other relevant investigations. A base deficit (*see p.82*) of lower than -4 mmol/L is significant, although in practice further investigation is not usually undertaken until it falls to below -8 mmol/L.

Arterial blood gas values in normal full term neonates

	$[H^+]$ nmol/L	pH	pCO_2 kPa	pO_2 kPa
Arterial — 1-6 hours	46-49	7.31-7.34	4.7-6.0	8.0-10.6
Arterial — 6-24 hours	37-43	7.37-7.43	4.4-4.8	9.3-10.0
Arterial — 2-7 days	42-44	7.36-7.38	4.4-4.8	9.3-11.3

Figure 5.5 Arterial $[H^+]$, pH and blood gas values in normal full term neonates

DIFFERENTIAL DIAGNOSIS OF ACID-BASE DISTURBANCES

(see Figures 5.6 and 5.7)

Acid-base disturbances may be simple, i.e. having an isolated respiratory or metabolic cause. Physiological compensation of the primary disorder, i.e. by changes in renal acid excretion in respiratory disorders, and in ventilation, and hence carbon dioxide excretion, in metabolic disorders, usually occurs. Absence of adequate compensation will result in persistent acidosis or alkalosis until the underlying cause is corrected. It should be noted that effective renal compensation is a slower process than respiratory mechanisms and there may be a time lag of several days before compensation is complete.

A simple approach to interpretation is to ask these questions:

1. Is the baby acidotic or alkalotic?

   i.e. $[H^+] < 38$ nmol/L ($pH > 7.42$) - alkalotic

   $[H^+] > 48$ nmol/L ($pH < 7.32$) - acidotic

2. If acidotic:

   if pCO_2 is high - respiratory cause

   if pCO_2 is low - metabolic cause

   If alkalotic:

   if pCO_2 is low - respiratory cause

   if pCO_2 is high - metabolic cause

3. Is the expected compensation present?

   e.g. in metabolic acidosis, a compensatory fall in pCO_2.

ACIDOSIS

The commonest causes of acidosis in neonates are hypoxia and poor tissue perfusion, which may derive from birth asphyxia or later illness. Infants with infections are particularly likely to be acidotic due to poor perfusion and overproduction of hydrogen ions.

Causes of acid-base disturbances in neonates

	$[H^+]$	pH	pCO_2	$[HCO_3^-]$	Causes
Respiratory acidosis	↑	↓	↑	N/↑*	Hypoventilation - CNS depression - lung disease - neuromuscular disease - obstruction of upper airways - inadequate artificial ventilation
Respiratory alkalosis	↓	↑	↓	N/↓*	Overventilation Hyperammonaemia
Metabolic acidosis	↑	↓	N/↓**	↓	Renal impairment Hypoxia Poor perfusion Loss of fluid from gastrointestinal tract Metabolic disorders
Metabolic alkalosis	↓	↑	N/↑**	↑	Bicarbonate administration Pyloric stenosis Hypokalaemia Diuretics Vomiting Nasogastric suction Chloride deficiency

*A small change in $[HCO_3^-]$ accompanies an acute respiratory disturbance; compensation causes a greater change in the same direction.

**Compensatory change.

Figure 5.6 Causes of acid-base disturbances in neonates

METABOLIC ACIDOSIS

The commonest cause of acidosis is lactic acidosis as a consequence of poor perfusion. If hypovolaemia is present, the primary management of such a baby would be administration of fluid (e.g. 0.9% saline) in adequate volumes (e.g. 15-20 mL/kg body weight).

The metabolic component of acid-base disturbances can be assessed from calculation of the bicarbonate and base excess in freely flowing blood. Base excess is a calculated parameter and provides an assessment of the metabolic component of an acid-base disturbance. It requires calculation of 'standard' bicarbonate, which is defined as the concentration of bicarbonate at a pCO_2 of 5.3 kPa (i.e. removal of any respiratory component). A negative base excess is referred to as a base deficit. A commonly used formula to assess the amount of base required for correction is the following:

Base required = 0.3 x body weight (kg) x base deficit (mmol)= mmol bicarbonate required

In practice, half this amount is given as sodium bicarbonate solution (maximum strength 4.2%) into a large vein and acid-base status reassessed.

Major changes in perfusion and cardiac output may follow such therapy. It should, therefore, only be used in situations where the acidosis is severe and likely to persist without treatment. The bicarbonate infusion should be given over at least one hour except in an acute emergency.

Metabolic acidosis in neonates caused by renal disease may be due to renal failure or renal tubular acidosis (RTA) (*see p.60*). The commonest cause of renal failure is poor renal perfusion secondary to asphyxia; it is usually reversible and only conservative methods of management are required. If plasma creatinine concentration is normal and there is hyperchloraemia with metabolic acidosis, then RTA is probable. There are many inherited metabolic disorders (*see Chapter 10*) that cause metabolic acidosis, e.g. methylmalonic acidaemia and propionic acidaemia.

Differential diagnosis of metabolic acidosis may be aided by calculation of the plasma anion gap, i.e. $([Na^+]+[K^+])-([HCO_3^-]+[Cl^-])$. A gap of greater than 20 mmol/L is suggestive of an organic acid disorder (*see p.174*) or lactic acidosis due to hypoxia. Biochemical investigations that may help with the differential diagnosis include urinary ketones, plasma glucose, ammonia and lactate concentrations, urine and plasma amino acids and urinary organic acids. If plasma chloride concentration is increased, with normal concentrations of amino acids and organic acids, renal tubular disease should be considered.

Differential diagnosis of acidosis	
Cause	**Supporting evidence**
Circulatory	↑ Plasma lactate, ↑ anion gap, ↓ blood pressure
Renal	N/↑ creatinine, ↑ [Cl^-], N/↑ urine pH, normal anion gap
Respiratory	Clinical signs, ↑ pCO_2
Metabolic	↑ Anion gap, +ve urinary ketones, N/↓ urine pH

Figure 5.7 Differential diagnosis of acidosis

ALKALOSIS

The commonest cause of alkalosis is iatrogenic respiratory alkalosis in ventilated babies. Excess administration of bicarbonate can also produce alkalosis when acidosis has been overestimated clinically. Metabolic alkalosis in a vomiting baby is highly suggestive of pyloric stenosis with loss of gastric acid.

HYPOXIA

The normal arterial pO_2 for term babies breathing air is 8-11 kPa. A pO_2 below 2-3 kPa will cause metabolic acidosis secondary to anaerobic metabolism and demands urgent attention.

A low pO_2 may be due to pulmonary disease, failure of circulatory adaptation at birth (persistent pulmonary hypertension) or an anatomical by-pass of the pulmonary circulation, e.g. persistent ductus arteriosus. It is important to diagnose an anatomical cause so that corrective surgery can be undertaken if appropriate. Most pulmonary causes of hypoxia can be differentiated by a combination of history, examination, chest X-ray and bacteriological investigation. Even with a normal pO_2, insufficient oxygen delivery to the tissues can be caused by cardiac failure, severe anaemia or low oxygen concentration (Figure 5.8). This leads to metabolic acidosis.

In severely hypoxaemic babies, the 'nitrogen washout' test can be used to separate the pulmonary causes from the failure of adaptation or 'by-pass' causes. The procedure is first to measure the pO_2 from the right radial artery, or to determine the oxygen saturation in the right arm (i.e. pre-ductal part of the circulation) using a pulse oximeter. The baby is then given as near to 100% oxygen as is practical, using a headbox. In hypoxia of pulmonary origin, this manoeuvre will cause a large increase in pO_2 and SaO_2. In pulmonary by-pass, pO_2 may increase but not by more than 1-2 kPa, and the baby will remain significantly hypoxic. Cardiac ultrasound examination will define any structural abnormality. If the heart is structurally normal and the lungs clear on chest X-ray, the baby probably has persistent pulmonary hypertension. This represents failure of pulmonary vasodilation at birth and can arise *de novo* or after asphyxia. Pulmonary vasodilators usually lead to steady improvement within the first week. Nitric oxide given by inhalation, or IV prostacyclin or tolazoline, can be used, together with attention to maintaining $[H^+] < 40$ nmol/L (pH > 7.40) if possible, until the pulmonary hypertension has resolved.

Causes of tissue hypoxia in newborn infants

Low cardiac output

- hypovolaemia
- sepsis
- cardiac defects

Low pO_2 (hypoxaemia)

- lung disease
  - respiratory distress syndrome
  - sepsis
- congenital heart disease with right to left shunt
- low haemoglobin (anaemia)
  - feto-maternal transfusion
  - haemolysis
  - blood sampling

Figure 5.8 Causes of tissue hypoxia in newborn infants

The aim of oxygen therapy is to maintain adequate oxygenation and thereby minimise cardiac work and respiratory effort. Premature infants should have pO_2 values of 7-11 kPa to optimise tissue oxygenation, but minimise the risk of blindness caused by retinopathy of prematurity (*see p.85*). By contrast, full term infants with diaphragmatic hernia, for example, may require pO_2 values of 11-13 kPa.

HYPEROXAEMIA

Excess oxygen carries significant hazards, particularly in immature infants. The major hazards are lung toxicity and retinopathy of prematurity.

Pulmonary Toxicity

This is related to the concentration of inspired oxygen and is a significant risk if a baby receives oxygen concentrations of 80% or more over a period of more than a few hours. Bronchopulmonary dysplasia, recognised as a severe complication following idiopathic respiratory distress syndrome in babies who have received mechanical ventilation, has many histopathological features in common with those produced by oxygen toxicity in animals. The earliest changes resemble exaggerated normal repair processes in the bronchiolar walls. The lungs become solid and oedema develops around the bronchioles, followed by fibroblastic proliferation if the high inspired oxygen is maintained. Foci of distorted, proliferated capillaries are seen in some areas, while in others there is a relative lack of a capillary bed. Organised secretions occlude bronchiolar lumina and there is hyperplasia and squamous metaplasia of the bronchial epithelium. These latter features are probably associated with the positive pressures used in ventilation and are difficult to disentangle from those related to oxygen administration.

These abnormalities develop most readily in very immature lungs, particularly in association with air leaks. Preventative measures include the use of adequate ventilation to reduce the ambient oxygen requirements, while avoiding high ventilatory pressures if possible. Avoidance of air leaks by appropriate ventilation, including patient-triggered ventilation, is equally important.

Retinopathy of prematurity (ROP)

This condition, previously known as retrolental fibroplasia, was first recognised in 1940 in the USA. It came to public notice in the 1940s and 1950s, when its occurrence and the major consequence – blindness – reached almost epidemic proportions in surviving premature infants, particularly in the USA. At that time, the condition was thought to be caused purely by oxygen toxicity. Since the 1970s, the frequency of the disease has increased again in the 'new' population of surviving very premature babies (i.e. < 28 weeks gestation or < 1000 g birth weight). It remains the commonest cause of blindness in the neonatal period, although it is now very unusual in infants of more than 32 weeks gestation.

The disease is recognised in the perinatal period by indirect ophthalmoscopy and this is now performed on at-risk babies in neonatal units. Milder grades of severity are common, and 80-90% regress spontaneously. They are probably of little importance. Occasionally, however, they progress to severe disease (cicatrical ROP), leading eventually to distortion and detachment of the retina. Treatment by cryotherapy or laser therapy may arrest progressive disease.

The relationship with oxygen appears to be a complex one. Retinal blood vessels grow out to the periphery during gestation but do not reach the temporal margin until after term. High levels of local tissue oxygenation cause spasm of these vessels and ischaemia of the retinal periphery. Subsequently, new, poorly organised blood vessels proliferate from remaining central vessels and attempt to vascularise the periphery. Bleeding and retinal detachment can follow, the time interval between initiation of disease and damage averaging 4-6 weeks.

The damaging effects of oxygen in preterm infants are probably exaggerated because of the poor function of oxygen-generated free radical scavengers in this population. Thus, the level of retinal pO_2 causing damage may vary. It is widely recommended that arterial pO_2 should be kept below 12 kPa as a precautionary measure and some previously accepted treatments, e.g. use of 100% oxygen instead of air for resuscitation, are now being questioned.

Factors other than oxygen are associated with ROP, possibly through direct effects on retinal vasculature: they include intraventricular haemorrhage, hypoxia, apnoeas, hypocapnia (producing intracerebral vasoconstriction) and the use of indomethacin to stimulate closure of a patent ductus arteriosus. A variety of potential preventative agents, particularly vitamin E, have not been proven to be effective.

Hypo- and hypercapnia

The normal pCO_2 in neonates after the first week of life is 4.0-5.5 kPa. A low pCO_2 is uncommon in a spontaneously breathing newborn baby. The commonest cause is over-ventilation secondary to metabolic acidosis. Over-ventilation can also occur in spontaneously breathing babies with cerebral irritability due to birth trauma or birth asphyxia. An increased pCO_2 is usually caused by hypoventilation, either primary or secondary to metabolic alkalosis.

OTHER ABNORMALITIES

Carboxyhaemoglobin is of relevance in mothers who smoke. Carbon monoxide crosses the placenta and binds strongly to fetal haemoglobin, making it unavalable for oxygen transport, causing a functional anaemia.

Inhaled nitric oxide is used to treat pulmonary hypertension in the newborn. The nitric oxide-haemoglobin complex is converted to methaemoglobin. High concentrations of nitric oxide can lead to methaemoglobinaemia. Patients receiving inhaled nitric oxide should be monitored to keep the methaemoglobin concentration below 5% of the total haemoglobin.

FURTHER READING

Brouillette RT, Waxman DH. Evaluation of the newborn's blood gas status. Clin Chem 1997; **43:** 215-21.

Duc G, Sinclair JC. Oxygen administration. In: Effective care of the newborn infant. Sinclair JC, Bracken MB (Eds). Oxford: Oxford University Press 1992, pp.178-99.

Fielder AR, Shaw DF, Robinson Ng YK. Natural history of retinopathy of prematurity: a prospective study. Eye 1992; **6:** 767-9.

Fielder AR, Levene MI. Screening for retinopathy of prematurity. Arch Dis Child 1992; **67:** 860-7.

Hanning CD, Alexander-Williams JM. Pulse oximetry: a practical review. BMJ 1995; **311:** 367-70.

Moyl JTB. Uses and abuses of pulse oximetry. Arch Dis Child 1996; **74:** 77-80.

Roberton MRC, Rennie JM. Intensive care monitoring. In: Textbook of Neonatology 3rd edn. Rennie JM, Roberton MRC (Eds). Edinburgh: Churchill Livingstone, 1999, pp 361-72.

Silverman WA. Retrolental Fibroplasia; A Modern Parable. Monographs in neonatology. New York: Grune and Stratton, 1980.

Stork JE, Stork EK. Acid-base physiology and disorders in the neonate. In: Neonatal-Perinatal Medicine: Diseases of the Fetus and Infant. Fanarff A, Avroy A (Eds). Saint Louis: Mosby Year Book, 1997, pp. 630-7.

Walter JH. Metabolic acidosis in newborn infants. Arch Dis Child 1992; **67:** 767-9.

Chapter 6

Jaundice

PHYSIOLOGICAL JAUNDICE

Thirty to seventy percent of normal babies develop 'physiological' jaundice after 48 hours of age. Total bilirubin does not usually increase above 200 µmol/L, with a peak at 3-4 days, and usually falls to normal by 7-10 days. Almost all the bilirubin is unconjugated, with conjugated bilirubin < 20 µmol/L (for 'direct reacting' bilirubin methods < 40 µmol/L). It is important to be aware of the methodology used for measuring conjugated bilirubin, as 'direct reacting' methods give higher results (*see p.73*). These babies with physiological jaundice are well and thriving, and require no investigation or treatment. A variety of factors may exacerbate the bilirubin concentration (Figure 6.1).

An exaggerated rise in bilirubin concentration may be seen if the baby is bruised or has, for example, a cephalohaematoma: each gram of haemoglobin yields 600 µmols of bilirubin on breakdown. Other causes include dehydration due to inadequate fluid intake, infection, polycythaemia at delivery, breast feeding or use of oxytocins during delivery.

Pathological factors exacerbating physiological jaundice		
Prematurity	Infections	Inadequate calorie intake
Dehydration	Hypoxia	Meconium retention
Haemolysis	Hypoglycaemia	Intestinal obstruction
Polycythaemia	Hypothyroidism	

Figure 6.1 Pathological factors exacerbating physiological jaundice

Although physiological jaundice is the commonest cause of jaundice in neonates, there are numerous potential underlying conditions that require diagnosis so that appropriate treatment can be given. Features suggesting a pathological cause are:

- early jaundice (< 24 hours)
- jaundice in a sick neonate

- high total bilirubin (> 300 μmol/L)
- rapid increase in bilirubin concentration (> 100 μmol/L in 24 hours)
- jaundice prolonged beyond 14 days
- conjugated bilirubin > 20 μmol/L.

Severe, unconjugated hyperbilirubinaemia incurs a risk of kernicterus: features of kernicterus include fits, lethargy and opisthotonic posturing, which may be seen if the plasma bilirubin concentration exceeds 500 μmol/L. Late consequences of untreated hyperbilirubinaemia, without the classic features of kernicterus, include progressive nerve deafness and, more rarely, athetoid cerebral palsy. Adequate hydration, which may involve tube feeding or an intravenous infusion, together with phototherapy, will usually avert the need for exchange transfusion in non-haemolytic jaundice. A balance needs to be struck between interfering with the normal care of well babies, who are at low risk of such complications, and protecting sick and vulnerable infants. Bilirubin will need to be monitored frequently (4-6 hourly initially). Treatment is often instituted according to guidelines and if the bilirubin rises above a predetermined concentration (see Figure 6.2) an exchange transfusion must be performed. Preterm babies are thought to be at greater risk of bilirubin toxicity, and, therefore, phototherapy is instituted at lower bilirubin concentrations in babies below 37 weeks, with a correspondingly lower threshold for exchange transfusion. All babies who have had a bilirubin concentration exceeding the threshold for exchange must have neonatal hearing screening.

EARLY JAUNDICE

Jaundice that appears unusually early (i.e. within first 24 hours) suggests haemolysis (Figure 6.3). A number of conditions can cause excessive breakdown of red cells in the fetus and neonate. These may present as early neonatal jaundice or, if more severe, so that the rate of haemolysis is greater than the rate of red cell production, as anaemia from birth. Early jaundice should always be investigated (Figure 6.4).

Intrinsic red cell abnormalities that cause anaemia and that can present at this time include spherocytosis, an autosomal dominant condition with excessive red cell fragility, and red cell enzyme abnormalities, the most common of which are glucose 6-phosphate dehydrogenase (G6PD) deficiency and pyruvate kinase (PK) deficiency. Haemoglobinopathies do not usually present as neonatal jaundice. Acquired defects producing haemolysis include both intrauterine and postnatal infections. However, the commonest causes of haemolytic disease of the newborn are blood group incompatibilities between mother and fetus.

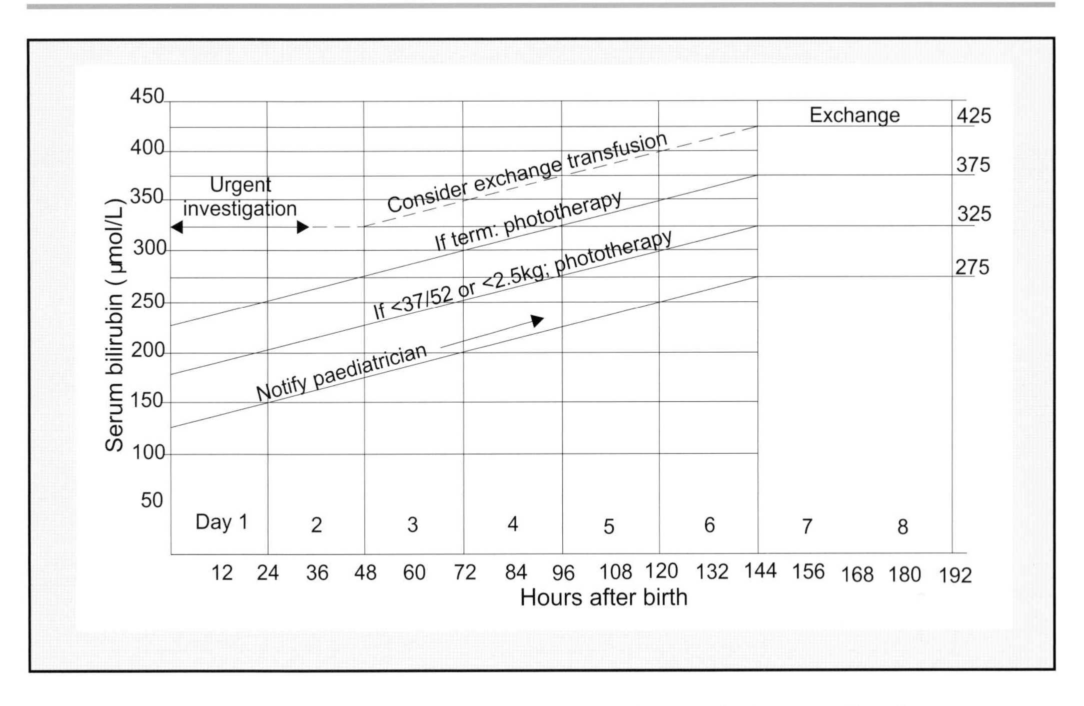

Figure 6.2 Action chart for management of non-haemolytic jaundice in neonates. *See Figure 6.4

Causes of early neonatal jaundice
Haemolysis - blood group incompatibility - red cell membrane defects - spherocytosis - bruising/haemorrhage G6PD deficiency PK deficiency Infection (intrauterine and perinatal) Genetic defects of bilirubin metabolism

Figure 6.3 Causes of early neonatal jaundice

Laboratory investigation of early neonatal jaundice

- Conjugated bilirubin
- Haematology
  - Hb, blood group, FBC (including reticulocytes), film
  - direct antiglobulin test
- G6PD deficiency screen
  - consider other red cell enzyme deficiencies
- Urine
  - infection screen
  - reducing sugars
  - bilirubin

Figure 6.4 Laboratory investigation of early neonatal jaundice

GLUCOSE 6-PHOSPHATE DEHYDROGENASE DEFICIENCY

Glucose 6-phosphate dehydrogenase (G6PD) deficiency is an X-linked disorder that is associated with drug-induced haemolytic crises and neonatal jaundice. The disease is expressed in males and homozygous females. Female heterozygotes are not usually affected clinically, although they can have mild symptoms. The disorder occurs most frequently in persons of Mediterranean, African and Asian origin, with an incidence as high as 20% in some populations. The incidence in Northern Europe and Japan is very low.

A significant number (20-30%) of G6PD deficient infants develop neonatal jaundice. The jaundice occurs spontaneously without drug contact, and can occur in the full term as well as the preterm infant. It usually occurs by the second or third day of life and subsides by the end of the first week. The timing of the jaundice may be later or extended if there is additional drug contact. Affected neonates may also become jaundiced after contact with one of the offending drugs through the placenta, in breast milk or after contact with clothes impregnated with naphthalene (mothballs). A large number of drugs, including antimalarials, antibiotics and analgesics, can precipitate haemolysis. The possibility of G6PD deficiency should be considered in jaundiced newborns of either sex with at-risk parents. Parents of affected babies should be provided with a list of drugs to be avoided.

BLOOD GROUP INCOMPATIBILITY

The most important causes of neonatal jaundice are fetal-maternal blood group incompatibility involving the ABO system, the Kell system and the rhesus system (*see Chapter 11*). This last group can present with very severe disease (hydrops fetalis) or even produce fetal death. All pregnant women who are rhesus negative should be screened for the presence of antibody at booking and again at 28 weeks gestation. If they have no rhesus antibodies, they are given rhesus immunoglobulin after delivery to prevent antibody development. If antibodies develop during pregnancy, or the concentration rises, this indicates that the fetus is likely to be rhesus positive and at risk of being affected (*see p.201*).

PROLONGED JAUNDICE

Jaundice presenting or persisting after 14 days in the term baby is abnormal. It is important to perform some measurement of bilirubin conjugation, and consider the possible causes (Figure 6.5). The presence of urinary bilirubin (which may be detectable by a urine dipstick) is indicative of conjugated hyperbilirubinaemia.

BILIRUBIN

There are four bilirubin fractions in plasma:

- unconjugated bilirubin (alpha)
- monoglucuronide conjugated bilirubin (beta)
- diglucuronide conjugated bilirubin (gamma)
- bilirubin that is covalently bound to albumin (delta).

Measurement of conjugated bilirubin

Laboratory measurement of bilirubin fractions is fraught with difficulties as there are numerous methods, which can give different results. There are generally two types of methods that are used to measure bilirubin. In direct methods, bilirubin is reacted with a dye (diazo reagent) and the resulting coloured compound is measured spectrophotometrically. Conjugated bilirubin reacts rapidly with the dye and is referred to as 'direct reacting'. Measurement of the unconjugated fraction requires the addition of a chemical 'accelerator'; unconjugated bilirubin is therefore termed 'indirect reacting'. Measurement of the direct reacting fraction is dependent on the exact conditions in the assay and different methods may give different results.

Routinely used methods for 'direct reacting' bilirubin overestimate the true conjugated fractions because other components also react, with the result that reference ranges are higher than with the more specific methods that measure 'true' conjugated bilirubin.

A direct reacting fraction of up to 40 µmol/L can be found in neonates with physiological jaundice; concentrations above this are abnormal. In a baby with prolonged jaundice, a concentration of 'direct reacting' bilirubin greater than 15% of the total bilirubin is abnormal.

Reference ranges are lower for methods that allow more specific measurement of the conjugated and unconjugated bilirubin fractions. In normal neonates with physiological jaundice there is very little true conjugated bilirubin (< 20 µmol/L).

It is very important to be aware of these differences, especially if a baby transfers between hospitals with different laboratory services.

Causes of prolonged jaundice

- Breast feeding
- Prematurity
- Congenital infection/immune disorders
- Parenteral nutrition (*see Chapter 15*)
- Biliary atresia (and other structural defects)
- Endocrine disorders
  - hypothyroidism (*see p.140*)
  - hypopituitarism
  - adrenal disorders
- Genetic disorders (*see Chapter 10*)
  - α_1-antitrypsin deficiency
  - cystic fibrosis (*see p.142*)
  - galactosaemia
  - Niemann-Pick type C
  - disorders of bilirubin metabolism
  - other inherited metabolic disorders

Figure 6.5 Causes of prolonged jaundice

LIVER FUNCTION TESTS

This is a group of biochemical tests that are frequently used to assess liver damage and function. Their value usually lies in the detection of an abnormality of liver function and/or monitoring disease progression and, generally, they are of limited use in making a diagnosis of a specific type of liver disease, although they can help in guiding the need for further investigations. Abnormalities in each of them can occur in non-hepatic disease; they are not specific for the liver. The normal values differ from those in infants and older children. Liver dysfunction also affects clotting factors (*see Chapter 11*) and clotting tests are included as part of liver function assessment. The liver function tests typically comprise measurements of plasma aminotransferases (transaminases), alkaline phosphatase and γ-glutamyl transferase activities, and the plasma concentrations of albumin and bilirubin.

Aminotransferases

Two aminotransferases are measured, aspartate aminotransferase (AST) and alanine aminotransferase (ALT). Both are widely distributed in body tissues. There are no tissue specific isoenzymes. Plasma activities are increased (approximately 2-fold) in the early months of life compared with later in infancy. Gross increases (more than 20-fold) of activity occur if there is liver cell necrosis, e.g. in acute hepatitis, significant trauma or tissue hypoxia, because the enzyme leaks out into the extracellular fluid. In chronic liver disease and with cholestasis, activities are also increased but usually to a lesser degree (e.g. 2 to 10-fold).

ALT and AST are usually increased to a similar degree in liver disease. AST, however, can be elevated in other conditions, e.g. muscle disease and cardiac damage, whereas ALT is raised to a lesser degree, if at all, in other conditions. ALT is, therefore, a more specific marker of liver disease.

Alkaline phosphatase (ALP)

ALP is present in liver, bone, intestine, placenta and kidney. Plasma total activity is, therefore, of poor specificity in detecting liver disease. Plasma ALP is high at birth (placental ALP) but falls rapidly (half life 3-4 days) within the first week. Increased activity is particularly associated with cholestatic liver disease and/or bone disease. Increased activity is a feature of osteopenia of prematurity (*see p.131*) and, therefore, ALP is not a particularly useful test for detecting liver dysfunction in the neonatal period.

Although ALP has tissue specific isoenzymes, and measurement can help determine the origin of an increased activity, in practice, specific isoenzyme measurement is not routinely available.

ALBUMIN

Low plasma concentration can occur as a result of reduced synthesis in chronic liver disease, but there are many other potential causes. This makes it a non-specific test of hepatic function; because of the reserve capacity of the liver, it is also insensitive.

γ-GLUTAMYL TRANSFERASE (γ-GT)

This enzyme is widely distributed in human tissue. Most of the activity in the blood appears to originate primarily from the hepatobiliary system, specifically the biliary tract. Increased activity may arise from enzyme induction by drugs (e.g. some anticonvulsants) or from damage to, or disease of, the bile ducts. Increased activities (e.g. 10-fold) occur in biliary atresia and other causes of cholestatic disease. In hepatitis, activities are usually normal or only slightly elevated. γ-GT can also be elevated in cholestatic liver disease complicating parenteral nutrition (*see Chapter 15*). In the inherited disorders of bile acid metabolism, plasma activities of γ-GT are normal or low (*see p.99*). Plasma activities of the enzyme are much higher in neonates than in older children. In normal, full term neonates, the activity at birth is approximately 6-7 times higher than in older children and adults. Activity declines after the first 1-3 months, reaching adult levels by 5-7 months.

JAUNDICE IN THE PRETERM INFANT

The aetiological factors for jaundice in the preterm population include all those found at term, compounded by the greater liver immaturity, tendency to more frequent bruising and delayed establishment of enteral feeding in this group. Polycythaemia, caused by delayed clamping of the umbilical cord or associated with intrauterine growth retardation, may also be seen. The effects of unconjugated bilirubin on the brain are thought to be more dangerous in preterm infants than in those born at term. There is reduced albumin binding of bilirubin owing to relative hypoproteinaemia; acidosis or hypoxia may reduce the effectiveness of the physiological blood-brain barrier, and the immature brain may itself be more vulnerable to bilirubin toxicity.

For these reasons, the plasma concentrations of bilirubin at which phototherapy or exchange transfusion are employed for preterm babies are lower in most units than those for term infants. The formulae used in many UK units (in non-haemolytic jaundice) are as follows :

threshold plasma bilirubin concentration (µmol/L)

- for phototherapy: (gestational age (weeks) x 10) - 100
- for exchange transfusion: (gestational age (weeks) x 10)

Physiological jaundice is frequently prolonged beyond ten days in the preterm population. In our unit we would not investigate prolonged jaundice in a well preterm baby until the age of 14 days, when we would check plasma total and conjugated bilirubin and aspartate aminotransferase (AST), urinary bilirubin, and send urine for culture and reducing substances.

SPECIFIC CAUSES OF JAUNDICE

BREAST FEEDING AND JAUNDICE (*see Chapter 14*)

Plasma bilirubin concentration tends to be higher in breast-fed than in bottle-fed infants, but usually the difference is minimal. However, in an estimated 2% of breast-fed infants, an unconjugated, moderately severe hyperbilirubinaemia persists beyond the second week and remains unchanged thereafter for up to 16 weeks. Affected infants are well and thriving and conjugated bilirubin is not increased.

This condition is completely benign; if breast feeding is discontinued for 24-48 hours, bilirubin concentration falls. A similar degree of jaundice occurs in 25% of siblings of affected infants; it appears to be due to factors in maternal milk that inhibit UDP-glucuronyltransferase activity.

PERINATAL INFECTIONS (*see Chapter 13*)

Neonatal hepatitis may be caused by a variety of infections (see Figure 6.6) that can be acquired *in utero*, during delivery, or early in the newborn period from the mother or from blood transfusions. These infections present as a sick infant with conjugated hyperbilirubinaemia, bilirubinuria, pale stools and increased plasma activities of liver enzymes. However, although a common problem worldwide, infective hepatitis accounts for only a small proportion of cases of conjugated hyperbilirubinaemia in developed countries.

BILIARY ATRESIA

Approximately 1 in 10-15,000 babies born in the UK has biliary atresia. Suspicion of the diagnosis should be raised by prolonged jaundice (due predominantly to conjugated bilirubin), pale stools and detectable urinary bilirubin. Liver enzymes are usually elevated and it may be difficult to distinguish this condition from neonatal hepatitis. Diagnosis is made by visualisation of the biliary tree by ultra-sound, radioisotope scans (Technetium-DISIDA (diisopropyliminodiacetic acid)) and liver biopsy. It is very important to make the diagnosis promptly, as surgery (Kasai hepato-portoenterostomy procedure) gives the best results if performed before eight weeks of age. As a result of increased publicity and professional awareness, late referral has become less common, but sadly still occurs, with consequent poorer outcome.

The other major cause of extrahepatic biliary disease in neonates is a choledochal cyst, which can be diagnosed by ultrasound.

Infections causing neonatal hepatitis

	Time of presentation	Diagnostic test(s)
Transplacental		
Rubella	Day 1	Serology, culture
Cytomegalovirus	Day 1	PCR, serology, culture
Toxoplasmosis	Day 1	PCR, serology
Syphilis	Day 1 - 12 weeks	Serology
Perinatally or postnatally acquired		
Herpes simplex virus	1-2 weeks	Culture from vesicles or swabs PCR antigen detection
Cytomegalovirus	4-8 weeks	PCR, serology, culture
Hepatitis B	6-12 weeks	Serology
Enteroviruses, e.g. coxsackie	Any	Culture (stool and throat swabs) PCR

Figure 6.6 Infections causing neonatal hepatitis

α_1-ANTITRYPSIN DEFICIENCY

α_1-Antitrypsin deficiency, with either the ZZ or SZ phenotypes, can present as prolonged neonatal cholestatic jaundice, although liver disease is by no means an invariable consequence (approximately 15% have persistent liver dysfunction). The incidence of these phenotypes is approximately 1 in 2000 births. The presentation is variable: some infants have evidence of only mild liver disease that resolves completely, while others progress rapidly to liver failure and, without liver transplantation, will die. The clinical picture can be indistinguishable from that of biliary atresia. Interpretation of plasma α_1-antitrypsin concentration is difficult in the newborn because of changing concentrations; plasma concentrations *per se* do not allow a definitive diagnosis to be made, although a concentration of <1.1 g/L during the first four weeks of life is suggestive of a possible deficiency. Phenotyping is required to establish the diagnosis.

BYLER DISEASE (PROGRESSIVE FAMILIAL INTRAHEPATIC CHOLESTASIS I)
Byler disease is one of several clinically similar congenital disorders characterised by progressive familial intrahepatic cholestasis (PFIC), and caused by a group of bile duct transport defects. In PFIC 1, presentation is with cholestatic jaundice and hepatomegaly. A prominent finding is a *low* plasma γ-GT activity. Pancreatitis and diarrhoea are common and plasma cholesterol concentration is normal or low, i.e. atypical of cholestasis. Patients with PFIC 2 have a different mutation but also a low γ-GT. A further variant (PFIC 3) has been identified with an elevated γ-GT.

ALAGILLE SYNDROME
This syndrome is characterised by cholestasis caused by a decreased number of intrahepatic bile ducts and various associated congenital malformations. Hepatomegaly is usually present, together with facial dysmorphism and congenital cardiac anomalies. It is very rare, with an incidence of approximately 1 in 100,000 births, and with equal sex incidence. The genetic defect has been identified to mutations of a transmembrane protein encoded on chromosome 20.

DISORDERS OF BILIRUBIN METABOLISM IN THE NEONATE
These are all rare inherited defects and, in the absence of a family history, should only be considered after exclusion of the more common causes.

Crigler-Najjar syndrome type I
This is caused by the absence of hepatic bilirubin UDP-glucuronyl transferase. It manifests as severe, unconjugated, non-haemolytic, hyperbilirubinaemia (> 340 µmol/L) in the first few days of life, which does not respond to phenobarbitone therapy. The jaundice is persistent, and lifelong phototherapy is required to prevent kernicterus. Liver transplantation has been successful in many cases.

A definitive diagnosis can be made by the measurement of glucuronyl transferase activity in liver tissue after 3-4 months of age, and by demonstrating the absence of bilirubin glucuronides in the bile. DNA technology is advancing and prenatal diagnosis is likely to be possible in the future.

Crigler-Najjar syndrome type II
This is a milder form of the disease, with plasma bilirubin concentration usually below 340 µmol/L. Although UDP-glucuronyl transferase activity is reduced, it is not completely deficient and jaundice can be significantly reduced by phenobar-

bitone treatment. The family, i.e. parents and siblings, should be investigated for jaundice. Some parents have a mild unconjugated hyperbilirubinaemia with no liver dysfunction; this may represent a heterozygous form of the disease.

Dubin-Johnson and Rotor syndromes

Presentation of both syndromes is with a benign conjugated hyperbilirubinaemia with normal liver size, normal plasma liver enzyme activities and abnormalities of coproporphyrin metabolism. The extent of jaundice is enhanced by stress, intercurrent illness or fasting. Both these disorders are benign, with an excellent prognosis. Although the two disorders are phenotypically similar, they differ with respect to urinary coproporphyrin excretion and the excretion of a test load of bromosulphthalein.

NEONATAL HAEMOCHROMATOSIS (NEONATAL IRON STORAGE DISEASE)

Although rare, this condition is an important cause of acute liver failure in neonates. Excess storage of hepatic and extrahepatic iron begins prenatally. The primary defect is unknown but it may be a secondary manifestation of fetal liver disease. There is an increased risk of recurrence in subsequent pregnancies of more than 90%, suggesting the involvement of a maternal factor. Presentation is with jaundice, hypoglycaemia and coagulopathy. Plasma ferritin concentration is greatly elevated. A chelation and/or antioxidant regimen should be commenced when the diagnosis is suspected, although most affected infants will require liver transplantation to survive.

NIEMANN-PICK TYPE C

Niemann-Pick type C is a lysosomal storage disease, caused by a defect of cholesterol esterification. 60-70% of infants present with prolonged cholestasis, hepatomegaly and splenomegaly. Some have fetal ascites. The liver has a characteristic histological appearance. In most infants, the jaundice and liver disease resolve spontaneously. Neurological symptoms usually develop after five years of age.

ENDOCRINE DISORDERS

Adrenal disorders, congenital hypothyroidism (*see Chapter 9*) and congenital hypopituitarism are recognised causes of prolonged neonatal jaundice and should always be considered. Endocrine investigations should include measurement of plasma free thyroxine, TSH and 09:00 h cortisol concentrations. Liver disease usually resolves within six weeks following appropriate treatment.

OTHER CAUSES OF PROLONGED JAUNDICE

Galactosaemia and other metabolic disorders are discussed in Chapter 10. Fructosaemia is unlikely to present in the neonate unless a sucrose-containing milk formula or medicines have been given. Although cystic fibrosis rarely causes cholestasis, in a few cases, biliary obstruction can be severe enough to resemble biliary atresia. G6PD deficiency (*see p.92*) should be considered in any jaundiced infant of Mediterranean descent. Long chain acyl-CoA dehydrogenase deficiency, mevalonate kinase deficiency, carbohydrate deficient glycoprotein syndrome, peroxisomal disorders and Smith Lemli Opitz syndrome can all present with jaundice. Defects in bile acid synthesis can be associated with prolonged neonatal jaundice, although liver disease may be delayed until infancy.

INVESTIGATION OF PROLONGED JAUNDICE

Any neonate with prolonged jaundice (i.e. continuing beyond 14 days) must be investigated (Figure 6.7).

It is particularly important to be alert to signs of liver dysfunction. These include:

- conjugated bilirubin > 20 µmol/L
- pale stools
- bilirubinuria
- bleeding/prolonged clotting
- failure to thrive
- hypoglycaemia
- abnormal liver function tests (including γ-GT).

Babies with biliary atresia are usually of normal birth weight and have hepatomegaly without splenomegaly. A baby with an intrauterine infection is more likely to be small for dates, to have failed to thrive and have splenomegaly in addition to hepatomegaly. Babies with inherited metabolic disorders may have associated signs or symptoms, e.g. dysmorphism. The definitive diagnosis of a metabolic disorder requires further biochemical investigations (see Figure 6.8). These analyses should be considered in the context of the history, clinical presentation and the results of other investigations, e.g. radiology, virology, bacteriology, haematology and histology. A significant delay in diagnosis or treatment of an infant with cholestasis can be devastating if the erroneous assumption is made that the jaundice is 'physiological' or due to breast feeding. *Unexplained conjugated hyperbilirubinaemia in the newborn must always be investigated.*

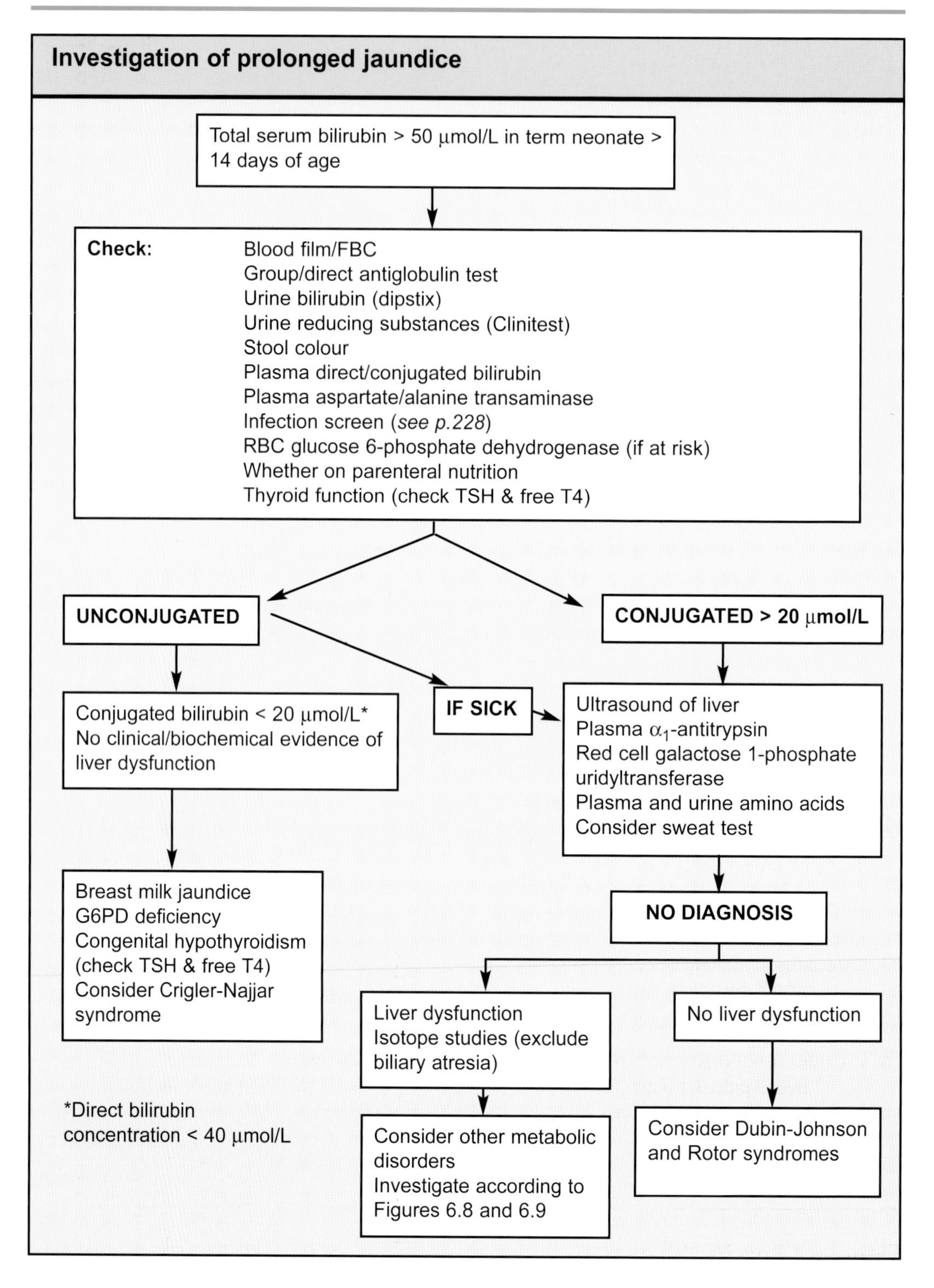

Figure 6.7 Investigation of prolonged jaundice

Investigations for metabolic disease in persistent neonatal jaundice

BLOOD

Acyl carnitines (plasma/dried blood spot)

Very long chain fatty acids (plasma)

Amino acids

Thyroid function tests – check that neonatal screening test has been performed

Galactose 1-phosphate uridyltransferase (qualitative screen) (erythrocytes)

Glucose 6-phosphate dehydrogenase – if high risk group, check that screening has been performed (erythrocytes)

URINE

Amino acids

Sugars

Organic acids

NOTES

1. If plasma amino acids show an increased tyrosine or methionine, second line tests should include: plasma α-fetoprotein, urine succinylacetone, erythrocyte porphobilinogen synthase or urine δ-ALA

2. If the baby is acutely ill, consider: urgent investigations for urea cycle defects (ammonia and orotic acid) and fatty acid oxidation defects (acyl carnitines and organic acids)

3. In babies with persistent cholestasis of unknown cause, consider: investigations for disorders of bile acid synthesis, neonatal haemochromatosis, peroxisomal disorders, cystic fibrosis, defects of cholesterol metabolism, Niemann-Pick type C and bile salt transport defects.

Figure 6.8 Specific biochemical investigation for metabolic disease in patients with persistent neonatal jaundice

Investigation of prolonged or late presenting jaundice in neonates

Cause	Type of jaundice	Supporting information	Further investigations
Breast feeding	U	Jaundice spontaneously resolves if breast feeding withdrawn. No clinical or biochemical evidence of liver dysfunction.	
Infection	C/U	Improves with treatment	Infection screen (see Figure 6.6). Urine culture
Rhesus/ABO isoimmunisation	C	History of early haemolytic jaundice.	
Parenteral nutrition (PN)	C	History of PN	Nil if resolves after PN has been discontinued
Biliary atresia	C	Pale stools	Liver ultrasound/Tc-DISIDA scan
α_1-antitrypsin deficiency	C		Plasma α_1-antitrypsin phenotyping
Hypothyroidism	U	Clinical signs	TSH, free T4
Alagille syndrome	C	Characteristic facies Congenital abnormalities Pulmonary artery hypoplasia	Hypoplasia or reduced intrahepatic bile ducts on liver biopsy
Galactosaemia	C	Cataracts Urine reducing substances positive	Erythrocyte galactose 1-phosphate uridyltransferase
Peroxisomal disorders	C	Hypotonia Dysmorphic features Neurological dysfunction	Plasma very long chain fatty acids
Glucose 6-phosphate dehydrogenase deficiency	U	Usually present early Drug related family history Mediterranean, Asian or African race	Erythrocyte glucose 6-phosphate dehydrogenase
Crigler-Najjar types I & II	U	No liver dysfunction Type II responds to phenobarbitone	Glucuronides in bile Glucuronyl transferase in liver

continued...

Investigation of prolonged or late presenting jaundice in neonates (cont.)			
Cause	**Type of jaundice**	**Supporting information**	**Further investigations**
Cystic fibrosis	C	Meconium ileus Family history	Plasma/bloodspot immuno-reactive trypsin Sweat chloride DNA testing
Hypopituitarism	C	Hypoglycaemia Dysmorphism Optic nerve hypoplasia Low free T4	Plasma free T4 and TSH Plasma cortisol
Lysosomal storage disorders, e.g. Niemann-Pick type C	C	Hepatomegaly Splenomegaly	Leucocyte or fibroblast enzyme activity
Bile acid synthesis defects	C	Normal γ-GT	Urine bile acids
Progressive familial intrahepatic cholestasis 1 (Byler disease)	C	Hepatomegaly Low γ-GT Low/normal cholesterol	γ-GT Serum bile acids Molecular biology

C = conjugated U = unconjugated

Figure 6.9 Investigation of prolonged or late presenting jaundice in the neonate

FURTHER READING

Chaudhury JR, Walkoff AW, Chowdhury NR, Arias IM. Hereditary jaundice and disorders of bilirubin metabolism. In: The Metabolic and Molecular Basis of Inherited disease, 8th edn. Scriver CR, Beaudet AL, Sly WS, Valle D, Childs B, Kinzler KW, Vogelstein B (Eds). New York: McGraw-Hill, 2001, pp. 3063-101.

Dennery PA, Seidman DS, Stevenson DK. Neonatal hyperbilirubinaemia. N Engl J Med 2001; **344:** 581-90.

Isherwood D. Neonatal jaundice. CPD Clinical Biochemistry 2001; **3:** 35-42.

McKiernan PJ, Roberts EA, Kelly DA. The acutely ill baby. In: Diseases of the Liver and Biliary System in Children. Kelly DA (Ed). Oxford: Blackwell Science, 1999, pp. 46-61.

Primhak RA, Tanner MS. $Alpha_1$ - antitrypsin deficiencies. Arch Dis Child 2001; **85:** 2-5.

Roberts EA. The jaundiced baby. In: Diseases of the Liver and Biliary System in Children. Kelly DA (Ed). Oxford: Blackwell Science, 1999, pp. 11-45.

Sykes E, Epstein E. Laboratory measurement of bilirubin. Clin Perinatol 1990; **17:** 397-435.

Chapter 7

Hypo- and hyperglycaemia

BLOOD GLUCOSE IN NEONATES

The major source of glucose for the brain is the blood supply. Low blood glucose concentrations can cause cellular energy failure and membrane depolarisation, resulting in neuronal necrosis and ensuing neurological dysfunction, manifesting as seizures and possible permanent brain injury. At birth, following the sudden discontinuation of nutrient supply from the mother, the neonate mobilises glucose and fatty acids to meet demands for energy.

Blood glucose concentration falls immediately after birth (2-3 hours) in most babies and there is a risk of hypoglycaemia (< 2.0 mmol/L), particularly in the first 12 hours; for healthy term babies this is 'normal' and transient, usually lasting no longer than 24 hours. This phenomenon is associated with developmental immaturity of gluconeogenesis and glycogenolysis in the liver in the perinatal period. Hypoglycaemia is particularly likely to develop if feeding is delayed. Transient moderate hypoglycaemia (i.e. blood glucose 1.0-2.0 mmol/L), in the first 48 hours of life in an otherwise healthy baby born at term who is normally developed and asymptomatic, is not harmful in the short term, as ketones are synthesised and provide an alternative energy source.

MEASUREMENT OF BLOOD GLUCOSE

Glucose can be measured in plasma or whole blood, with the obvious advantage of whole blood not requiring centrifugation. Whole blood glucose concentration is approximately 15% lower than plasma glucose, the exact figure depending on the haematocrit.

Neonatal units commonly use 'stix' based methods as a rapid means of assessing approximate concentrations of glucose in whole blood. There are several point-of-care instruments for measuring blood glucose concentration. These must be assessed for use in neonates, paying particular attention to the effect of haematocrit and accuracy at low concentrations. At high haematocrits, the blood glucose reading may be misleadingly low. Whilst it is important not to delay treatment of hypoglycaemia or hyperglycaemia based on a stix measurement in a symptomatic baby, it is also important to recognise that they may not be reliable, and diagnosis depends on an accurate laboratory glucose measurement.

Hypoglycaemia or hyperglycaemia that is *suspected* from these screening tests, or any glucose screening measurement that does not fit with the clinical circumstances, must always be confirmed by an accurate glucose measurement before management changes are instituted. Laboratory specimens must be taken into appropriate tubes with an antiglycolytic agent, e.g. fluoride and oxalate. Storage, if required, should be at 4°C.

Responsibility and accountability for ward-based glucose measurements must be clear, with written protocols for operation, internal quality control and external quality assurance, training, review of performance and audit.

HYPOGLYCAEMIA

Hypoglycaemia is a common metabolic problem in neonatal medicine. In the majority of healthy neonates, the frequently observed low blood glucose concentration is a reflection of normal metabolic adaptation to extrauterine life.

DEFINITION

It is unclear what concentration of blood glucose results in neurological damage and, for this reason, the definition of hypoglycaemia in the neonate has been widely debated, has been a cause of confusion, and remains a contentious issue. It is not possible to accurately define a 'safe' glucose concentration, as it will differ on an individual basis dependent on maturity and the protection derived from the supply of alternative fuels, i.e. ketones. Most paediatricians use a working definition of < 2.0 mmol/L in whole blood as a pragmatic intervention threshold with a margin of safety. There is no good evidence that the preterm baby is less neurologically vulnerable to hypoglycaemia than the term infant. Similar values should be aimed at in both groups.

CLINICAL FEATURES

Neonates without associated risk factors can tolerate very low blood glucose concentrations in the immediate postnatal period without any apparent clinical symptoms, by using ketones as alternative fuels. However, vulnerable groups may not use such fuels effectively (e.g. preterm, growth restricted, asphyxiated or septic babies).

The clinical signs of hypoglycaemia include:

- changes in levels of consciousness (e.g. irritability, lethargy, stupor, coma)
- apnoea, cyanotic spells
- feeding poorly, after feeding well

- hypothermia
- hypotonia, limpness
- tremor
- seizures.

Clinical signs caused by hypoglycaemia should be alleviated by correction of the blood glucose concentration.

CAUSES

Hypoglycaemia can be a consequence of impaired glucose supply because of inadequate glycogen stores and/or conditions associated with hyperinsulinism. These conditions are summarised in Figure 7.1. After the first 24 hours of life, hyperinsulinism is the most common cause of resistant hypoglycaemia.

Preterm or small for gestational age (SGA) infants

Infants who are preterm or who are small for gestational age following intrauterine malnutrition are particularly at risk from hypoglycaemia. Fetal growth in the last trimester includes the deposition of energy stores as glycogen in the liver and fat in adipose tissue. Therefore, babies born prematurely or with poor growth in the last trimester are deficient in these energy stores. They are likely to become hypoglycaemic and less likely to be able to mount a ketotic response. A proportion of SGA infants also have an inappropriately raised plasma insulin concentration, which exacerbates the risk of hypoglycaemia. There is a risk of permanent neurological sequelae in this group.

These infants tend to have well preserved head growth but absent adipose tissue. They have inadequate hepatic glycogen stores and are also thought to have impaired gluconeogenesis, despite having elevated plasma glucagon, growth hormone and cortisol concentrations.

Well babies whose weight is below the 10th centile for age, particularly those who look thin, should be milk fed as soon as possible after birth, with frequent monitoring of blood glucose. If glucose infusion is needed initially, weaning onto milk feeds can usually be achieved after 2-3 days. Occasionally, very high glucose administration rates are necessary to maintain euglycaemia.

Causes of hypoglycaemia in neonates

INADEQUATE GLUCOSE SUPPLY

- Decreased glucose production
  - Prematurity
  - Sepsis
  - Small for gestational age
  - Inadequate nutrition
  - Birth asphyxia
  - Congenital heart disease
  - Hypothermia
- Inherited metabolic disorders
  - Disorders of carnitine transport/cycle
  - Disorders of gluconeogenesis (e.g. pyruvate carboxylase deficiency, fructose bisphosphatase deficiency)
  - Disorders of fat oxidation (e.g. medium chain acyl CoA dehydrogenase deficiency)
  - Glycogen storage disorders, especially type I
  - Amino acid disorders (e.g. tyrosinaemia type I)
  - Organic acid disorders (e.g. methylmalonic acidaemia)
  - Galactosaemia
- Hormone deficiencies/imbalance
  - Congenital hypopituitarism
  - Congenital glucagon deficiency (short chain 3-hydroxyacyl CoA dehydrogenase deficiency)
  - Growth hormone deficiency
  - Congenital adrenal hyperplasia
  - Adrenal hypoplasia/insufficiency

HYPERINSULINISM

Acquired
Maternal diabetes
Maternal glucose infusion
Erythroblastosis fetalis
Insulinoma (adenoma)
Munchausen syndrome by proxy
Birth asphyxia
Small for gestational age

Genetic

Recessive	*Dominant*
SURI	Glucokinase deficiency
KIR 6.2	Glutamate dehydrogenase deficiency

Sporadic
Beckwith syndrome
Focal lesions

OTHER

Exchange transfusion
Parenteral nutrition

Figure 7.1 Causes of hypoglycaemia in neonates

HYPERINSULINISM

After the first 24 hours of life, hyperinsulinism is the commonest cause of persistent or recurrent neonatal hypoglycaemia. Most affected infants present with severe intractable hypoglycaemia within the first 72 hours. Neurological outcome depends on the promptness and adequacy of management of the hypoglycaemia. A requirement for glucose infusion rates of greater than 10 mg/kg/min to maintain euglycaemia is consistent with inappropriate insulin activity. The hypoglycaemia is non-ketotic. Hyperinsulinism before birth leads, in most cases, to physical resemblance at birth to the infant of a mother with poorly controlled diabetes, with macrosomia, increased adipose tissue and signs of hyperinsulinism, including high birth weight and greater length.

Maternal or gestational diabetes mellitus

Although most infants of mothers with diabetes mellitus are of normal size and well, they should all have blood glucose screening before feeds for the first 24 hours.

Hyperinsulinism in the neonate is inversely related to the adequacy of maternal control of blood glucose in the third trimester. The fetus can be as severely affected in gestational diabetes as in established maternal diabetes. If maternal diabetes is recognised, fetal growth will be closely monitored and the mother will usually be treated with insulin. An unexpectedly large infant with early hypoglycaemia may result when the mother has hitherto unrecognised glucose intolerance. In such cases, a maternal glucose tolerance test should be performed at six weeks to see whether or not this has resolved. Hypoglycaemia can present within an hour of birth. Usually, such severely affected infants are large for gestational age. They may have had a traumatic delivery, shoulder dystocia being a particular hazard since the head size is relatively small. Polycythaemia, congenital defects, jaundice, lung immaturity and hypocalcaemia all occur more frequently in infants of mothers with diabetes mellitus. The majority of these infants, however, are of appropriate weight for gestational age and, with early and frequent (2-3 hourly) feeds from birth and appropriate (3 hourly) monitoring of blood glucose, never become hypoglycaemic. Symptomatic infants or those who become hypoglycaemic despite early feeding require admission to a neonatal unit and i.v. dextrose infusion (*see p.115*). Hyperinsulinism is the primary cause of their hypoglycaemia, but they may also have failure of the normal increase in plasma glucagon concentration at two hours of age.

Genetic causes of hyperinsulinism

Hypoglycaemia associated with inappropriately high circulating concentrations of insulin from birth was, until recently, referred to as 'nesidioblastosis'. This term refers to the histological observation of an overgrowth of insulin-producing β cells in the pancreas. Another rare (though not genetic) cause is a discrete islet cell tumour of the pancreas (insulinoma); these tumours are benign and hypoglycaemia resolves after resection.

Beckwith's syndrome is associated with a deletion within the short arm of chromosome 11. Features, some or all of which may be present, include macrosomia, macroglossia, exomphalos, visceromegaly, horizontal creases on the earlobe and hyperinsulinaemic hypoglycaemia. The syndrome can usually be recognised at birth. Hypoglycaemia is a feature in 50% of cases and is associated with islet cell hypertrophy. It may be transient or, occasionally, persistent for several months and is associated with later learning difficulties. Screening for neonatal hypoglycaemia is therefore important in infants with any features of this condition. There is an association with renal tumours in later childhood and ultrasound monitoring is required. The genetics are complex with familial and sporadic forms.

Advances in molecular genetics have shown that 30-50% of cases of hyperinsulinism are caused by abnormalities in genes controlling metabolic processes of membrane cation transport. These genetic forms of congenital hyperinsulinism are responsible for 'nesidioblastosis'. In most cases, there is diffuse involvement of the β cells, but in some there is focal involvement.

Recessive mutations of the genes (located on chromosome 11) for the sulphonylurea receptor (SUR I) and the ATP dependent potassium channel (KIR6.2) in the plasma membrane of the pancreatic β cells have been described. Neonates with either of these two disorders have high birth weights because of the growth-promoting effects of insulin *in utero*. These conditions manifest with severe hypoglycaemia that cannot be controlled with diazoxide; near total pancreatectomy is necessary to prevent hypoglycaemia. These mutations cause the most severe type of hyperinsulinism.

Two dominantly inherited mutations, in the genes for glucokinase and glutamate dehydrogenase, have been described, which cause hypoglycaemia. Generally this is milder than in the SUR I mutations. Neonates with glutamate dehydrogenase deficiency have an associated mild hyperammonaemia because glutamate dehydrogenase also regulates the urea cycle. They exhibit a worsening of hypoglycaemia after a high protein intake. This disorder probably explains what was formerly called 'leucine sensitive hypoglycaemia'.

Sporadic forms of genetically-determined hypoglycaemia are associated with focal lesions causing hyperinsulinism; these are due to loss of the maternal allele from the chromosome, leading to imbalanced expression of imprinted paternal alleles.

The expanding genetic information about the causes of neonatal hypoglycaemia is allowing more specific diagnosis and appropriate treatment. Neonates with hyperinsulinism that does not respond to diazoxide therapy are likely to have SUR I mutations. Prompt consultation with an endocrinologist/metabolic specialist is essential so that the neonate can benefit from the new advances in diagnosis and management.

Transhepatic pancreatic catheterisation and venous sampling enable localisation of the site of the focal insulin hypersecretion. Neonates with focal hyperinsulinism can be treated with partial pancreatectomy if the region of islet cell hyperplasia can be identified.

Prompt and appropriate management is necessary in order to avoid neurological damage and life-long handicap. The aim of management is to prevent symptomatic hypoglycaemia. Glucose infusion alone, even at very high rates, may be insufficient. Intramuscular glucagon may be a useful short term measure, as may somatostatin (octreotide), together with diazoxide and chlorothiazide. Surgery becomes urgent if these measures fail. A localised adenoma may be demonstrable by arteriography of the coeliac axis and its removal will then be curative. Prompt referral to a centre with experience in the management of hyperinsulinism is important.

Suitable regimens include:

- high glucose infusion (15-20 mg/kg/min)
- glucagon (200 µg/kg s.c, i.m. or i.v.)
- diazoxide (5 mg/kg orally or i.v. b.d.)
- chlorothiazide (10 mg/kg orally b.d.)
- somatostatin (5 µg/kg octreotide s.c. 6-8 hourly).

Exogenous hyperinsulinism
Hyperinsulinism of exogenous origin (e.g. Munchausen's syndrome by proxy) can be confirmed by demonstrating a high plasma insulin concentration, without an increase in C-peptide, in the presence of hypoglycaemia.

Endocrine Defects

Hypoglycaemia can result from defects of the glucoregulatory hormones. These can be permanent primary congenital defects or secondary consequences of hormone imbalance.

The congenital defects are all rare and include:

- growth hormone deficiency (hypoglycaemia is rare)
- adrenal hyperplasia (steroid synthesis defects)
- hypopituitarism (including septo-optic dysplasia)
- isolated ACTH deficiency.

Inherited Metabolic Disorders

Hypoglycaemia is a feature of several inherited metabolic disorders (Figure 7.1). For further details, see Chapter 10.

PREVENTION

Hypoglycaemia is dangerous if prolonged and/or very severe, and requires prompt management. Because of the risks associated with hypoglycaemia, all neonatal units have a protocol to screen for hypoglycaemia in certain situations.

Healthy full term infants, born after a normal pregnancy and delivery, with no abnormal clinical signs nor known risk, do not require monitoring of blood glucose.

Neonates with clinical signs compatible with hypoglycaemia (see above) should be screened. If the value is 2.0 mmol/L or less, clinical intervention is indicated.

Neonates with risk factors for hypoglycaemia, including particularly those who are preterm or small for gestational age (SGA), have inadequate fuel storage and are less likely to be able to mount an adequate ketotic response. They can, therefore, experience a crisis in energy supply and possible neurological sequelae. Birth asphyxia, infections, maternal diabetes and Rhesus haemolytic disease all predispose to neonatal hypoglycaemia.

Glucose monitoring should be initiated in all neonates with a known risk factor, including preterm babies, (see Figure 7.2) within 2-3 hours after birth. If plasma glucose is < 2.0 mmol/L, closer surveillance is required (*see p.115*). For monitoring of infants receiving parenteral nutrition, see p.272.

Risk factors for hypoglycaemia

Associated with changes in maternal metabolism

- Intrapartum administration of glucose
- Drug treatment
  - terbutaline, ritodrine, propranolol
  - oral hypoglycaemic agents
- Maternal diabetes

Associated with neonatal problems

- Idiopathic condition or failure to adapt
- Perinatal hypoxia-ischaemia
- Infection
- Hypothermia
- Hyperviscosity
- Erythroblastosis fetalis, hydrops fetalis
- Other
  - iatrogenic causes
  - congenital cardiac malformations

Other factors

Intrauterine growth retardation
Preterm
Hyperinsulinism
Endocrine disorder
Inherited metabolic disorder

Figure 7.2 Risk factors for hypoglycaemia

MANAGEMENT

Once hypoglycaemia is confirmed, management should follow a schedule such as that shown in Figure 7.3. The therapeutic objective is to maintain the blood glucose concentration greater than 2.5 mmol/L, to give a margin of safety. A baby with symptomatic hypoglycaemia, who is not tolerating feeds, requires immediate admission to a neonatal unit and intravenous dextrose administration. If administration of 7 mg/kg/min dextrose (4 mL/kg/h 10% dextrose) fails to lead to an adequate stable glucose concentration, the infusion is increased progressively to 12 mg/kg/min. If this fails, the use of i.v. or i.m. hydrocortisone (5 mg/kg stat and then 1 mg/kg 6 hourly) should be considered. Glucagon (20 µg/kg) can be tried, even in small-for-dates babies, when there is a sudden, severe fall of blood glucose concentration that cannot be raised with i.v. dextrose. Most hypoglycaemia that is caused by substrate depletion will respond to these measures.

In the asymptomatic baby, milk feeds of a preterm formula (79 kcal/100 mL) may produce a more rapid increase in blood glucose than the usual formula (67 kcal/100 mL) or human milk.

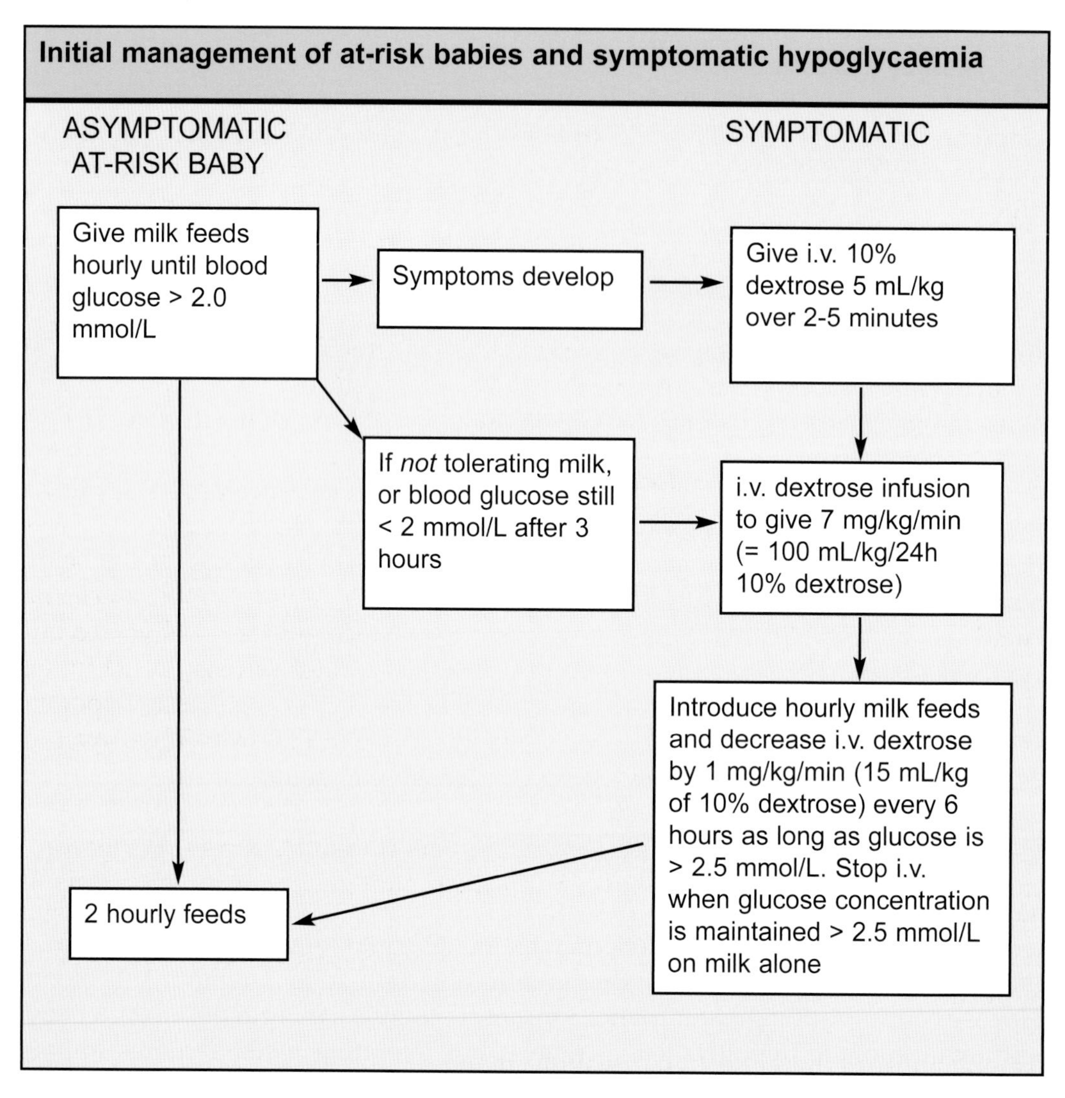

Figure 7.3 Initial management of at-risk babies and symptomatic hypoglycaemia

PERSISTENT HYPOGLYCAEMIA

If hypoglycaemia persists or the baby requires a glucose infusion in excess of 10 mg/kg/min to maintain a normal plasma concentration, hyperinsulinism, metabolic and endocrine disorders must be considered and appropriate investigations undertaken (*see p.117*). Consultation with an endocrinologist/specialist metabolic paediatrician is desirable.

INVESTIGATION OF PERSISTENT HYPOGLYCAEMIA (Figure 7.4 and Figure 7.5)

Hypoglycaemia must always be confirmed by an accurate laboratory test. DO NOT rely on a ward-based stix result.

Neonates presenting acutely with hypoglycaemia are often dangerously ill and may be moribund. However, if blood is not taken for further investigations before glucose is administered, it may be very difficult to establish a diagnosis subsequently. It is very important to collect specimens of blood *at the time* of the acute event. Failure to do this may necessitate long and difficult invasive investigations.

Initially, it can be very helpful to measure plasma free fatty acids (FFA) and 3-hydroxybutyrate. In most circumstances, as blood glucose falls, lipolysis and subsequently ketogenesis are stimulated; thus the plasma concentration of FFA and 3-hydroxybutyrate increase in approximately equimolar fashion. In patients who have hyperinsulinism, FFA and 3-hydroxybutyrate concentrations will be low because insulin suppresses lipolysis. This pattern of low FFA and 3-hydroxybutyrate at the time of hypoglycaemia is not diagnostic of hyperinsulinism, being also observed in patients with hypopituitarism. However, hyperinsulinism can be ruled out by the demonstration of ketosis, i.e. elevated FFA and 3-hydroxybutyrate in the presence of hypoglycaemia. These metabolites can also assist in the diagnosis of inherited defects of fatty acid oxidation. In these patients, hypoglycaemia is accompanied by a disproportionate increase in FFA over 3-hydroxybutyrate: in fact, there may be little increase in 3-hydroxybutyrate at all.

C-peptide provides an indication of overall insulin production and its measurement in plasma can be useful to confirm endogenous hyperinsulinism. Measurement of blood ammonia concentration is important to diagnose the condition of hyperammonaemia with hyperinsulinism (due to glutamate dehydrogenase deficiency).

The diagnostic criteria for hyperinsulinism are:

- blood glucose < 2.5 mmol/L (laboratory measurement)
- absence of ketonuria
- glucose requirement > 10 mg/kg/min to maintain blood glucose above 2.5 mmol/L
- inappropriately low blood free fatty acid and ketone body concentrations at the time of hypoglycaemia

- glycaemic response after the administration of glucagon when hypoglycaemic
- measurable plasma insulin concentration at the time of hypoglycaemia.

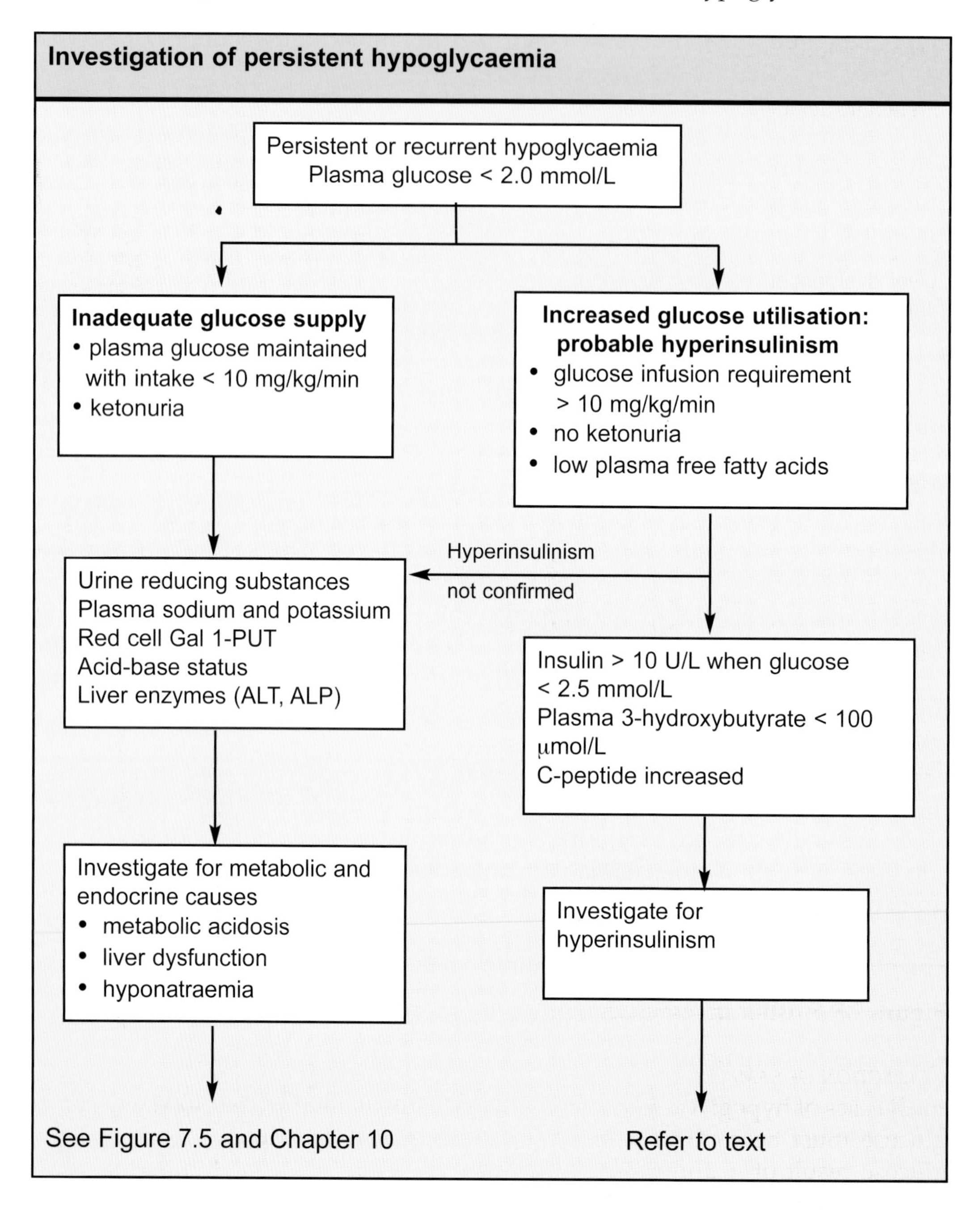

Figure 7.4 Investigation of persistent hypoglycaemia

Further investigation of neonatal hypoglycaemia		
Associated presentation/problem	**Probable disorders/diagnosis**	**Investigations**
Metabolic acidosis	Glycogen storage disorders Congenital lactic acidosis Disorders of gluconeogenesis Fatty acid oxidation defects Organic acid disorders	Plasma lactate Plasma 3-hydroxybutyrate Plasma free fatty acids Urine organic acids Plasma acyl carnitines
Liver dysfunction Jaundice	Tyrosinaemia type I Galactosaemia Glycogen storage disorders Hereditary fructose intolerance Fatty acid oxidation defects Disorders of gluconeogenesis	Plasma/urine amino acids Galactose 1-phosphate uridyl transferase Urine sugars Urine organic acids Plasma acyl carnitines
Hyponatraemia	Adrenal hyperplasia Adrenal insufficiency Hypopituitarism	Plasma 17-hydroxy-progesterone Plasma cortisol Plasma growth hormone, TSH and fT4
Hyperammonaemia	Hyperinsulinism	See p.112 See Chapter 10
Absence of acidosis and liver dysfunction	Adrenal insufficiency Adrenal hyperplasia Hypopituitarism Growth hormone deficiency ACTH deficiency Hyperinsulinism	Plasma cortisol Plasma 17-hydroxy-progesterone Plasma growth hormone, TSH and fT4 Plasma insulin (when hypoglycaemic)

Figure 7.5 Further investigation of neonatal hypoglycaemia

COLLECTION OF SAMPLES

In all cases of hypoglycaemia suggested by a 'stix' test result, the blood or plasma glucose must be confirmed by an accurate laboratory test. A ward measured glucose result of < 2 mmol/L is an unreliable result on which to base further investigations. Measurement of metabolites and hormones in plasma and screening for urinary ketones in specimens taken at the same time as hypogly-

provide important diagnostic information. It is, therefore, of great importance to collect appropriate specimens when the baby is hypoglycaemic. Store urine (5 mL ideally, 1-2 mL is useful) and plasma (2 mL in fluoride ideally) at -20°C for further investigation. The extent of investigation may be limited by the small specimen of blood likely to be available and hence must be individualised.

Specimen requirements should be checked with the local laboratory. Investigations should include:

- blood (collected before administration of glucose)
    - glucose (laboratory measurement)
    - ammonia
    - insulin
    - C-peptide
    - growth hormone
    - cortisol
    - 3-hydroxybutyrate
    - free fatty acids
    - lactate
    - amino acids (quantitative)
    - acyl carnitine species (blood spots and plasma).

All specimens should be sent to the laboratory immediately. They can be stored and analysed later if the cause of hypoglycaemia remains unclear.

Further investigations, which may be done on samples collected after administration of glucose, include:

- urine (collect the first urine passed once hypoglycaemia is suspected, preferably 5-10 mL; glucose should not be withheld if indicated clinically before urine can be collected)
    - organic acids
    - reducing substances
    - ketones (Acetest or Ketostix)
    - amino acids
- blood
    - acid-base status
    - sodium, potassium

- liver function tests
- phosphate
- urate
- cholesterol
- triglycerides
- creatine kinase
- galactosaemia screen
- 17-hydroxyprogesterone
- DNA studies for fat oxidation defects.

Ketonuria

Ketosis is a normal physiological response to hypoglycaemia, being due to production of ketone bodies in the liver (acetoacetate, 3-hydroxybutyrate) from fatty acids released from adipose tissue. *Absence of ketonuria* at the time of severe hypoglycaemia is abnormal and strongly suggests hyperinsulinism or a fat oxidation defect. Ketotic hypoglycaemia points to hormone deficiency or an inherited metabolic disorder.

Fasting/fed profile of metabolites

If hypoglycaemia relates specifically to starvation or feeding, then useful diagnostic information can sometimes be obtained by measuring metabolites in the fed or fasted states. This approach requires careful planning between the clinician and clinical biochemist so as to maximise data obtained from the precious, usually small, blood specimens. Careful clinical supervision is essential as the risk of hypoglycaemia is obviously great.

Metabolites which it can be useful to measure include plasma lactate, 3-hydroxybutyrate, free fatty acids and alanine, in addition to glucose. In the authors' experience, pyruvate is not recommended, as current methodologies have limitations, and only rarely does the knowledge of the concentration contribute to the diagnosis.

HYPERGLYCAEMIA

Neonatal hyperglycaemia (see Figure 7.6) is defined as a blood glucose > 8 mmol/L (irrespective of whether glycosuria is present). As with hypoglycaemia, accurate laboratory measurement of blood glucose is essential to confirm the diagnosis. Hyperglycaemia with glycosuria causes an osmotic diuresis, leading to intravascular dehydration, weight loss and hypotension. It may be associated with acidosis and/or ketosis.

Neonatal hyperglycaemia is usually a transient phenomenon that resolves spontaneously. It is often associated with the use of parenteral nutrition (PN) solutions and corticosteroid therapy in low birth weight babies. Insulin infusion may be required over several weeks in this situation until steroid therapy/PN are discontinued.

Neonatal diabetes mellitus is very rare (1 in 500,000) and in about a third of cases is transient and resolves in the neonatal period.

Causes of hyperglycaemia

- IUGR or preterm babies given an excess glucose load
  - 10% dextrose infusion
  - parenteral nutrition
  - introduction of steroid therapy
- Neonatal diabetes mellitus
- IUGR babies with ineffective glycaemic central mechanisms on milk feeds
- Sick/septic babies (↑ cortisol ↓ insulin)

Figure 7.6 Causes of hyperglycaemia

The management of neonatal hyperglycaemia may include:

- reduction of glucose intake
- screening for underlying cause, e.g. sepsis
- correction of fluid balance with 4.5% albumin infusion or 0.45% saline if acidotic (and possibly i.v. insulin)
- i.v. insulin infusion in very low birth weight infants, starting with 0.05 units/kg/h and increase as tolerated; up to ten times this amount may be required.

FURTHER READING

Aynsley-Green A, Hawden JM. Hypoglycaemia in the neonate: current controversies. Acta Paediatr Japonica 1997; **39 (suppl 1):** 512-6.

Aynsley-Green A, Hussain K, Hall J, Saudubray JM, Nihoul-Fékété C *et al.* Practical management of hypertension in infants. Arch Dis Child Fetal Neonatal Ed 2000; **82:** F98-F107.

Cornblath M, Hawdon JM, Williams AF, Aynsley-Green A, Ward-Platt MP, Schwartz R, Kalhan SC. Controversies regarding definition of neonatal hypoglycaemia: Suggested operational thresholds. Pediatrics 2000; **105:** 1141-5.

Cowett RM, Farrag HM. Neonatal glucose metabolism. In: Principles of Perinatal-neonatal Metabolism, 2nd edn. Cowett RM (Ed). New York: Springer, 1998.

Glaser B, Thornton P, Otonkoski T, Junien C. Genetics of neonatal hyperinsulinism. Arch Dis Child Neonatal Ed 2000; **82:** F79-F86.

Hawdon JM, Aynsley-Green A. Disorders of blood glucose homeostasis in the neonate. In Textbook of Neonatology, 3rd edn, Rennie JM, Robertson NRC (Eds). London: Churchill Livingstone, 1999.

Henderson M. Neonatal hypoglycaemia. CPD Bulletin Clinical Biochemistry 1999; **1:** 45-8.

Morris AAM, Thekakara A, Wilks Z, Clayton PT, Leonard JU, Aynsley-Green A. Evaluation of fasts for investigating hypoglycaemia or suspected metabolic disease. Arch Dis Child 1996; **75:** 115-9.

Saudubray J-M, de Lonlay P, Touati G, Martin D, Nassogne MC *et al.* Genetic hypoglycaemia in infancy and childhood: Pathophysiology and diagnosis. J Inherit Metab Dis 2000; **23:** 197-214.

Stanley CA Baker L. The causes of neonatal hypoglycaemia. New Engl J Med 1999; **340:** 1200-1.

Williams AF. Hypoglycaemia of the newborn – a review. Bull World Health Org 1997; **75:** 261-90.

Chapter 8

Calcium, magnesium and phosphate

CALCIUM

INTRODUCTION

The body content of calcium in infants is about 400 mmol/kg – less than half that of an adult – of which 99% is in bone. There is active placental transport of calcium to the fetus throughout the latter part of pregnancy at an estimated rate of 3.2 mmol/kg/24h, which results in fetal plasma concentrations of total and ionised calcium higher than those in the mother.

Fetal 25-hydroxycholecalciferol concentrations correlate with those of the mother, although absolute concentrations are lower. 1,25-dihydroxycholecalciferol (calcitriol) does not cross the placenta to a significant extent; it is synthesised in the placenta itself and in the fetal kidney. Parathyroid hormone (PTH) and calcitonin do not cross the placenta and are also synthesised by the fetus. There is a massive increase in fetal bone mineralisation in the third trimester.

Plasma calcium concentration falls after birth to a nadir at 1-2 days, after which there is a slow rise to a constant level. Thereafter, plasma calcium concentration is kept constant at 2.1-2.7 mmol/L, despite it being in free exchange with the bony reservoir. Sixty percent of plasma calcium is ultrafiltrable and 40% is protein bound; 80-90% of the bound calcium is bound to albumin, so that a decrease of plasma albumin concentration results in a decreased total calcium concentration. Twenty-five percent of ultrafiltrable calcium is complexed with phosphate and citrate, the remainder being free calcium ions. It is changes in this ionised fraction that produce clinical effects. Acidosis increases, and alkalosis decreases, the proportion of ionised calcium. In hypoalbuminaemia, it can be assumed that each 1 g/L decrease in plasma albumin concentration decreases total plasma calcium concentration by approximately 0.025 mmol/L. Alternatively, ionised calcium can be measured directly.

REGULATION

The daily requirement of calcium in neonates is 1-2 mmol/kg/24h. Calcium homeostasis is complex. Total body calcium is mainly determined by intestinal absorption and renal excretion of calcium. Intestinal absorption, mainly in the duodenum and jejunum, is an efficient active transport system, stimulated by

1,25-dihydroxycholecalciferol. Parathyroid hormone influences calcium absorption by increasing renal production of calcitriol. Renal calcium excretion is regulated, partly in parallel with sodium, in the proximal convoluted tubule and partly independently in the distal tubules. Parathyroid hormone promotes calcium reabsorption in the loops of Henle and distal convoluted tubules and thus reduces calciuria. Some extraneous factors, such as loop diuretics, can greatly increase urinary calcium, as does an increase in plasma phosphate concentration.

The distribution of calcium between bone and extracellular fluid is hormonally regulated. Parathyroid hormone and calcitriol both stimulate the release of calcium from bone. Calcitonin inhibits bone resorption and increases urinary calcium excretion; the physiological relevance of these latter effects is not well understood.

HYPOCALCAEMIA

Definition and clinical features

In neonates, small decreases in plasma calcium concentration below normal are usually asymptomatic. Total plasma calcium concentrations below 1.8 mmol/L, or ionised calcium concentrations of less than 0.7 mmol/L, can cause clinical effects. These include twitching, apnoeas, fits and, characteristically, a prolonged QT interval on ECG. Chvostek's sign (of hypocalcaemia) can be demonstrated easily in a baby (tapping the facial nerve over the parotid gland in front of the ear causes a unilateral facial twitch). Symptomatic hypocalcaemia occurs more commonly in preterm infants, infants of diabetic mothers, and following perinatal hypoxia-ischaemia.

Causes

Infants may be predisposed to 'early' hypocalcaemia if there is low maternal vitamin D, e.g. in Asian or Vegan mothers. The major causes of neonatal hypocalcaemia are summarised in Figure 8.1.

Investigation

Initial investigations in unexplained, persistent hypocalcaemia in a term baby should include measurement of plasma phosphate, magnesium, alkaline phosphatase, albumin and creatinine, and assessment of acid-base status. The mother should be investigated for vitamin D deficiency by measurement of plasma 25-hydroxycholecalciferol. Further investigation, including measurement of PTH and calcitriol, may be required (see Figures 8.2 and 8.3).

Conditions associated with neonatal hypocalcaemia	
Pathogenesis	**Cause**
Exaggerated physiological fall (in the first 1 to 3 days)	Prematurity Infants of diabetic mothers
Low intake	Inadequate oral/enteral nutrition Inadequate parenteral nutrition
Pathological	
• related to parathyroid hormone	Hypoparathyroidism, transient or genetic Maternal hyperparathyroidism Di George syndrome Hypomagnesaemia
• related to vitamin D	Maternal vitamin D deficiency Fat malabsorption 1α-hydroxylase deficiency
• multifactorial (related to chronic disease or inherited metabolic disease)	Liver or renal disease Organic acid disorders Hypoxic-ischaemic encephalopathy
Iatrogenic	
• increased losses	Loop diuretics
• insoluble calcium salts formation	High phosphate intake Exchange transfusion

Figure 8.1 Conditions associated with neonatal hypocalcaemia

MANAGEMENT

Asymptomatic hypocalcaemia requires no treatment. Seizures respond to slow i.v. injection of 2 mL/kg 10% calcium gluconate under ECG control, followed by oral supplements of calcium gluconate (200-500 mg/kg/24h) and appropriate management of the underlying cause.

Typical biochemical findings in neonatal hypocalcaemia				
Cause	**Presenting age**	**Plasma phosphate**	**Plasma alkaline phosphatase**	**Other plasma investigations**
Physiological	24-48 h	N	N	
Maternal vitamin D deficiency	24-48 h	N/↓	↑	PTH ↑/N
1α-hydroxylase deficiency	Infancy (rarely neonatal)	N/↓	↑	PTH ↑/N
Malabsorption	Any	N/↓	↑	PTH ↑/N
Hypoparathyroidism	Any (rarely neonatal)	↑	N	PTH ↓↓
Pseudohypopara-thyroidism	Any (rarely neonatal)	↑	N	PTH ↑/N
Hypomagnesaemia	>5 days	N	N	Mg^{++} <0.4 mmol/L
Iatrogenic	>5 days	N/↑	N	

Figure 8.2 Typical biochemical findings in neonatal hypocalcaemia

HYPERCALCAEMIA

This is defined as a total calcium concentration greater than 2.70 mmol/L in a sample derived from free-flowing venous blood. Hypercalcaemia in the neonatal period is less common than hypocalcaemia. Clinical features include irritability, constipation, failure to thrive, polydipsia, polyuria (caused by reduced renal concentrating ability) and nephrocalcinosis with renal failure.

The causes of hypercalcaemia include immobilisation, malignancy, hyperparathyroidism, hyperthyroidism, familial hypocalciuric hypercalcaemia, the use of thiazide diuretics and William's syndrome. The latter is a serious, sporadic disorder in which hypercalcaemia, thought to be caused by hypersensitivity to vitamin D, is associated with typical 'elfin' facies, developmental delay and supravalvular aortic stenosis. Treatment of the hypercalcaemia does not appear to affect the other features of this condition.

Hypercalcaemia can occur with hypophosphataemia and hypercalciuria in phosphate-depleted preterm infants. Hypercalciuria without hypercalcaemia can occur in preterm infants with poorly acidified urine, particularly when there is low urine flow rate, and can lead to temporary nephrocalcinosis. Over 20% of babies that are less than 32 weeks gestation are affected. This condition can also complicate long-term administration of frusemide for congenital heart disease or in the management of bronchopulmonary dysplasia. In this situation, frusemide should be replaced by a thiazide.

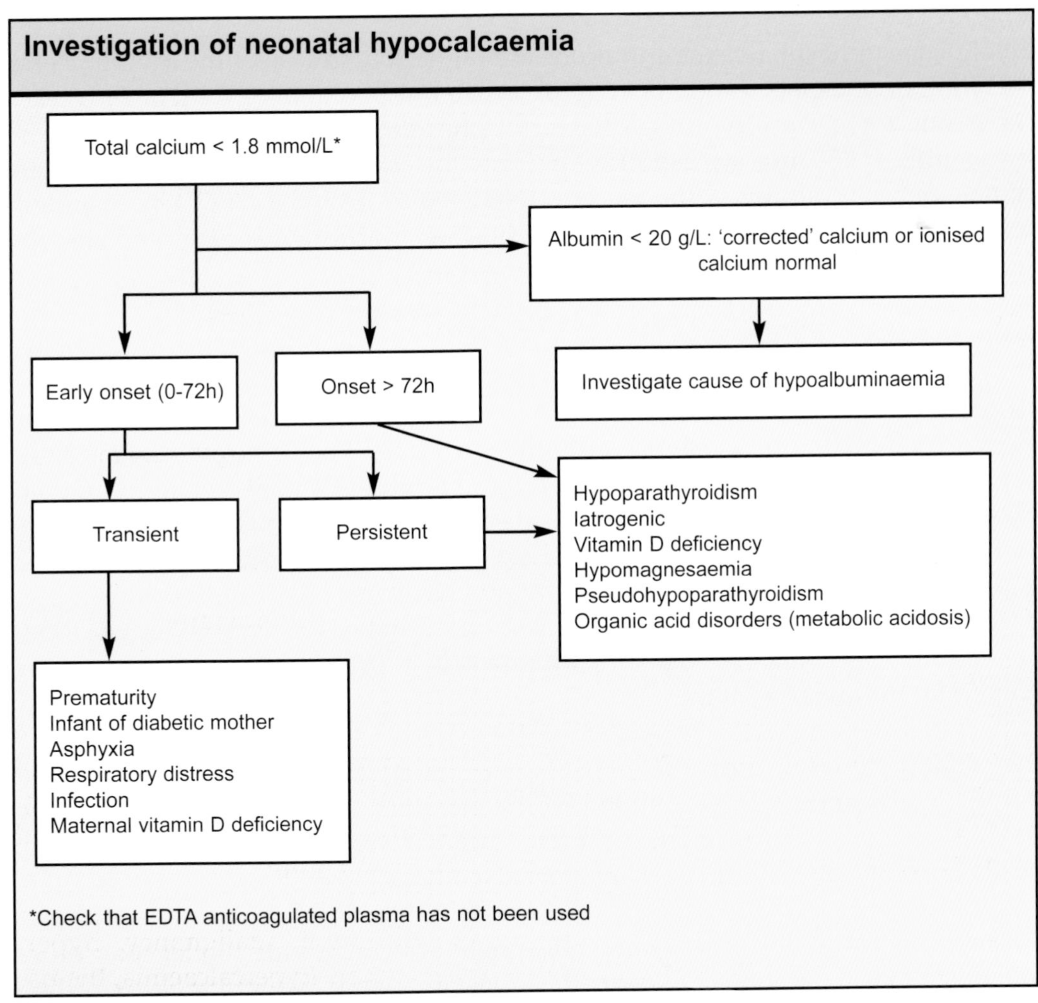

Figure 8.3 Investigation of neonatal hypocalcaemia

MAGNESIUM

HYPOMAGNESAEMIA

Hypomagnesaemia can lead to hypocalcaemia by reducing parathyroid hormone secretion or the responsiveness of the parathyroids to calcium: thus, the parathyroid hormone concentration may be low or normal. The hypocalcaemia is typically refractory to calcium replacement. Hypomagnesaemia is particularly common in infants of mothers with diabetes. Intramuscular 50% magnesium sulphate (0.2 mL/kg), should be given to babies who develop hypocalcaemia and whose plasma magnesium concentration falls to 0.4 mmol/L or below.

PHOSPHATE

Fetal plasma phosphate concentrations are higher than those of the mother. Fetal accretion of phosphorus occurs at approximately 2.0 mmol/kg/24 h at 28 weeks, increasing further up to term. After birth, phosphorus accretion is less. Human breast milk at 150 mL/kg/24h provides only the equivalent of 0.9 mmol/kg/24h of phosphorus, and this is almost completely (90%) absorbed. Similarly, standard term formula milks provide less phosphorus than is acquired *in utero*, and absorption is also less good, being estimated to be about 25%.

More than 80% of body phosphorus in neonates is extracellular, mainly in bone, the rest being distributed throughout all soft tissues and body fluids. Phosphorus in body fluids is either inorganic – the commonly measured component – or organic, mainly in phospholipids and phosphoesters. Body phosphorus per kilogram body weight doubles between birth and adult life; infants retain more than 50% of ingested phosphorus, which is absorbed throughout the small intestine, partly under the control of calcitriol. When dietary inorganic phosphate is restricted, as in enterally fed preterm infants receiving breast milk or unsupplemented formula, fractional intestinal absorption increases. This is largely independent of calcitriol. The daily requirement is 1-2 mmol/kg at term, and 2-3 mmol/kg for preterm infants.

Regulation of plasma inorganic phosphate is mainly through the control of renal tubular reabsorption. This is limited by the maximal reabsorptive capacity of the tubules. Parathyroid hormone decreases tubular reabsorption, and, therefore, leads to an increase in urinary phosphate excretion.

Plasma concentrations of inorganic phosphate in neonates are higher than those in adults. Plasma inorganic phosphate values are a little lower in breast-fed than in bottle-fed babies. Mean plasma phosphate concentration at seven days is around 2.0 mmol/L.

NEONATAL OSTEOPENIA

Chronic deficiency of calcium or phosphorus intake results in poor mineralisation of new bone or demineralisation of existing bone, leading to osteopenia. In severe cases, this can produce radiological changes and a risk of fracture after minimal trauma of ribs or long bones. In such babies, plasma calcium concentration is normal, plasma phosphate is less than 2.0 mmol/L (sometimes less than 1.0 mmol/L) and alkaline phosphatase activity is grossly elevated. Tubular reabsorption of phosphate is typically greater than 90%, giving a low urinary phosphate:creatinine ratio. In some very small infants, low plasma phosphate concentrations (less than 1 mmol/L) can co-exist with active demineralisation of bone, hypercalciuria, and development of nephrocalcinosis.

This situation of prolonged insufficient mineral intake is particularly likely to affect preterm babies. This condition was formerly known as 'rickets of prematurity', but is now referred to as 'osteopenia of prematurity', as vitamin D deficiency is not thought to have a primary role. Affected babies are usually less than 30 weeks gestation at birth. They are clinically and radiologically normal at birth, but bony changes develop over the first 6 to 12 weeks, and there is a fall off of longitudinal growth. In more severe disease, radiological changes of loss of bone density are seen first, followed, if the condition continues, by flaring and cupping of the bone ends, and fractures of ribs or long bones. These babies can have prolonged oxygen dependency related to increased compliance of the chest wall. Fractures can be mis-attributed to non-accidental injury.

The management of osteopenia of prematurity includes adequate provision of vitamin D (800 IU daily) and dietary phosphate supplementation. Preventative measures such as increased mineral provision in parenteral nutrition solutions, and the widespread use of calcium and phosphate supplemented preterm milk formulae and commercially available breast milk additives have made this condition less common than formerly in babies without a gut abnormality. For a baby taking 150 mL/kg/24h of preterm formula or appropriately supplemented human milk, phosphorus retention rates of 1.6-1.7 mmoL/kg/24h can be achieved. Because of the interactions between calcium and phosphate, molar ratios of 1.3-1.4:1 Ca:P are recommended in milks and parenteral nutrition solutions.

FURTHER READING

Bishop NJ. Metabolic bone disease. In: Textbook of Neonatology 3rd edn. Rennie JM, Roberton NRC (Eds). London: Churchill Livingstone, 1999, pp 1002-8.

Mimouni F, Tsang RC. Pathophysiology of neonatal hypercalcaemia. In: Fetal and Neonatal Physiology 2nd edn. Polin RA, Fox WA (Eds). Philadelphia: WB Saunders, 1997, pp 2329-35.

Namgung R, Tsang RC. Neonatal calcium, phosphorus and magnesium homeostasis. In: Fetal and Neonatal Physiology, 2nd edn. Polin RA, Fox WA (Eds). Philadelphia: WB Saunders, 1997, pp 2308-29.

Chapter 9

Neonatal screening

INTRODUCTION

The aim of neonatal screening is to detect and diagnose disorders before symptoms first appear, so that treatment or management can be instituted early and outcome improved. There are well established criteria for selecting those disorders which justify a screening programme (Figure 9.1) and it may be appropriate to screen for some conditions only in particular populations. Universal programmes for phenylketonuria (PKU) and congenital hypothyroidism (CHT) exist in most developed countries. Programmes for cystic fibrosis and sickle cell disorders are established in some parts of the UK and there are plans to extend these on a national basis. Elsewhere in Europe, North America and Australasia there are programmes for other conditions (Figure 9.2).

Criteria for selection of disorders for neonatal screening	
Definition of the abnormality	Is the abnormality adequately defined?
Population to be screened	What is considered to be the appropriate population to screen?
Incidence	Are there data on the incidence of the condition in the population?
Screening methods	Is a suitable, efficient and cost-effective method available?
Follow-up procedures	Are confirmatory diagnostic tests available and is there an acceptable treatment/management protocol?
Monitoring the effects	Is the natural history of the disease favourably affected by the screening procedure? Are there any adverse effects?
Costs	What are the resource implications: education, operating costs, follow-up?
Equivocal results	What is to be done about 'borderline' results?

Figure 9.1 Criteria for selection of disorders for neonatal screening

Disorders that can be detected by neonatal screening programmes	
Disorders	**Incidence * Approximate cases per 100,000**
Congenital hypothyroidism (1)	10-25
Phenylketonuria (1)	11
Cystic fibrosis (2)	40
Sickle cell disorders (2)	25
Duchenne muscular dystrophy (2)	22-28
Galactosaemia (2) **	2.5
Homocystinuria (2)	1-2
Maple syrup urine disease (2)	0.5
Tyrosinaemia (3) **	1-5
Congenital adrenal hyperplasia (3)	5-10
Medium chain acyl CoA dehydrogenase deficiency (3)	5-10
Biotinidase deficiency (3)	Unknown in UK (1-2 elsewhere)
Organic acidaemias (3)	3
Urea cycle disorders (3)	2.5
Glucose 6-phosphate dehydrogenase deficiency (3)	Population dependent

(1) National programme exists throughout the UK and Ireland
(2) Screening carried out in some parts of the UK and Ireland
(3) Currently not carried out in the UK and Ireland
* Incidence data is from the UK population where known (see Further Reading Pollitt *et al* 1997)
**Some cases of tyrosinaemia and galactosaemia may be detected via the PKU screening programme
Significant population differences may occur for some disorders

Figure 9.2 Disorders that can be detected by neonatal screening programmes

Babies are screened by testing a capillary sample of blood obtained by a heel-prick stab; this is usually taken on to card to form dried blood spots. In the UK, testing is currently done at about 6-10 days, although in many other countries the practice is to test earlier.

Screening is usually undertaken on a large scale and most laboratories test a newborn population in excess of 50,000. This offers advantages of cost-effectiveness associated with large scale testing and, more importantly, concentrates experience and information, facilitates audit and promotes development of expertise for these relatively rare disorders.

A laboratory screening programme not only involves specimen collection and analytical procedures, but also an advisory service and clinical audit. An important part of the programme is the teaching and education of health professionals (e.g. midwives, health visitors, clerical officers) involved in the service.

A specification for the service should include standards against which the performance of the programme can be monitored; some countries have national standards covering process, systems and outcome measures. A national programme centre for the UK is currently being established. Data on age of babies when tested, the number of cases diagnosed, false positives and negatives, age at diagnosis and start of treatment are all important measures of performance. It is important to be able to identify, in a timely manner, any babies who have not been screened, in order to prevent missed cases or delayed diagnoses.

PHENYLKETONURIA (PKU)

NEONATAL SCREENING AND MANAGEMENT IN CHILDHOOD

Phenylketonuria is an autosomal recessively inherited disorder caused by deficiency of the enzyme phenylalanine hydroxylase (Figure 9.3). The gene resides on the long arm of chromosome 12 and molecular biology techniques have allowed the characterisation of more than 400 different mutations causing this enzyme deficiency. The extent of the enzyme deficiency varies from complete absence to residual activity as high as 25%, depending on the particular mutation. A high proportion of affected individuals are compound heterozygotes, although a few specific mutations may account for the majority of cases in a particular population. The incidence of phenylketonuria varies widely, but in most countries with screening programmes it lies between 1 in 5000 and 1 in 20,000 live births. In the UK, the average incidence is 1 in 10,000 with a carrier frequency of 1 in 50.

When phenylalanine hydroxylase is deficient, phenylalanine accumulates rapidly following commencement of normal milk feeding. Within the first few days a very high blood concentration of phenylalanine develops that, if untreated, will cause severe and irreversible learning difficulties. The phenolic acid metabolites of phenylalanine, i.e. *p*-hydroxyphenylpyruvate, phenyllactate and *o*-hydroxyphenylacetate also accumulate and are excreted in large quantities in the urine. The diagnosis is confirmed by the finding of a plasma phenylalanine concentration above 200 µmol/L and usually in excess of 1000 µmol/L (normal <100 μmol/L), with other amino acids not increased, normal liver enzymes and normal biopterin investigations (*see p. 139*). A baby who is found to have a gross increase in plasma phenylalanine, which is confirmed by quantitative analysis, may be given a 'presumptive' diagnosis of classic PKU. Dietary treatment is commenced whilst awaiting the results of the biopterin investigations.

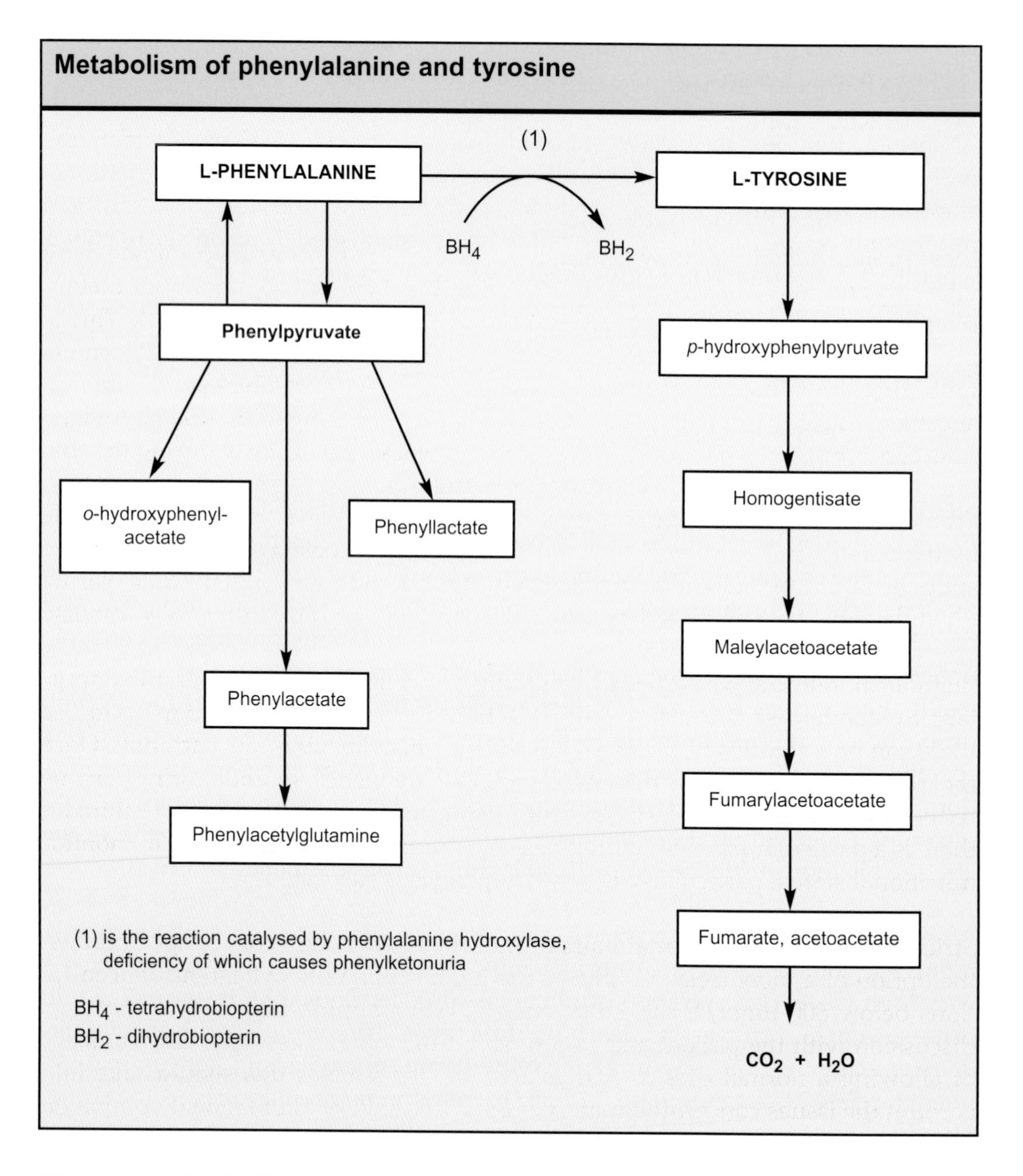

Figure 9.3 Metabolism of phenylalanine and tyrosine

It is important that the diet should commence as soon as possible to ensure optimal outcome. The basis of the diet is a low phenylalanine content, supplemented with a 'protein substitute', which is either a mixture of free L-amino acids or a protein hydrolysate free from phenylalanine. Several products are available and those suitable for neonates include:

XP Analog LCP® (Scientific Hospital Supplies)
XP Analog® (Scientific Hospital Supplies)
PKU1® (Milupa)
Lofenalac® (Mead Johnson)
Phenex 1® (Ross)

Most protein substitutes now generally available are nutritionally complete, with vitamins and minerals added to them. A small and controlled amount of dietary phenylalanine intake is essential for normal growth and development. This is provided as 50 mg 'exchanges' and in the neonate is provided as breast or formula milk. Breast feeding can continue by giving the baby the protein substitute first and then 'topping up' with breast milk. Regular monitoring of plasma phenylalanine concentration is required (at least twice a week), particularly during the first few weeks of treatment. Dietary phenylalanine is then increased or decreased according to the plasma concentration. Blood sampling can be performed at home by the parents and specimens sent to the laboratory by post, either as dried blood spots or liquid blood. Current practice in the UK is to recommend that plasma phenylalanine be maintained between 120 and 360 μmol/L during early infancy.

Regular monitoring continues to be required throughout childhood. It is important to standardise the blood sampling time for individuals, i.e. a.m./p.m., as there can be a significant diurnal variation of phenylalanine concentration. Once the plasma concentration has stabilised, the frequency of monitoring can be reduced to once a week. More frequent monitoring of phenylalanine is required if there is a particular problem with illness or compliance. It is important to monitor nutritional status, particularly if non-compliance is suspected.

Strict dietary treatment is maintained until the child is ten years of age and then the option of a more 'relaxed' diet to maintain plasma phenylalanine concentrations below 800 μmol/L can be discussed. When approaching 17 years of age, discussion with the patient and family about the advantages and disadvantages of allowing a normal diet should take place; for females this should take into account the issues concerning maternal PKU (see below). Professional opinion on the optimal plasma phenylalanine concentration and the desirability of dietary relaxation may differ, although there is an increasing tendency to maintain stricter control with more frequent monitoring and to allow less relaxation. The dietary regimen is not easy, and expert dietetic support is essential.

With early treatment and good dietary management, the outcome for patients with phenylketonuria is good, with normal growth and development. Although most children probably come close to their full intellectual potential, there is some evidence that a few children, even though treated early, suffer a mild degree of neurological impairment.

With the advance of molecular biology, carrier detection and prenatal diagnosis using mutation analysis are now theoretically possible for most families. However, for most couples who already have a child with PKU, this has rarely been undertaken because of the good outcome from dietary treatment.

Siblings of confirmed cases of PKU have a 1 in 4 risk of having PKU. In the UK, early testing of these 'at-risk' babies can be done on day 2 or 3.

PREGNANCY AND PHENYLKETONURIA

Pregnancy in women with phenylketonuria who are not on a strictly controlled diet is associated with a high incidence of severe fetal damage. Without treatment, learning difficulties resulting in severe handicap will occur in a large percentage (95%) and there is also a high risk of microcephaly, intrauterine growth retardation and congenital heart disease. The risk of these congenital abnormalities can be greatly reduced by strictly controlling plasma phenylalanine prior to conception and throughout pregnancy.

As most neonatal screening programmes commenced in the early 1970s, there are still women of childbearing age who were not screened as neonates. In addition, some countries will have a population of young immigrants who may not have been screened. Mothers of babies with unexplained microcephaly and/or congenital heart disease should therefore be tested for PKU, particularly if these are present in more than one sibling.

Phenylketonuria is a complex metabolic disorder and the patients and families need regular and on-going support for blood-sampling, dietary management, genetic counselling and liaison with schools and community services. Care is best provided by a multi-disciplinary team that includes a clinical nurse specialist, dietitian, clinical biochemist and metabolic paediatrician.

BIOPTERIN VARIANTS

Tetrahydrobiopterin is an essential coenzyme for phenylalanine hydroxylase (Figure 9.4) and also tyrosine and tryptophan hydroxylases.

Inherited defects of dihydropteridine reductase (DHPR) or biopterin synthesis result in tetrahydrobiopterin deficiency and hence defective hydroxylation of phenylalanine, thus causing hyperphenylalaninaemia. In addition to defective hydroxylation of phenylalanine, there is also defective hydroxylation of tyrosine and tryptophan, and hence failure to produce the neurotransmitters dopamine and serotonin. These biopterin defects can result in severe neurological disorders that are not effectively treated with a low phenylalanine diet alone but require treatment by supplementation with neurotransmitters.

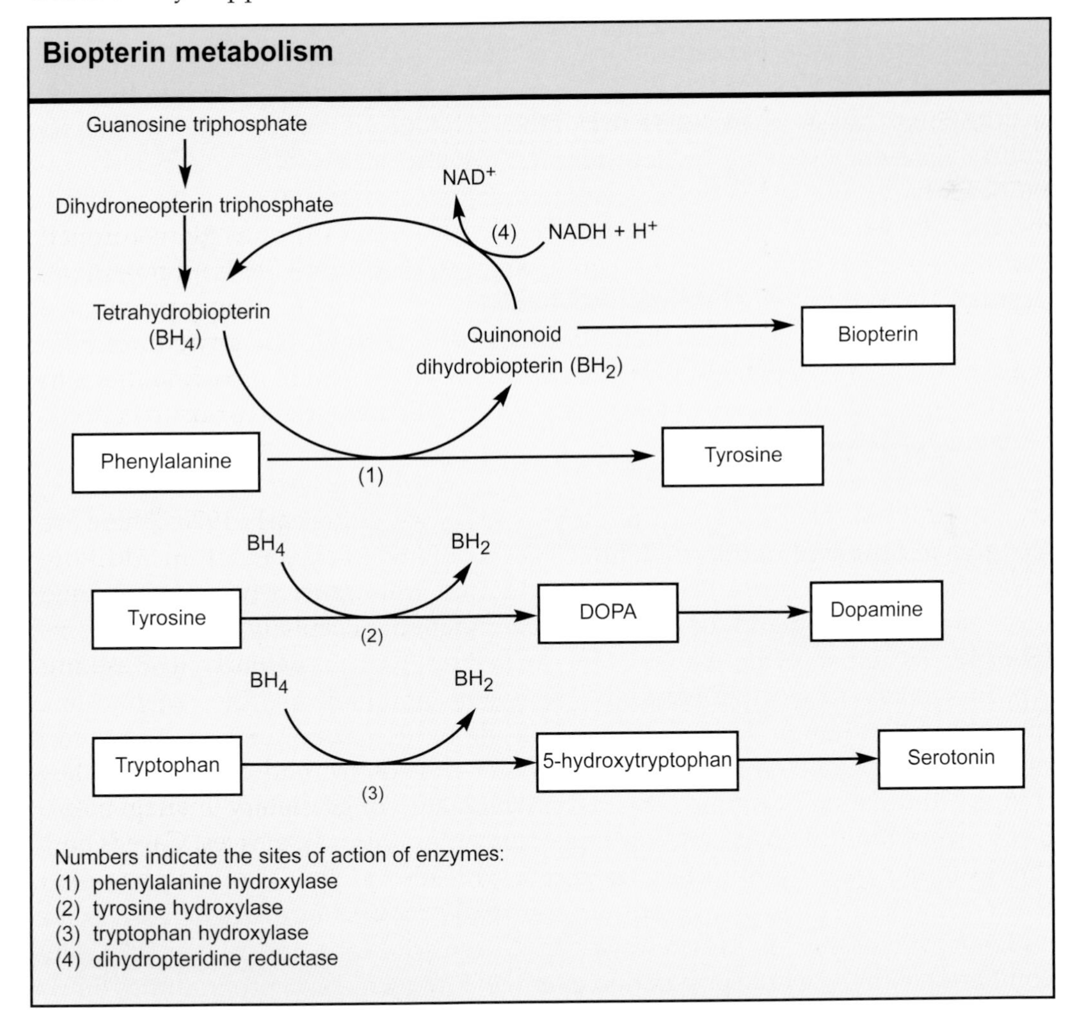

Figure 9.4 Biopterin metabolism

Although they are rare (1-3% of all cases of inherited hyperphenylalaninaemia), it is essential that every baby found to have hyperphenylalaninaemia is tested for these defects so that appropriate therapy can be initiated if necessary. The tests involve measurement of erythrocyte or whole blood dihydropteridine reductase activity, total plasma or whole blood biopterin and urinary biopterin species.

OTHER CAUSES OF HYPERPHENYLALANINAEMIA

Liver dysfunction, e.g. in neonatal hepatitis, galactosaemia and biliary atresia, may cause a significant elevation of several plasma amino acids, including phenylalanine. In this situation, increased phenylalanine is usually associated with abnormally high plasma tyrosine and, possibly, methionine and threonine, concentrations. Some babies on parenteral nutrition develop hyperphenylalaninaemia, although this is usually milder than in classic phenylketonuria, with plasma phenylalanine concentrations well below 1000 µmol/L.

In addition to classic phenylketonuria, other genetic variants of the phenylalanine hydroxylase enzyme may be detected and are characterised by a persistent but milder increase of plasma phenylalanine (i.e. greater than 100 µmol/L), typically around 250-400 µmol/L. Most of the affected individuals do not require dietary treatment as their plasma phenylalanine concentrations are within or close to the desirable treated range. They are usually clinically well and, apart from an occasional (e.g. annual) check of their plasma phenylalanine, do not require more regular follow-up. Females will require counselling as they approach child-bearing age and may need to go on a low phenylalanine diet to ensure optimal outcome for pregnancy.

CONGENITAL HYPOTHYROIDISM

Congenital primary hypothyroidism (CHT) is defined as defective function of the thyroid gland from birth. Primary hypothyroidism is caused by a defect at the level of the thyroid gland. In regions where iodine deficiency is not endemic, the disorder is most often caused by an ectopic or absent thyroid gland. Approximately 15% of patients have recessive inherited disorders of hormone biosynthesis, although this will depend on the particular population. The failure of the thyroid gland to produce thyroxine (T4) leads to high concentrations of thyroid stimulating hormone (TSH). Early replacement treatment with thyroxine can prevent brain damage and optimise outcome. Secondary hypothyroidism is the result of a defect in pituitary function and leads to inappropriately low TSH. It is rare, with an incidence of around 1 in 40,000 where iodine deficiency is not endemic. Prevalence of CHT is lower in Afro-Caribbeans and higher in Asians compared with the whole population average. Most screening programmes detect an elevation of thyroid stimulating hormone rather than a reduction in thyroxine, as the former is the more sensitive measure. However, the few screening programmes that use thyroxine measurement as the primary screen may also pick up the hypopituitary cases, which will not be detected by the programmes that use TSH. Plasma TSH concentration is high at birth and declines over the first week. It has usually stabilised by day 6, when screening is undertaken in the UK. Programmes that test earlier may have poorer sensitivity and specificity.

Following a positive screening test, the diagnosis of hypothyroidism is confirmed by the finding of grossly elevated plasma TSH (in the majority of cases > 200 mU/L) and a low concentration of free T4. The baby should be examined by a paediatrician as soon as possible Classic clinical features, e.g. lethargy, slow feeding, jaundice and constipation, are absent in many cases. Treatment should not be delayed if there are any symptoms, however minimal, and L-thyroxine (typically 25 µg/24h) should be given once a blood specimen has been taken for definitive tests (i.e. quantitative plasma TSH and free T4). Thyroxine is administered orally by crushing and mixing the tablet with a little milk. If there are absolutely no clinical signs, it is prudent to wait for confirmation of the high TSH test result on a repeat blood specimen before starting treatment. The repeat test for TSH should be arranged urgently and, if the diagnosis is confirmed, treatment should be commenced without further delay.

Not all cases of biochemical hypothyroidism detected by the neonatal screening programme are persistent and it is important in such cases to avoid unnecessary long-term treatment. For these reasons, withdrawal of the treatment should be considered when the child is two years of age unless a thyroid scan has revealed complete agenesis.

For persistent CHT, treatment with thyroxine is continued throughout life with regular checks of plasma free T4 and TSH concentrations to ensure optimal replacement. The checks should be frequent during the first two years, and the results interpreted using appropriate reference ranges for age. Longitudinal prospective studies commenced in the 1980s have shown that, although the outcome overall for treated CHT is good with good growth, IQ in some cases is below average. It is likely that those babies with the most severe hypothyroidism at birth have been compromised prenatally and are at the greatest risk of suffering long-term impairment.

Some babies have mild but significant elevation of TSH in the newborn period, which returns to normal within a few weeks. In our experience in the UK, this transient phenomenon tends to occur particularly in Asian babies. Premature babies, particularly if they are 'sick' or have had surgery, often have higher TSH concentrations associated with low or low-normal thyroxine concentrations. It may be beneficial to supplement such infants with thyroxine for a period. Conditions that are associated with abnormalities of plasma thyroid hormone concentrations in the neonatal period are listed in Figure 9.5.

Thyroid hormone abnormalities in neonates

	TSH	T4
Primary congenital hypothyroidism	↑↑↑	↓
Secondary congenital hypothyroidism	Inappropriately ↓	↓
Maternal medication (inorganic iodine or anti-thyroid drugs)	↑↑	↓
Transient hypothyroidism	↑ or ↑↑	N/↓
Iodine excess (e.g. topical iodine)	↑	N/↓
Iodine deficiency	↑	↓
Prematurity	N/↑	N/↓

Figure 9.5 Conditions leading to abnormalities of plasma thyroid hormone concentrations in neonates

OTHER CONDITIONS

CYSTIC FIBROSIS

Cystic fibrosis (CF) is the commonest single gene disorder in Caucasians. It is caused by mutations in the cystic fibrosis transmembrane conductance regulator gene (CFTR) on chromosome 7. Over 800 different mutations have been found. In the UK, a single mutation (ΔF508) accounts for about 75% of defective genes. The clinical effects of untreated CF are caused by progressive lung disease and pancreatic insufficiency. The case for screening has usually rested on the fact that most patients with CF have a pre-symptomatic stage before diagnosis.

Neonatal screening is undertaken in several countries (including parts of the UK, France, Australia and the USA), using the same heel-prick blood specimen for PKU and CHT testing, during the first week of life. Several screening protocols have been used: most rely on measurement of dried blood spot immunoreactive trypsin (IRT) at approximately one week of age as the first test. IRT has a low discriminating power in the first 1-2 days of age since transient hypertrypsinaemia in some unaffected neonates is indistinguishable from that seen in neonates with CF. Babies with CF who have meconium ileus may give a false negative result.

A two-tier approach using IRT followed by DNA analysis for the ΔF508 and other common mutations in the same specimen is used in some centres, whereas others request a second, i.e. repeat, specimen for IRT. Depending on the protocol and the DNA results, a sweat test may be required to make a definitive diagnosis.

Although newborn screening programmes for cystic fibrosis reduce the age at diagnosis and the time spent in hospital in the first year of life, uncertainty remains as to whether newborn screening improves long-term prognosis, and the issue remains under debate. Early diagnosis of CF in a baby or young infant will, however, allow the parents the opportunity of prenatal diagnosis for the next pregnancy, whereas previously, diagnosis of the propositus often came too late to prevent the birth of an affected sibling.

A decision has been made to provide a national newborn screening programme for CF in the UK.

SICKLE CELL DISORDERS (SCD)

In normal term newborns, 70-90% of total haemoglobin is fetal haemoglobin (HbF) with 10-30% adult haemoglobin (HbA) (*see p.193*). Sickle cell disease is caused by a single mutation in the β globin gene, which causes the production of sickle haemoglobin (HbS). Aggregation of HbS in low oxygen tensions leads to sickling of the red cells with consequent vaso-occlusion and red cell destruction, leading to pain, anaemia and damage to various organs. The sickle cell disorders include homozygous HbSS, mixed heterozygous HbSC and HbSD, and HbS/β thalassaemia. Sickle cell disorders (SCD) are particularly common in the black Afro-Caribbean ethnic groups. In these populations, the incidence of SCD is approximately 1 in 100-300 births. Infants with SCD are at risk of pneumoccocal septicaemia, and there is a high risk of death from this infection. It is important to screen for sickle cell disorders in at-risk populations. Early diagnosis improves morbidity and mortality through the use of prophylatic penicillin, pneumoccocal vaccination and open access to appropriate inpatient care.

Screening can be done using the heel-prick blood specimen by using HPLC or isoelectric focusing to separate the different haemoglobins. Great care must be taken in interpretation owing to the large percentage of fetal haemoglobin present at the time of screening. Presumptive positives should be confirmed by repeat analysis at a later age (e.g. 3-6 months), together with family studies.

The diagnosis of carrier status allows couples to be counselled about the risks for future pregnancies. It is uncertain whether knowledge of the carrier status of the newborn is beneficial for the individual.

A national screening programme for SCD is planned to be introduced across the UK by 2004.

CONGENITAL ADRENAL HYPERPLASIA

Congenital adrenal hyperplasia (CAH) (*see p.60*) due to 21-hydroxylase deficiency is screened for by measurement of 17-hydroxyprogesterone in heel-prick blood. Screening programmes are provided in some countries, but not the UK. Presentation ranges from early neonatal death, gender misassignment and salt losing adrenal crises, to the later onset forms presenting at or after puberty.

The aim of screening for CAH is to provide an earlier diagnosis and treatment. Plasma 17-hydroxyprogesterone concentration is high at birth and declines over the first week. Very early testing can cause problems, with poor specificity in premature and low birth weight babies, and 'sick' babies who are stressed. By detecting cases of CAH with screening programmes, it is claimed that adrenal crises can be avoided and morbidity and mortality reduced.

Greater awareness of the possibility of CAH in babies with ambiguous genitalia or unexplained hyponatraemia or salt loss (*see p.53*) has reduced the number of missed and late diagnoses without the need for whole population screening, and is currently the approach to diagnosis in the UK and some other countries.

FAT OXIDATION DEFECTS

Screening for medium chain acyl CoA dehydrogenase (MCAD) deficiency, by measuring acyl carnitine species in blood spots using tandem mass spectrometry (*see p.149*) is provided in several countries including Australia, Germany and parts of the USA. In the UK, there is some concern that a proportion of biochemically affected individuals will never experience any significant ill effects, and that universal screening might provoke unnecessary anxiety in some families. A national study is planned for the UK. The case for screening for other fat oxidation defects is currently less clear than for MCAD deficiency, as the performance of the screening test has not been adequately assessed.

ORGANIC ACID DISORDERS

Methylmalonic acidaemia, propionic acidaemia and isovaleric acidaemia can also be detected by acyl carnitine analysis and are included in some tandem mass spectrometry screening programmes. The impact of screening on patient outcome is unknown.

UREA CYCLE DISORDERS

Acute forms of these conditions present very early with life-threatening illness, and neonatal screening is therefore required early, i.e. at 1-3 days of age, if it is to be of benefit. Some pilot programmes using tandem mass spectrometry exist in the USA, Australia and Germany. It is important that these are evaluated to assess potential benefits. Screening for urea cycle disorders is not practised in the UK. Early suspicion of these disorders with measurement of plasma ammonia is therefore important.

MAPLE SYRUP URINE DISEASE

This is a very rare disorder of branched chain amino acid catabolism, although there are some specific populations with a higher incidence owing to consanguineous marriages. Neonatal screening is performed in many parts of the USA and some other countries. Phenylketonuria screening programmes that screen for several amino acids (and not just phenylalanine), will also detect maple syrup urine disease.

HOMOCYSTINURIA

Neonatal screening is usually based on detection of increased methionine in blood spots. The case for screening is good but unfortunately the current tests have poor sensitivity, and the milder pyridoxine-responsive cases are missed.

BIOTINIDASE DEFICIENCY

The serious effects of late or untreated biotinidase deficiency, and the success and ease of treatment, make it a good candidate for neonatal screening. Suitable methods are available for testing dried blood spots. However, data from several programmes suggest a low incidence, and detection of partial deficiencies complicates the screening. There are no incidence data or programmes in the UK.

DUCHENNE MUSCULAR DYSTROPHY

The primary test is measurement of creatine kinase with confirmation by molecular analysis. There are several programmes in existence, including one in Wales. Neonatal screening for Duchenne muscular dystrophy is contentious as there is currently no treatment. The main aims are to provide counselling to families and increase the effectiveness of prenatal diagnosis. There may also be some benefits in planning care for the affected individual.

GLUCOSE 6-PHOSPHATASE DEFICIENCY

Screening for glucose 6-phosphatase deficiency is provided in certain countries including Greece, Italy, and China. In others, including the UK, whole population screening is not indicated, although it is important to test specifically at-risk babies, particularly those with early jaundice or jaundice precipitated or prolonged by drugs.

GALACTOSAEMIA

Galactosaemia is a relatively rare condition with an estimated incidence in the UK of approximately 1 in 45,000 births. The justification for screening is based on prevention of neonatal mortality. Recent evidence suggests that, in spite of early treatment, long-term outcome is poor, with neurological dysfunction and a high incidence of ovarian failure in females.

Screening is carried out in some parts of Europe and the USA and is usually performed by measurement of red cell galactose 1-phosphate by a microbiological method (Paigen method) or galactose 1-phosphate uridyl transferase (gal 1-PUT) (Beutler method). Screening using the Beutler assay may produce a false negative result if the child has had a significant blood transfusion. Application of one of these assays to the blood screening samples that have slightly raised phenylalanine on the PKU screen may detect some cases of galactosaemia; increased phenylalanine (with or without an increase in tyrosine) is a feature of the liver dysfunction. Galactosaemia caused by epimerase deficiency (*see p.180*) will not be detected by those methods that measure gal 1-PUT. A false positive gal 1-PUT result may occur if there is glucose 6-phosphate dehydrogenase deficiency, as this enzyme is required as part of the test.

Clinical awareness of the possibility of galactosaemia in a jaundiced or sick baby should trigger prompt investigation and diagnosis without the need for a whole population screening programme. In the situation where there is a newborn sibling of a known case of galactosaemia, the baby should be fed on a lactose-free formula (e.g. a soya-based formula) from birth until the result of the screening test becomes available.

TYROSINAEMIA TYPE I

A few centres specifically screen for tyrosinaemia: an example is Quebec, where there is a particularly high incidence of this disorder. Programmes to screen for PKU may also detect tyrosinaemia type I.

INFECTIOUS DISEASES

Neonatal screening for infectious diseases is difficult because it is often impossible to distinguish between antibodies of maternal and neonatal origin. In any case, therapeutic interventions are generally more effective when infections are diagnosed during pregnancy (*see Chapter 12*). Nevertheless, antibody testing on dried blood spots from neonates is used in many countries to obtain data on the prevalence of important infections in women of childbearing age, e.g. HIV, hepatitis B, hepatitis C.

PRACTICAL ASPECTS OF NEONATAL SCREENING

In the UK, screening tests are performed on a heel-prick blood specimen collected when the baby is between about 6-10 days old. Most babies are at home at this age and the specimen is usually collected by the Community Midwife. For those babies still in hospital, it is important that there is a system in place to ensure that these screening tests are not missed. This is particularly important for those babies still in special care units because of 'prolonged jaundice', and those in specialist intensive care units for whatever reason. There are reports of late diagnosis of congenital hypothyroidism because a screening test was not done while the baby was in hospital.

SCREENING TESTS

PKU is screened for by measuring phenylalanine, usually in dried blood spots. Four methods are in current use, these being the Guthrie microbiological assay, paper or thin layer chromatography of amino acids, an automated chemical method with fluorimetric detection and tandem mass spectrometry. The Guthrie method has, until recently, been the most commonly used method worldwide; tandem mass spectrometry is now increasingly being introduced. The Guthrie method depends on excess phenylalanine to overcome the inhibition of growth of a particular strain of *Bacillus subtilis* by β-2-thienylalanine. The method can be used semi-quantitatively and will give an approximate phenylalanine concentration. The chromatographic method can be performed on paper (Scriver) or thin-layer plates and differs from the other two methods in that it potentially allows some other disorders of amino acid metabolism (e.g. maple syrup urine disease, tyrosinaemia) to be detected, as well as PKU. The fluorimetric method is specific for phenylalanine. Tandem mass spectrometry uses a single dried blood spot to screen for amino acids and acyl carnitines. Although the instruments are expensive, the method is sensitive, specific and very rapid, and is suitable for large-scale screening.

SPECIMEN REQUIREMENT AND INTERPRETATION OF RESULTS

Blood specimens for neonatal screening are usually collected as spots on to thick absorbent cards, which are allowed to dry before being transported to the screening laboratory.

The cut-off concentration for a positive result will depend on the age at screening. In the UK, it is current practice to take the sample for screening at about 6-10 days and to recommend that the baby has received normal milk feeds for 72 hours prior to the blood being taken. PKU can be successfully detected much earlier than six days, as evidenced by practice in other countries, and, in certain situations where there is a high risk, e.g. sibling of a known PKU patient, special arrangements can be made to test for phenylalanine at three days of age. In such a situation, it is important that the routine screening test for CHT and PKU (if the three day test is negative) is repeated at six days.

If a baby is not receiving milk feeds, the screening test should still be taken at the normal time to allow detection of CHT. In this situation, it is unlikely that PKU will be missed, but it is prudent to re-test for PKU after milk feeding has been established.

The Guthrie method has the problem of possible false negative results for babies receiving antibiotics. It is usually apparent from the plate that there is inhibition of growth. In such a situation, the test should be repeated by another method (e.g. chromatography) or a repeat specimen collected. Antibiotic therapy does not interfere with the CHT screening procedure. Screening should never be delayed because of antibiotic therapy nor for any other reason.

In most screening programmes, CHT is detected by measurement of thyroid stimulating hormone (TSH) and in most centres the same blood spot card is used as for PKU screening. There are a few exceptions where thyroxine (T4) is the primary screening test. Although, potentially, T4 has the advantage of detecting secondary hypothyroidism, it has poor sensitivity and some babies with CHT will have a T4 concentration within the neonatal reference interval. For this reason, T4 programmes require high cut-off points and the protocol usually includes a second stage TSH test on a fixed percentage of the batch. TSH is, therefore, the test of choice, although secondary hypothyroidism will be missed.

There are a variety of well-proven and robust TSH methodologies, with a trend to non-isotopic methods (e.g. fluoroimmunoassay).

There is a surge of TSH during the first 24 hours of life (up to 20-50 mU/L in whole blood) with a return to normal concentrations (i.e. less than 10 mU/L) by day five. Most screening methods have an upper limit of normal of 10 mU/L for blood spot assays. TSH is not present in red blood cells and, therefore, plasma concentrations of TSH are approximately twice those found in dried blood spots.

FOLLOW-UP PROCEDURES

For both the PKU and CHT screening tests, rapid and effective follow-up procedures are required. The follow-up system will depend on the health care system in place. The type of protocol in use in the UK (Figure 9.6) involves immediate referral to a paediatrician for neonates with positive results. Equivocal results may turn out to be negative on re-test and it is important to minimise anxiety for parents. There are many causes for repeat specimens being requested (e.g. insufficient blood, specimen being lost in the post, unsatisfactory analysis). The reason for a repeat specimen being requested should be communicated to community services and, where appropriate, hospital paediatricians, for onward transmission to the parents.

Referral mechanisms are essential to ensure that blood is taken for confirmatory testing, clinical examination and, above all, communication of accurate and detailed information to anxious parents. Close cooperation between the screening laboratory and other health care professionals involved is, therefore, important for successful follow-up. The finding of a positive case, although of great interest to health care professionals, is devastating news to the family of a newborn baby.

FUTURE DEVELOPMENTS

Tandem mass spectrometry has significantly changed the potential for neonatal screening programmes. This technique allows the simultaneous detection of numerous metabolic disorders by analysis of amino acids and acyl carnitines in a single dried blood spot. Many countries, in particular, parts of the USA, Australia and Germany, have introduced tandem mass spectrometry programmes. Although the criteria for selection of disorders for neonatal screening have not changed (Figure 9.1) and the ability to screen for a disorder is not a reason in itself for screening, the availability of treatments and improved mortality and morbidity for many of these disorders is a powerful influence. However, caution and restraint are essential. Neonatal screening programmes must be critically evaluated to assess screening performance and outcome measures, including their impact on the families involved.

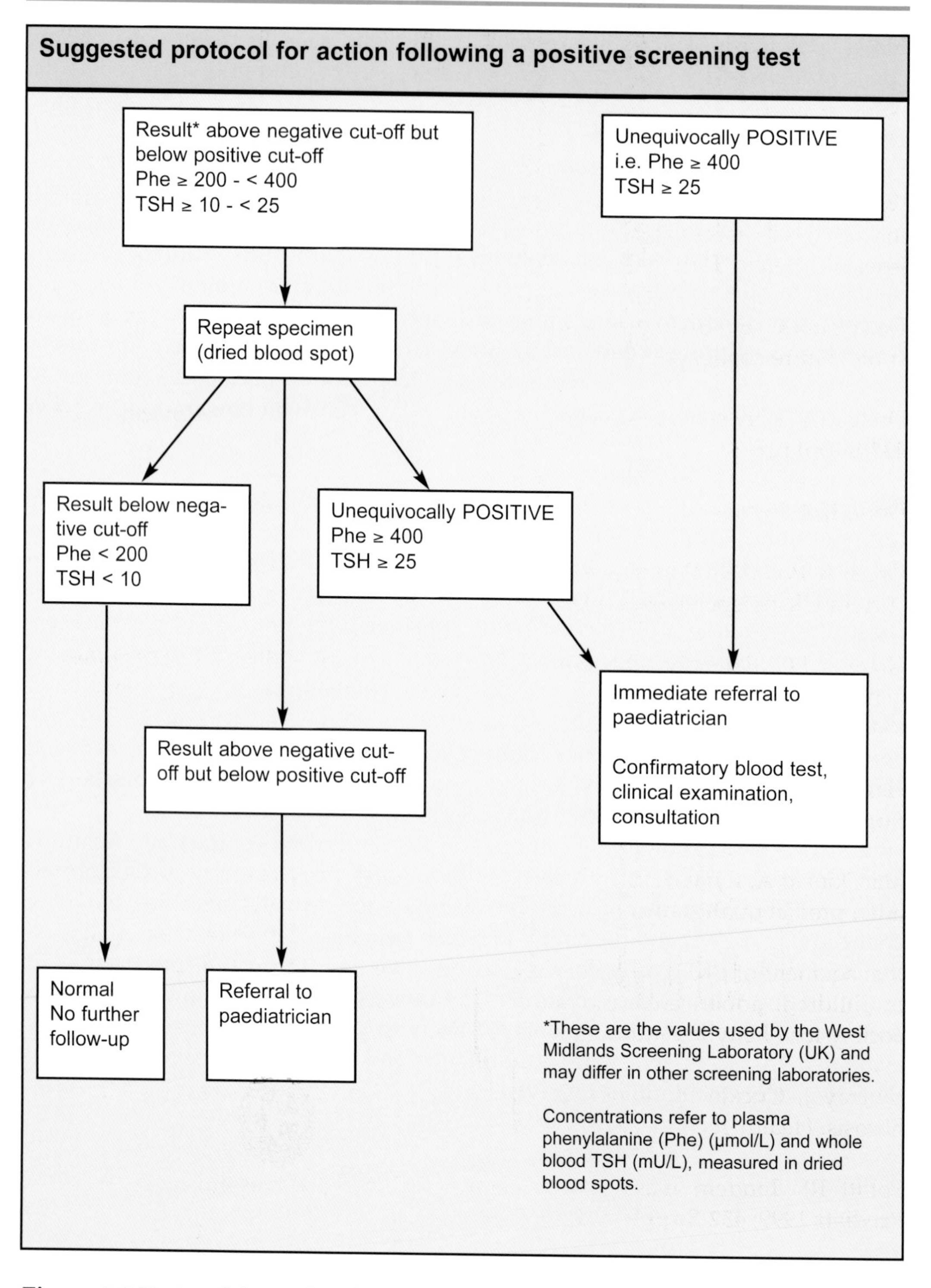

Figure 9.6 Protocol for action following a positive screening test

FURTHER READING

Anon. Screening newborn infants for cystic fibrosis. (Editorial). J Med Screening 2001; **8:** 57-60.

Davies SC, Cronin E, Gill M, Greengross P, Hickman M, Normand C. Screening for sickle cell disease and thalassaemia: a systematic review with supplementary research. Health Technol Assess 2000; Vol. 4 No.3.

Dezateaux C. Evaluating newborn screening programmes based on dried blood spots: future challenges. Br Med Bull 1998; **54:** 877-90.

Dodge JA. Why screen for cystic fibrosis? A clinician's view. Acta Paediatr 1999; **432 Suppl :** 28-32.

Doull IJM. Recent advances in cystic fibrosis. Arch Dis Child 2001; **85:** 62-6.

Green A, Pollitt RJ. Population newborn screening for inherited metabolic disease: current UK perspectives. J Inher Metab Dis 1999; **22:** 572-9.

Greeves LG, Patterson CC, Carson DJ, Thom R, Wolfenden MC *et al.* Effect of genotype on changes in intelligence quotient after dietary relaxation in phenylketonuria and hyperphenylalaninaemia. Arch Dis Child 2000; **82:** 216-21.

Hermesen G. Neonatal screening: ethical aspects. Acta Ped Scand 1999; **432 Suppl:** 99-103.

MacDonald A, Rylance G, Hall SK, Asplin D, Booth IW. Does a single blood specimen predict quality of control in PKU? Arch Dis Child 1997; **78:** 122-6.

Management of PKU. A consensus document for the diagnosis and management of children, adolescents and adults with phenylketonuria. London: National Society for Phenylketonuria (UK) Ltd, 1999.

Murray J, Cuckle H, Taylor G, Littlewood J, Hewison J. Screening for cystic fibrosis. Health Technol Assess 1999; **3:** 1-104.

Pollitt RJ. Tandem mass spectrometry screening: proving effectiveness. Acta Paediatr 1999; **432 Suppl:** 40-4.

Pollitt RJ, Green A, McCabe CJ, Booth A, Cooper NJ *et al.* Neonatal screening for inborn errors of metabolism: cost, yield and outcome. Health Technol Assess 1997; **1:** 1-202.

Rashed MS. Clinical applications of tandem mass spectrometry: ten years of diagnosis and screening for inherited metabolic disease. J Chromatog B Biomed Sci Appl 2001; **758:** 27-48.

Sweetman L. Newborn screening by tandem mass spectrometry: gaining experience. Clin Chem 2001; **47:** 1937-8.

Wilcken B, Travert G. Neonatal screening for cystic fibrosis: present and future. Acta Paediatr 1999; **432 Suppl:** 33-5.

Zeuner D, Ades AE, Karnon J, Brown J, Dezateux C, Anionwu EN. Antenatal and neonatal haemoglobinopathy screening in the UK: review and economic analysis. Heath Technol Assess 1999; **3:** 1-186.

Zytkovicz TH, Fitzgerald EF, Marsden D, Larson CA, Shih VE *et al*. Tandem mass spectrometry for amino, organic and fatty acid disorders in newborn dried blood spots: a two year summary from the New England newborn screening programme. Clin Chem 2001; **47:** 1945-55.

Chapter 10

Inherited metabolic disorders

INTRODUCTION

There are many individually rare, inherited metabolic disorders (IMDs) that present clinically in the neonatal period. Good data on the incidence of individual IMDs are not available, except where whole population screening programmes have been introduced. The incidence of different disorders can range between 1 in 10,000 to 1 in 500,000 and, for some, there is a wide variation between different populations. In spite of the relative rarity of individual disorders, collectively they present a sizeable problem and are important conditions to consider in certain patients, particularly in desperately sick neonates for whom there is no obvious diagnosis.

The IMDs that are most likely to present acutely in the neonate are those caused by defects in energy metabolism and intermediary metabolism, i.e. disorders of amino acid, organic acid or carbohydrate metabolism, urea cycle defects and electron transport chain defects. In addition, there are a few specific disorders of other areas of metabolism, e.g. purine and pyrimidine metabolism, and peroxisomal and lysosomal storage disorders, which may present in the newborn. The disorders listed in Figure 10.1 represent those that, in the authors' experience, are most likely to be encountered, although it is not an exhaustive list and other, rarer disorders have been reported in infants of this age.

Most babies with an IMD are born at or near term, with normal birth weight and no abnormal features, as the fetus has been protected during pregnancy. Symptoms usually develop within the first week of life, typically in the first 24-48 hours after full milk feeding is instituted.

Some IMDs may result in adverse effects on fetal development. In particular, some lysosomal storage disorders can present during pregnancy with fetal ascites and as hydrops fetalis. A history of more than one pregnancy presenting in this way is suggestive of such a disorder. It is therefore important to consider metabolic disease when other, commoner, causes of hydrops have not been found. Dysmorphism should also trigger consideration of an IMD (*see p.188*).

Inherited metabolic disorders that present in the neonate	
Amino acid disorders	Maple syrup urine disease Non-ketotic hyperglycinaemia Tyrosinaemia type I Homocystinuria (methylene tetrahydrofolate reductase deficiency)
Urea cycle disorders	Carbamoyl phosphate synthase deficiency Ornithine carbamoyl transferase deficiency Citrullinaemia Argininosuccinic acidaemia
Organic acid disorders	Methylmalonic acidaemia Propionic acidaemia Isovaleric acidaemia Glutaric aciduria type II (multiple acyl-CoA dehydrogenase deficiency)
Fatty acid oxidation disorders	Short chain defects Medium chain defects (e.g. MCAD) Long chain defects Carnitine transport/cycle defects
Carbohydrate disorders	Galactosaemia Glycogen storage disease type I Fructose 1,6-bisphosphatase deficiency Hereditary fructose intolerance
Energy production defects	Phosphoenolpyruvate carboxykinase deficiency Pyruvate dehydrogenase deficiency Pyruvate carboxylase deficiency Electron transport chain defects Mitochondrial defects (Pearson's syndrome)
Peroxisomal disorders	Zellweger's and pseudo-Zellweger's syndromes Neonatal adrenoleucodystrophy
Purine and pyrimidine disorders	Sulphite oxidase and xanthine oxidase deficiency (molybdenum cofactor deficiency) Adenosine deaminase deficiency

continued...

Inherited metabolic disorders that present in the neonate (cont.)	
Lysosomal storage disorders	G_{M1} gangliosidosis Niemann-Pick disease type C Krabbe's leucodystrophy Wolman's disease Pompe's disease Sly's disease (MPS 7) Gaucher's disease
Others	Menke's syndrome Congenital adrenal hyperplasia Sulphite oxidase deficiency (isolated) Smith-Lemli-Opitz syndrome Carbohydrate deficient glycoprotein syndrome Mevalonate kinase deficiency
Note: this list is not exhaustive	

Figure 10.1 Inherited metabolic disorders that present in the neonate

The biochemical basis of these disorders is wide ranging, and, for the non-specialist, there is a bewildering array of tests. The best approach to investigation is to take careful note of any clues from the history, presentation and preliminary biochemical tests, and then proceed to the more specific investigations after discussion with a specialist laboratory. If the baby is acutely ill (*see p.156*) urgent investigation is essential. Rapid recognition of an IMD is important to enable prompt treatment, and thereby prevent or limit damage to the CNS or other organs. Where treatment is not available, diagnosis is still important to enable prenatal diagnosis for subsequent pregnancies.

PRESENTATION

CLUES FROM THE HISTORY

Consanguinity and family history of a similar illness or unexplained deaths are important. A history of deaths in males particularly suggests an X-linked disorder such as ornithine carbamoyl transferase (OCT) deficiency. It is particularly important to note if a previous sibling has died following a 'Reye-like' illness, as amino acid, urea cycle, organic acid and fatty acid oxidation defects can present in this way.

If the child is likely to die before a diagnosis can be made, additional sampling is required – see Appendix B for guidelines on collecting specimens in an emergency.

CLINICAL FEATURES

The classic clinical presentation of an IMD is as a full-term baby, born after a normal pregnancy and delivery, who, after an initial symptom-free period, begins to deteriorate for no obvious reason. The time interval between birth and presentation may range from a few hours to weeks, depending on the nature of the defect, the feeding regimen and the presence of other stress factors, particularly infection or surgery. The observation of a relationship between symptoms and a change in feeding regimens, e.g. changing to glucose/saline, a non-lactose milk formula or reduced protein load, adds support to the possibility of an IMD and may suggest a particular diagnosis (e.g. galactosaemia, hereditary fructose intolerance).

In most cases, however, clinical features are non-specific, e.g. poor feeding, lethargy, vomiting, hypotonia, fits, and so do not suggest a particular diagnosis. Features that are particularly suggestive of an IMD include:

- abnormal smell, e.g. sweet, musty, cabbage-like, sweaty (amino acid and organic acid disorders)
- cataracts (galactosaemia)
- hyperventilation, secondary to metabolic acidosis (organic acid disorders)
- ambiguous genitalia ± hyponatraemia (congenital adrenal hyperplasia)
- neurological dysfunction with respiratory alkalosis ± low plasma urea (urea cycle disorders)
- metabolic acidosis with a high anion gap (organic acid disorders).

It is important to be aware that diagnosis of an infection does not preclude an associated IMD and that sepsis is a common accompaniment to an underlying metabolic defect.

INVESTIGATION OF A SICK NEONATE FOR A POSSIBLE IMD (Figure 10.2)

PRELIMINARY LABORATORY INVESTIGATIONS – CLUES TO AN IMD

Most sick neonates will have had basic biochemical and haematological investigations carried out as part of their clinical care. If an IMD is suspected, it can be particularly useful to review the results of these preliminary investigations before deciding to undertake the more specialised tests, as certain biochemical abnormalities are suggestive of a possible IMD. These include:

- hyperammonaemia
- hypoglycaemia
- lactic acidosis
- acid-base disturbance (metabolic acidosis/respiratory alkalosis)
- high anion gap
- inappropriate ketonuria/absence of ketones
- high or low plasma urate
- high or low plasma cholesterol, with or without high triglycerides.

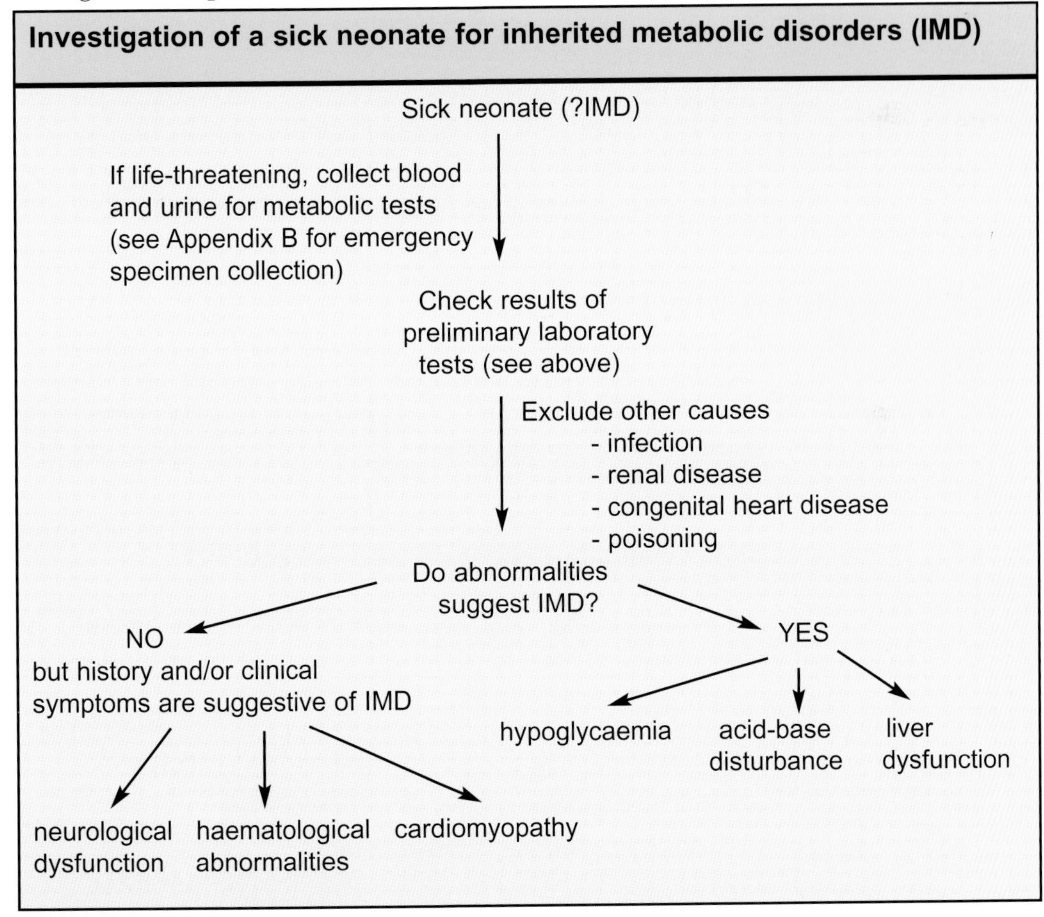

Figure 10.2 Investigation of a sick neonate for inherited metabolic disorders (*see also Figures 10.3 and 10.4*)

Guidance on the investigation of unexplained hypoglycaemia is included in Chapter 7.

In a neonate with metabolic acidosis, calculation of the anion gap, i.e. ($[Na^+]$ + $[K^+]$) – ($[Cl^-]$ + $[HCO_3^-]$), can be helpful: a gap > 20 mmol/L suggests an organic acidaemia, whereas a normal gap is more likely to be associated with renal tubular acidosis or bicarbonate loss from the gastrointestinal tract. A urine pH below 5.5 is suggestive of an organic acid disorder, although higher values do not exclude the possibility of such a disorder.

In normal neonates on regular feeds, the urine test for ketones should be negative, but may be slightly positive if in a fasting state. A strong positive result is abnormal and indicates a need for investigation, particularly for organic acid defects. An absence of ketones in a baby who is catabolic (e.g. prolonged period without adequate feeds, stress) is suggestive of a fatty acid oxidation defect.

A normal blood hydrogen ion concentration does not exclude an elevated plasma lactate concentration and measurement of plasma lactate should always be considered if there is hypoglycaemia or neurological dysfunction, as well as in acidotic states. Unexplained haematological abnormalities may occur in some IMDs (Figure 10.3).

SPECIFIC METABOLIC INVESTIGATIONS

If any clinical and/or biochemical abnormalities suggest a particular disorder or group of metabolic disorders, the patient should be investigated accordingly. When there is any doubt as to how to proceed, consultation with a specialist laboratory is essential to ensure optimal investigation.

In the situation where the neonate is acutely ill, then the following investigations should be considered and, when indicated, undertaken urgently:

- ammonia (plasma)
- lactate (plasma)
- amino acids (urine and plasma)
- organic acids (urine)
- galactose 1-phosphate uridyl transferase (erythrocytes)
- acyl carnitines (dried blood spots and plasma).

Haematological abnormalities associated with IMDs	
	Disorder(s)
Neutropenia	Glycogen storage disease type I (excluding IA) Organic acidurias (methylmalonic, propionic and isovaleric) Lysinuric protein intolerance Congenital orotic aciduria
Haemolytic anaemia	Neonatal haemochromatosis Cobalamin defects (haemolytic ureamic syndrome) Glycolytic enzyme defects, e.g. pyruvate kinase, glucose 6-phosphate dehydrogenase and phosphofructokinase Pearson's syndrome
Megaloblastic anaemia	Cobalamin defects Methylmalonic acidaemia Homocystinuria (combined with methylmalonic acidaemia) Congenital orotic acidaemia
Coagulation defects	Tyrosinaemia type I Galactosaemia Neonatal haemochromatosis Carbohydrate deficient glycoprotein syndromes

Figure 10.3 Haematological abnormalities associated with IMDs

If the baby is in a non-specialist hospital, some of these tests may not be available on site and arrangements to send specimens away for urgent investigation will be necessary. Plasma ammonia and lactate should, however, be available locally. Figure 10.4 suggests specialist investigations for sick neonates on the basis of the major presenting abnormality.

Specialist investigations for IMD in a sick neonate

Presentation	Possible metabolic disorders	Suggested investigations
Unexplained hypoglycaemia	Organic acid disorders Fatty acid oxidation disorders Amino acid disorders Glycogen storage disorders (especially type I) Disorders of gluconeogenesis Congenital adrenal hyperplasia Galactosaemia	Organic acids (U) Amino acids (U, P) 3-hydroxybutyrate (FP) Free fatty acids (FP) Carnitine and acyl carnitines (P) Lactate (FP) Insulin (P) Cortisol (P) 17-hydroxyprogesterone (P) Galactose 1-phosphate uridyl transferase (B)
Acid-base imbalance -metabolic acidosis (exclude primary cardiac and respiratory disorders)	Organic acid disorders Lactic acidosis	Organic acids (U) Lactate (FP) Amino acids (U, P) Carnitine and acyl carnitines (P)
-respiratory alkalosis	Urea cycle disorders	Ammonia (P) Orotic acid (U) Amino acids (U, P)
Liver dysfunction (often associated with hypoglycaemia and galactosuria) (see Chapter 6 for the investigation of prolonged jaundice)	Galactosaemia Fructose 1,6-bisphosphate deficiency Hereditary fructose intolerance Tyrosinaemia type I Glycogen storage disorders (type I) Disorders of gluconeogenesis α_1-antitrypsin deficiency Neonatal haemochromatosis Niemann-Pick disease type C	Galactose 1-phosphate uridyl transferase (B) Sugars (U) Amino acids (U, P) Succinylacetone (U) α-fetoprotein (P) Lactate (FP) Oligosaccharides (U) Organic acids (U) α_1-antitrypsin concentration and phenotype (S)
Neurological dysfunction: - seizures (*see p.188*) - depressed consciousness - hypotonia (see p.188 for disorders associated with dysmorphia)	Non-ketotic hyperglycinaemia Urea cycle disorders Xanthine/sulphite oxidase deficiency Homocystinuria (remethylation defect) Congenital lactic acidosis Peroxisomal disorders Organic acid disorders Lysosomal storage disorders	Amino acids (U, P, C) Orotic acid (U) Ammonia (P) Urate (P, U) Thiosulphate (U) Sulphite (U) Lactate (FP) Organic acids (U) Very long chain fatty acids (P) Leucocyte enzymes (B)

continued...

Specialist investigations for IMD in a sick neonate (cont.)

Presentation	Possible metabolic disorders	Suggested investigations
Cardiomyopathy	Glycogen storage disease type II (Pompe's) Fatty acid oxidation disorders Tyrosinaemia type I Electron transport chain disorders Carbohydrate deficient glycoprotein syndromes	Lactate (FP) 3-hydroxybutyrate (FP) Free fatty acids (P) Oligosaccharides (U) Organic acids (U) Carnitine and acyl carnitines (P) Amino acids (U, P) Transferrin isoforms (P)

Key:
U = urine B = heparinised blood P = plasma C = CSF
S = serum FP = fluoride-oxalate plasma

Sample requirements for specialist investigations should be checked with the laboratory

Figure 10.4 Specialist investigations for IMD in a sick neonate

SPECIMEN COLLECTION FOR SPECIALIST METABOLIC INVESTIGATIONS

If the baby has an episodic illness (e.g. related to a feeding regimen or associated infection) it is particularly important to collect blood and urine specimens during the acute phase, as the diagnosis may be missed if specimens are collected only when the infant is apparently well. As a minimum, random urine (ideally 5 mL, but smaller quantities are valuable) and blood (at least 1 mL heparin and 1 mL fluoride-oxalate) specimens should be collected, the plasma being separated and stored at -20°C as soon as possible after collection (i.e. within 30 minutes). This is especially important for ammonia (*see p.169*). The packed red cells should be stored unfrozen at +4°C. If the child is severely ill and deteriorating, more rigorous specimen collection is indicated (*see below and Appendix B*).

For all specimens, an accurate record of date and time of collection, together with the following information, should be provided:

- feeding regimen at the time of and immediately prior to sampling (this is particularly important if amino acids, organic acids and sugars are requested)
- details of all drug therapy and other treatments (including blood transfusions)
- full clinical details, the results of any preliminary biochemical and haematological investigations and degree of urgency.

Details of drug therapy are particularly important for amino acid investigations as several antibiotics produce ninhydrin-positive spots.

LIFE-THREATENING ILLNESS

If an illness is progressing rapidly and death seems inevitable, it is important to consider that appropriate specimens (blood, urine, skin and tissues) should be taken for biochemical analysis to enable reliable post-mortem investigation (*see Appendix* C). Blood and urine should be taken pre-mortem whenever possible. Results obtained from blood taken around the time of death or post-mortem may be difficult to interpret, as lactic acidosis, hyperammonaemia and hyper-aminoacidaemia due to protein autolysis are likely to confuse the picture. The opportunity for and potential value of a post-mortem investigation should be discussed with the parents and, if consent is obtained, this should be undertaken as soon as possible after death to minimise specimen deterioration. For those families where a diagnosis can be made, genetic counselling and the opportunity for prenatal diagnosis for future pregnancies can be of paramount importance. In these situations, great efforts should be made, in a sensitive manner, to obtain these important specimens.

SUDDEN UNEXPLAINED DEATH IN INFANCY AND METABOLIC DISEASE

A small percentage of cases of sudden unexplained death in infancy (SUDI) have been associated with metabolic disorders, particularly fatty acid oxidation defects. These include medium chain acyl CoA dehydrogenase deficiency (MCAD), long chain defects and disorders of carnitine metabolism (*see p.176*). It is therefore important to consider the possibility of metabolic disorders in infants who die suddenly and unexpectedly. Suggested investigations for such situations are provided elsewhere (*see Appendix* C).

INVESTIGATION OF SIBLINGS

When there are no samples for biochemical investigation from the index case but there is a high degree of suspicion (e.g. fatty change in the liver, family history), further children in the family can be investigated immediately after birth for disorders of fatty acid oxidation. Blood spot or plasma acyl carnitines and urinary organic acids collected during the first two days of life usually show the characteristic metabolites of a fat oxidation defect, although a negative result does not completely exclude the possibility of such a disorder. If tissue is available, extracted DNA can be tested for the common mutations associated with MCAD and LCHAD deficiencies. Alternatively, for other defects, a skin biopsy for fibroblast culture may be required.

MANAGEMENT OF THE ACUTE SITUATION

Whilst awaiting results of specific investigations, management should be supportive and geared to correcting electrolyte and acid-base imbalance, and maintaining adequate gas exchange. Regimens should be instituted to try to reduce the load on the affected metabolic pathway and induce an anabolic state as quickly as possible. Replacement of milk feeds with 10% dextrose infusion (oral or i.v.) is appropriate for most disorders, i.e. amino acid, organic acid, fat oxidation, urea cycle disorders and galactosaemia. However, this is not appropriate for the congenital lactic acidoses, which are likely to be exacerbated by a high carbohydrate load.

Severe hyperammonaemia should be treated without delay (*see p.173*).

Several IMDs have vitamin-responsive variants and the approach in some units is to give a vitamin cocktail whilst awaiting laboratory results. If this approach is used, it is crucial that appropriate specimens (blood and urine) are taken before the vitamins are given. In practice, it is rare for an IMD presenting acutely in the neonate to be one of these vitamin-responsive types and this approach is not generally recommended.

If more rigorous treatment is considered, e.g. dialysis or haemofiltration, this will usually require that the baby be transferred to a specialised centre that is experienced in the treatment of metabolic disorders.

ANTENATAL DIAGNOSIS

Increasing numbers of metabolic disorders can be tested for in high risk families by obtaining fetal tissue. Usually, the risk of an affected fetus for each pregnancy will be 1 in 4, as most IMDs are inherited in an autosomal recessive manner. Extensive counselling of the family, ideally before pregnancy, is essential before embarking on high risk investigations. Tissue can be obtained by chorionic villus biopsy, either transcervically or transabdominally, at about 10-11 weeks gestation, or by amniocentesis at 14-16 weeks. Chorionic villus sampling (CVS) has about a 1.5-2% risk of leading to miscarriage compared with a risk of approximately 1% for amniocentesis. CVS has the obvious advantage of providing a diagnosis at an earlier stage of gestation.

Diagnosis usually requires measurement of the specific enzyme (or other functional biochemical test) in a cultured or uncultured (direct) sample. DNA analysis is useful as an alternative where a specific mutation has been identified for the particular at-risk pregnancy and offers advantages in certain disorders. Amniocentesis enables measurement of enzymes in the cultured amniocytes or measurement of metabolites in the supernatant. This latter approach is of particular value when a specific enzyme or molecular defect has not been demonstrated, e.g. methylmalonic aciduria. Chromosomal analysis is usually also performed on the antenatal specimen. The outcome of such investigations is usually a decision to terminate the pregnancy if the fetus is found to be affected. However, in some situations, knowledge of an affected fetus is used to prepare the parents for the future. Treatment may also be started *in utero* or promptly after birth, e.g. biotin for biotinidase deficiency.

DISORDERS PRESENTING AS A SICK NEONATE

AMINO ACID DISORDERS

Those defects that cause accumulation of specific amino acids in blood, urine or CSF can be diagnosed by amino acid analysis. Quantitative plasma amino acid analysis is usually essential.

Maple syrup urine disease (MSUD)

The characteristic presentation is with feeding difficulties, lethargy and failure to thrive, with progressive CNS dysfunction. Biochemical abnormalities include metabolic acidosis and hypoglycaemia. In the classic form, urine and sweat have the characteristic sweet odour of maple syrup. The disorder is severe, with a progressive downhill course, that, if untreated, leads to early death. Milder variants have been described but these usually present later in infancy or early childhood, with mild developmental delay. MSUD is caused by defective decarboxylation of the branched chain oxo acids (Figure 10.5). If this disorder is particularly suspected, a positive dinitrophenylhydrazine screening test for oxo acids in urine provides a useful supporting clue.

The definitive diagnosis is made by the finding of grossly increased concentrations of branched chain amino acids (leucine, isoleucine and valine) in plasma, together with the presence of alloisoleucine and an increase in the corresponding oxo acids in urine. Plasma amino acid measurement may also show a reduced alanine concentration. Treatment involves a special diet that is low in branched chain amino acids. In patients with the severe form of MSUD, the initiation of correct dietary therapy may be life-saving. The longer term outlook, however, is not good, as there is a tendency for episodic bouts of illness, usually precipitated by an infection, resulting in impaired development and a poor long-term neurological outcome. In patients with the milder/atypical form of the disorder, good dietary management may prevent these bouts of episodic illness and improve the outcome.

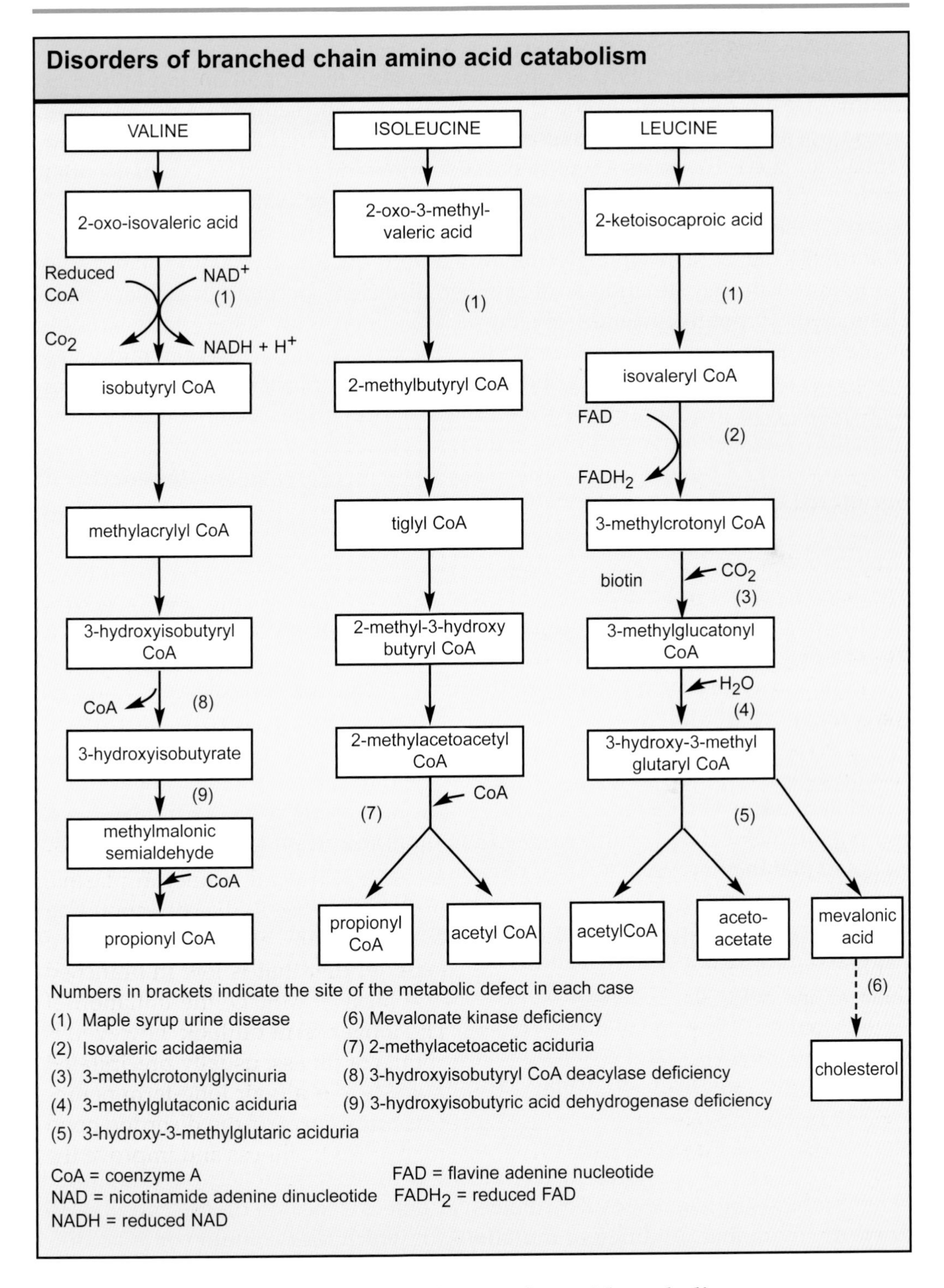

Figure 10.5 Disorders of branched chain amino acid catabolism

NON-KETOTIC HYPERGLYCINAEMIA (NKH)

Preliminary biochemical tests are usually normal in this condition and indication for investigation is based on the characteristic clinical picture of a neonate with severe uncontrollable seizures, respiratory failure and hypotonia. The electroencephalogram (EEG) shows a typical burst-suppression pattern and the baby often has hiccups. The basic defect lies in the glycine cleavage system, and diagnosis is based on the finding of elevated plasma and CSF glycine concentrations with an abnormally high CSF:plasma glycine ratio. Rapid quantitative amino acid results are required in this situation so that other disorders, perhaps treatable, can be eliminated. Hyperglycinaemia/glycinuria associated with ketonuria is strongly suggestive of an organic acid disorder (e.g. methylmalonic acidaemia) and investigation of urinary organic acids and blood spot or plasma acyl carnitines is therefore essential in this situation. At the time of writing, there is no effective treatment for NKH. Definitive diagnosis requires measurement of the glycine cleavage enzyme in liver. Prenatal diagnosis is possible by measurement of this enzyme in uncultured CVS.

TYROSINAEMIA TYPE I

The acute form of tyrosinaemia type I presents with severe liver disease and renal tubular dysfunction. The disease is due to a defect of the enzyme fumarylacetoacetase (Figure 10.6), which causes accumulation of succinylacetone and secondary increase of tyrosine, methionine, *p*-hydroxyphenylpyruvate and *p*-hydroxyphenyllactate due to inhibition of *p*-hydroxyphenylpyruvate oxidase.

In a neonate, the presenting feature may be hypoglycaemia progressing to fulminant liver failure. Characteristically, there is an increased plasma tyrosine concentration, often associated with increased methionine and phenylalanine. It should be noted that the finding of a raised plasma tyrosine concentration is only suggestive of tyrosinaemia type I. Other causes of acute liver disease, both metabolic and non-metabolic, e.g. galactosaemia and congenital viral infections, can cause increased plasma tyrosine concentrations of similar magnitude. Useful biochemical clues to support the diagnosis include a high plasma α-fetoprotein concentration, a very high plasma alkaline phosphatase activity (>2000 IU/L) and evidence of renal tubular dysfunction. The important tests to perform in this situation are measurement of urinary succinylacetone and erythrocyte porphobilinogen synthase.

Definitive diagnosis requires measurement of fumarylacetoacetase in cultured skin fibroblasts or leucocytes. The molecular defect is located on chromosome 15. There are more than 30 different mutations, of which four common ones account for more than 50% of cases. Certain mutations are more common in particular ethnic groups. For antenatal diagnosis, molecular genetic analysis may be a more useful investigation than enzyme assay in some families, particularly when it is to differentiate from the pseudodeficiency state (*in vitro* enzyme deficiency with no disease expression).

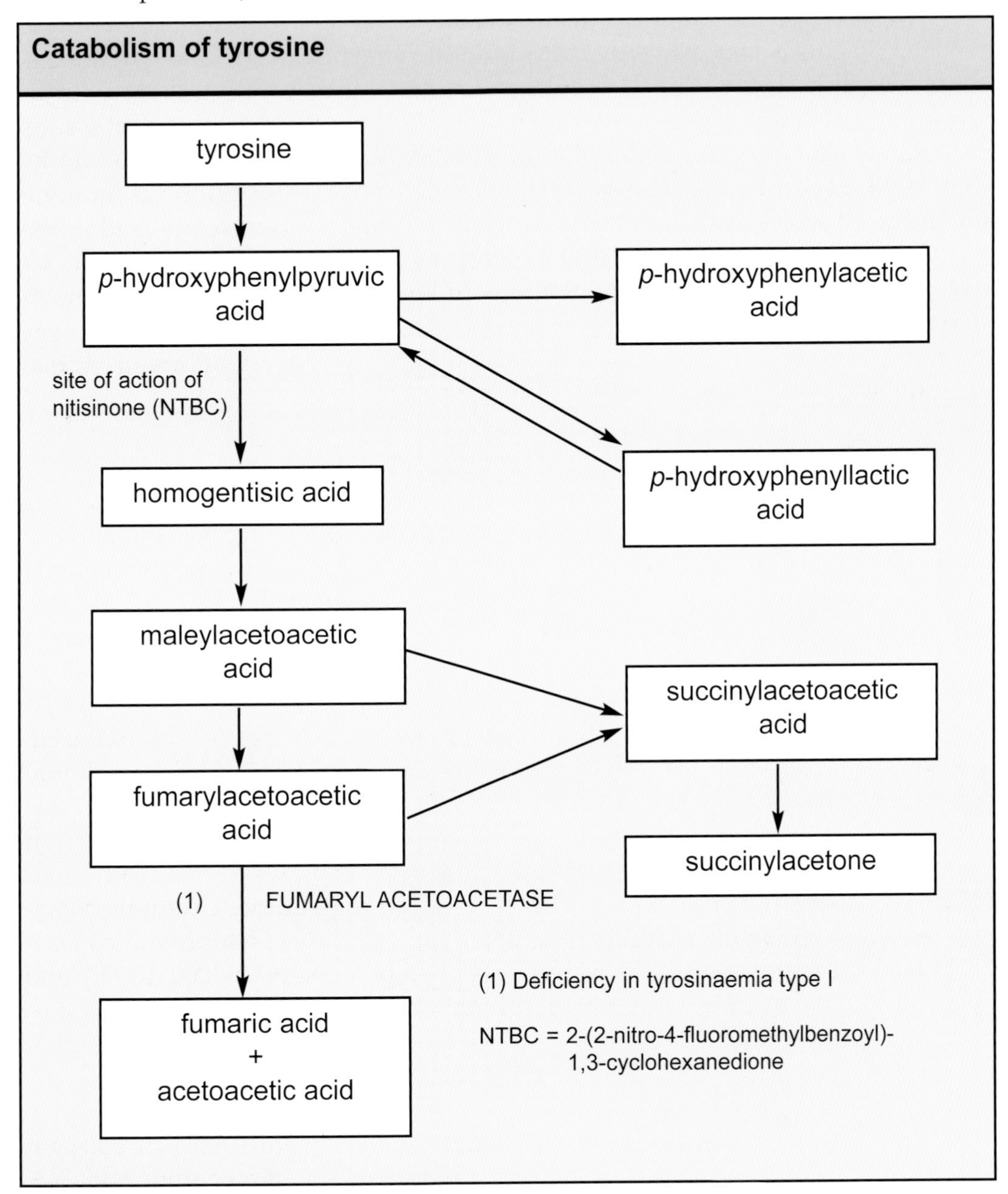

Figure 10.6 Catabolism of tyrosine

Immediate treatment is with the drug nitisinone, with the possibility of liver transplantation at a later stage. Nitisinone (NTBC, Figure 10.6) acts by inhibition of *p*-hydroxyphenylpyruvate oxygenase. Without treatment, a large percentage of patients will develop hepatoma. The outcome after treatment is much improved; it is not yet clear if treatment with nitisinone alone will prevent hepatoma. Prenatal diagnosis is possible by measuring the enzyme, or by DNA analysis, in chorionic villus biopsy (direct) or cultured amniotic fluid cells.

HOMOCYSTINURIA (DUE TO 5,10 METHYLENE TETRAHYDROFOLATE REDUCTASE DEFICIENCY)
Classic homocystinuria, due to cystathionine synthase deficiency, does not present in neonates, although some neonatal screening programmes may detect the disorder. The variant form, due to defective remethylation (Figure 10.7) can, however, present in the neonatal period with apnoeic episodes, fits and progressive CNS dysfunction.

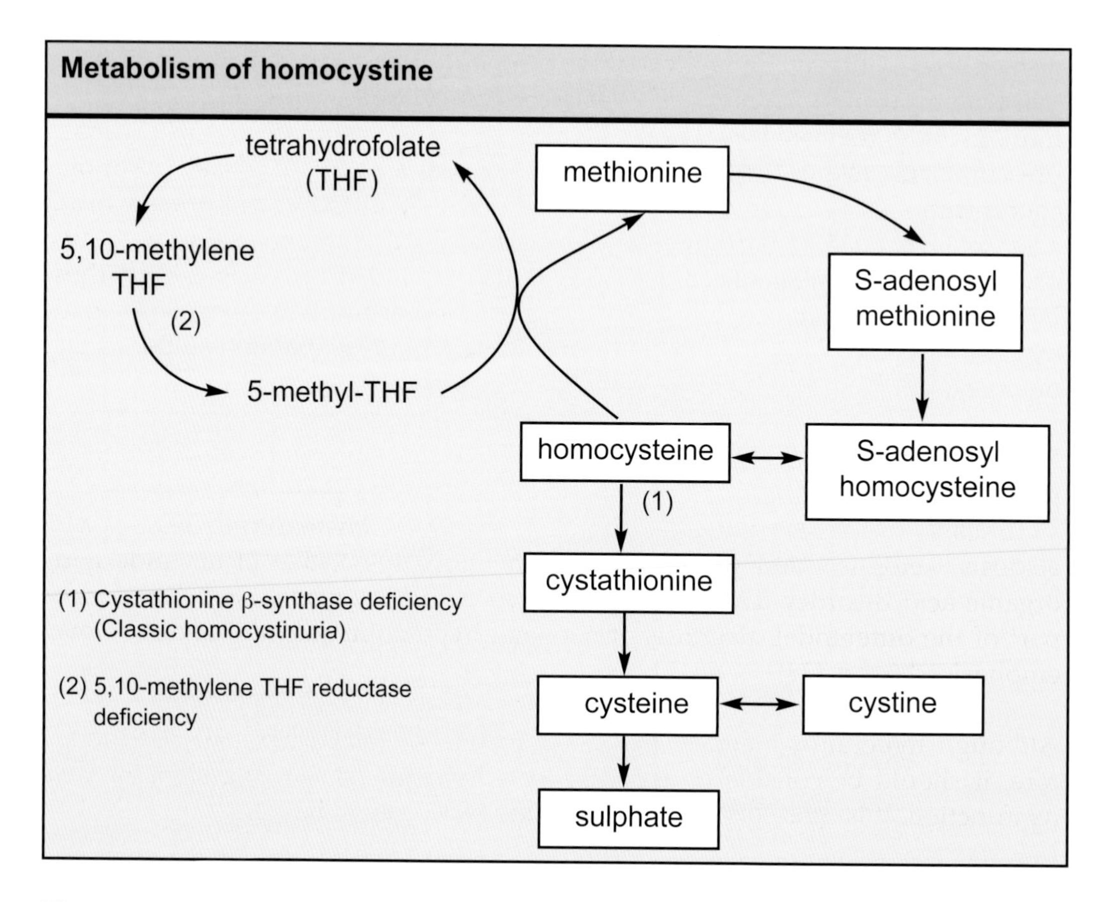

Figure 10.7 Metabolism of homocystine showing the defective enzymes in homocystinuria

Diagnosis of the variant form requires measurement of homocystine in plasma and urine. Free or total homocystine can be measured in plasma; plasma must be deproteinised promptly for the measurement of free homocystine. Total homocystine measurement has the advantage of simpler sample preparation without deproteinisation. The finding of a low or low-normal plasma methionine concentration, and the presence of homocystine in urine and plasma, is consistent with this defect. The diagnosis can be confirmed by demonstrating the enzyme defect in cultured skin fibroblasts. Prognosis can be improved by betaine therapy, particularly if started early in the neonatal period.

HYPERAMMONAEMIA

Causes of hyperammonaemia in neonates (Figure 10.8)

The commonest cause of a raised plasma ammonia concentration is contamination or deterioration of a specimen. Great care must be taken in sample collection, transport and analysis. In addition to the inherited disorders, there is a condition termed 'transient hyperammonaemia of the newborn', which can present as an overwhelming life-threatening illness in the first 48 hours of life. This condition is more likely to occur in the preterm baby (< 36 weeks gestation) and then usually presents with respiratory distress within 24 hours of birth. Plasma ammonia concentration is very high, usually in excess of 1500 µmol/L, and urinary orotic acid concentration is normal. The outcome is good if the condition is treated promptly and aggressively. Presentation may be indistinguishable from those IMDs presenting with hyperammonaemia, and a presumptive diagnosis is made by exclusion after careful assessment of plasma and urinary amino acids, urinary organic acids and orotic acid.

In addition to the urea cycle disorders (UCDs), some organic acid disorders, in particular methylmalonic and propionic acidaemias, can present in neonates with significant hyperammonaemia (400-800 µmol/L). Hyperammonaemia with acidosis, ketonuria and glycinuria is particularly suggestive of an underlying organic acid disorder. The importance of considering organic acid disorders as part of the differential diagnosis of neonatal hyperammonaemia cannot be over emphasised (*see p.174*).

Although hyperammonaemia as a complication of total parenteral nutrition is rare, it should be considered if the baby is lethargic or showing signs of CNS dysfunction. It is more likely to occur in low birth weight babies.

Causes of hyperammonaemia in neonates
Specimen contamination - poor specimen quality - difficult venepuncture - skin contamination - contaminated tube - delay in analysis
Sick baby - asphyxia, infection
Liver disease
Parenteral nutrition
Drugs affecting mitochondrial functioning, e.g. valproate
Inherited defects of the urea cycle
Inherited organic acid disorders
Transient hyperammonaemia of the newborn
3H syndrome (hyperammonaemia, hyperornithinaemia with homocitrullinuria)
Lysinuric protein intolerance
Hyperinsulinism (glutamate dehydrogenase deficiency)

Figure 10.8 Causes of hyperammonaemia in neonates

It is important to note that sick preterm neonates, in the absence of an inherited metabolic disorder, may have moderate elevation of plasma ammonia concentrations (up to 200 μmol/L), particularly if there is infection or hypoxia.

Urea cycle disorders

There are six inherited disorders of the urea cycle (Figure 10.9). With the exception of argininaemia, these disorders can present in a neonate with hyperammonaemia. The most common is ornithine carbamoyl transferase (OCT) deficiency, which has a prevalence of approximately 1 in 40,000. Plasma ammonia concentrations in excess of 800 μmol/L in the first 1-3 days of life are characteristic of the severe forms of UCD, although the ammonia concentration is dependent on protein intake and catabolic state, and may be much lower than this if full milk feeding has not commenced or has been reduced or withdrawn.

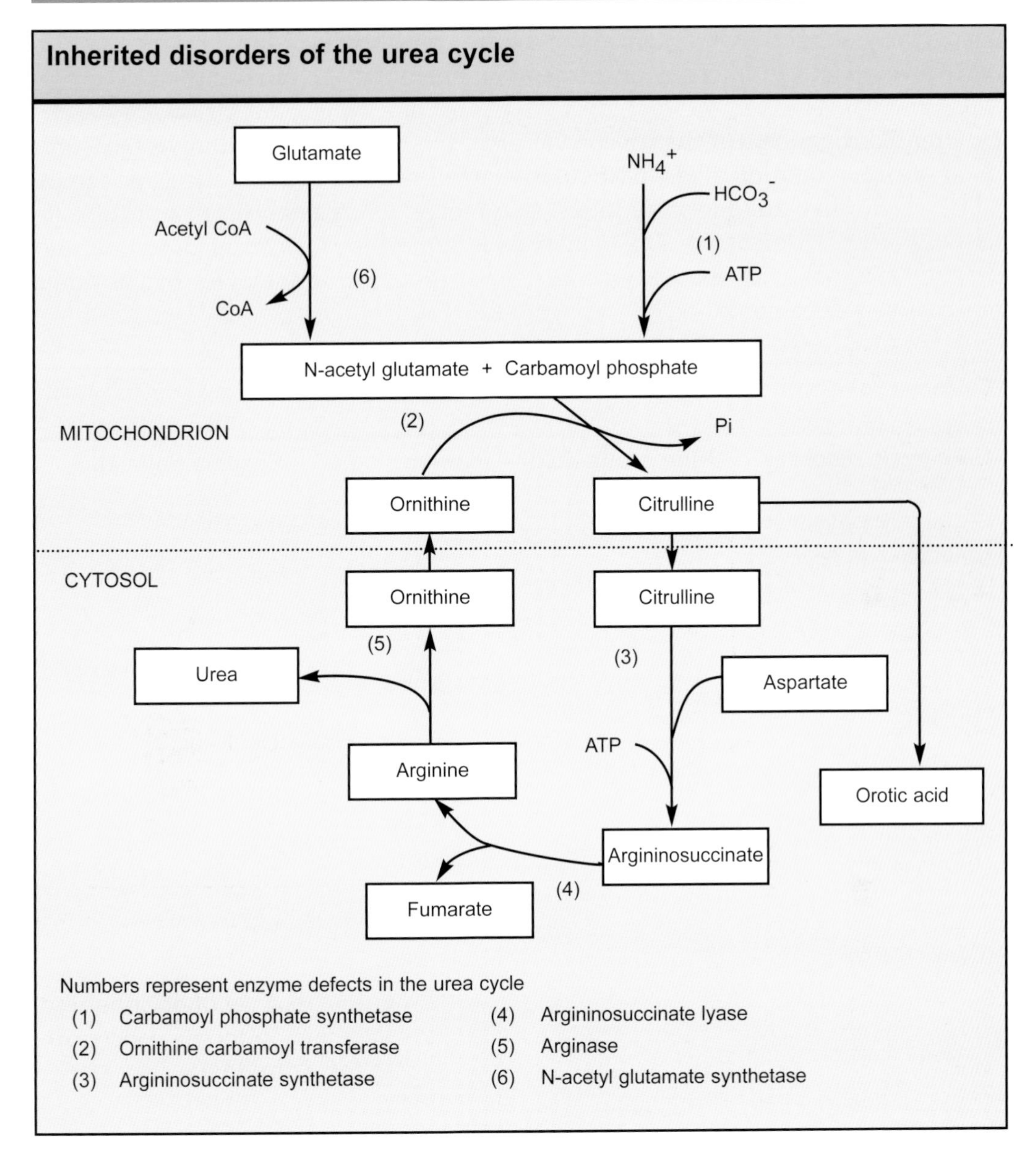

Figure 10.9 Inherited disorders of the urea cycle

Although babies with these conditions are well at birth, onset is usually very early (i.e. within 48 hours of birth), with a rapidly progressive encephalopathy. Initial features include lethargy, refusal of feeds, vomiting, irritability, seizures and tachypnoea. Ammonia is a respiratory stimulant, and the presence of a respiratory alkalosis is an important diagnostic clue. Like many other IMDs, the conditions may be misdiagnosed as sepsis. A family history of male neonatal deaths particularly suggests OCT deficiency, as the condition is X-linked. Liver failure may develop and pulmonary or intracranial haemorrhage can occur.

Differential diagnosis of the urea cycle disorders requires quantitative measurement of plasma amino acids, particularly citrulline, and urine orotic acid (Figure 10.10). Definitive diagnosis requires enzyme or DNA analysis in appropriate tissue. For OCT deficiency, DNA analysis is important for carrier detection and prenatal diagnosis, as the enzyme is not expressed in amniocytes or chorionic villus biopsy specimens.

Differential diagnosis of the urea cycle disorders

Urea cycle disorder	Urine orotic acid	Plasma	Enzyme deficiency
Carbamoyl phosphate synthetase deficiency	N	↑ glutamic acid/ glutamine ↑ alanine ↓ citrulline ↓ arginine	Liver
Ornithine carbamoyl transferase deficiency	↑	↑ glutamic acid/ glutamine ↑ alanine ↓ citrulline ↓ arginine	Liver
Citrullinaemia	↑	↑ citrulline ↓ arginine	Liver Fibroblasts
Argininosuccinic aciduria	↑	↑ argininosuccinate ↑ citrulline ↓ arginine	Liver Fibroblasts Erythrocytes
Argininaemia	↑	↑ arginine	Liver Erythrocytes
N-acetyl glutamate synthetase deficiency	N	↑ glutamine ↑ alanine	Liver

Figure 10.10 Differential diagnosis of the urea cycle disorders

INVESTIGATION OF NEONATAL HYPERAMMONAEMIA

Hyperammonaemia is not in itself a diagnosis. A detailed clinical history should be ascertained (particularly details of family history) to establish the cause, and additional tests should be performed:

- tests for liver dysfunction: alanine aminotransferase, alkaline phosphatase, bilirubin (total and conjugated or direct), albumin, prothrombin time
- plasma amino acids
- urine amino acids
- urine organic acids
- urine orotic acid
- plasma acyl carnitines.

TREATMENT OF HYPERAMMONAEMIA

Treatment is dictated by the plasma ammonia concentration. In severe OCT deficiency (and some other urea cycle disorders) ammonia concentrations can rise very rapidly to greater than 500 μmol/L. Hyperammonaemia (greater than 150 μmol/L) requires prompt and aggressive treatment to minimise the risks of permanent neurological handicap.

Until the results of investigations become available, dietary protein should be withdrawn or reduced while ensuring the provision of adequate calories from other sources. Treatment with sodium benzoate and/or sodium phenylbutyrate is useful in promoting excretion of nitrogen containing compounds. If the situation deteriorates, with worsening of the clinical state and/or rising ammonia concentrations or grossly elevated concentrations (> 500 μmol/L) that fail to fall significantly, aggressive therapy such as filtration or dialysis should be considered. The method of choice is continuous veno-venous haemofiltration or haemodiafiltration. Acute haemodialysis is also effective, but the benefit may be short lived. Peritoneal dialysis is less effective but can be used if haemodialysis is not immediately available. Even with early treatment, some patients with the severest types of UCD have a poor outcome, and discussion with the family about the pros and cons of embarking on aggressive treatment is required. These patients require long-term treatment. Prenatal diagnosis options may be particularly important.

The basis of long-term treatment of the UCD is dietary protein restriction (0.8-1.5 g/kg/24h). Sodium benzoate and/or sodium phenylbutyrate therapy may also be necessary to keep plasma ammonia concentrations down to an acceptable level (< 80 μmol/L). Benzoate conjugates with glycine to form hippurate, which is excreted and thereby diverts nitrogen away from the urea cycle. Sodium phenylbutyrate (or sodium phenylacetate) is converted to phenylacetylglutamine and excreted, thereby removing two nitrogen atoms. In severe cases, both benzoate and phenylbutyrate can be given. Benzoic acid may be hepatotoxic and, theoretically, could displace bilirubin from albumin: its use, therefore, may be a particular risk in a jaundiced neonate. With the exception of argininaemia, arginine becomes an essential amino acid in patients with a UCD and supplements are required. Treatment regimens require regular monitoring of plasma ammonia concentration and relevant amino acids (quantitative). The outcome with treatment depends on the individual disorder, the severity of the defect and compliance with the treatment regimen. For many, outcome is poor. For those patients who survive the initial hyperammonaemia, liver transplantation is an option.

ORGANIC ACID DISORDERS

Defects of branched chain amino acid and propionyl CoA catabolism

Organic acids are carboxylic acids of low molecular weight and are metabolites of amino acids, carbohydrates and fats. Organic acid disorders can affect several intermediary metabolic pathways, in particular the catabolism of the branched chain amino acids, leucine, isoleucine and valine (Figure 10.5), and of propionyl CoA (Figure 10.11). The intermediates that accumulate in these disorders, with the exception of MSUD, do not react with ninhydrin and cannot be diagnosed by amino acid analysis. Specific methods for organic acids using gas chromatography-mass spectrometry are essential. Over 50 disorders caused by a primary biochemical defect of organic acid metabolism have been described and their combined incidence is probably at least as great as that of the amino acid disorders.

Presentation in the neonatal period is usually as a severe metabolic acidosis with lethargy, vomiting and hypotonia. There are often other metabolic abnormalities associated with the acidosis, for example:

- hypoglycaemia
- hyperammonaemia
- hypocalcaemia
- ketonuria
- hyperlactataemia
- hyperuricaemia
- neutropenia
- increased plasma and urine glycine.

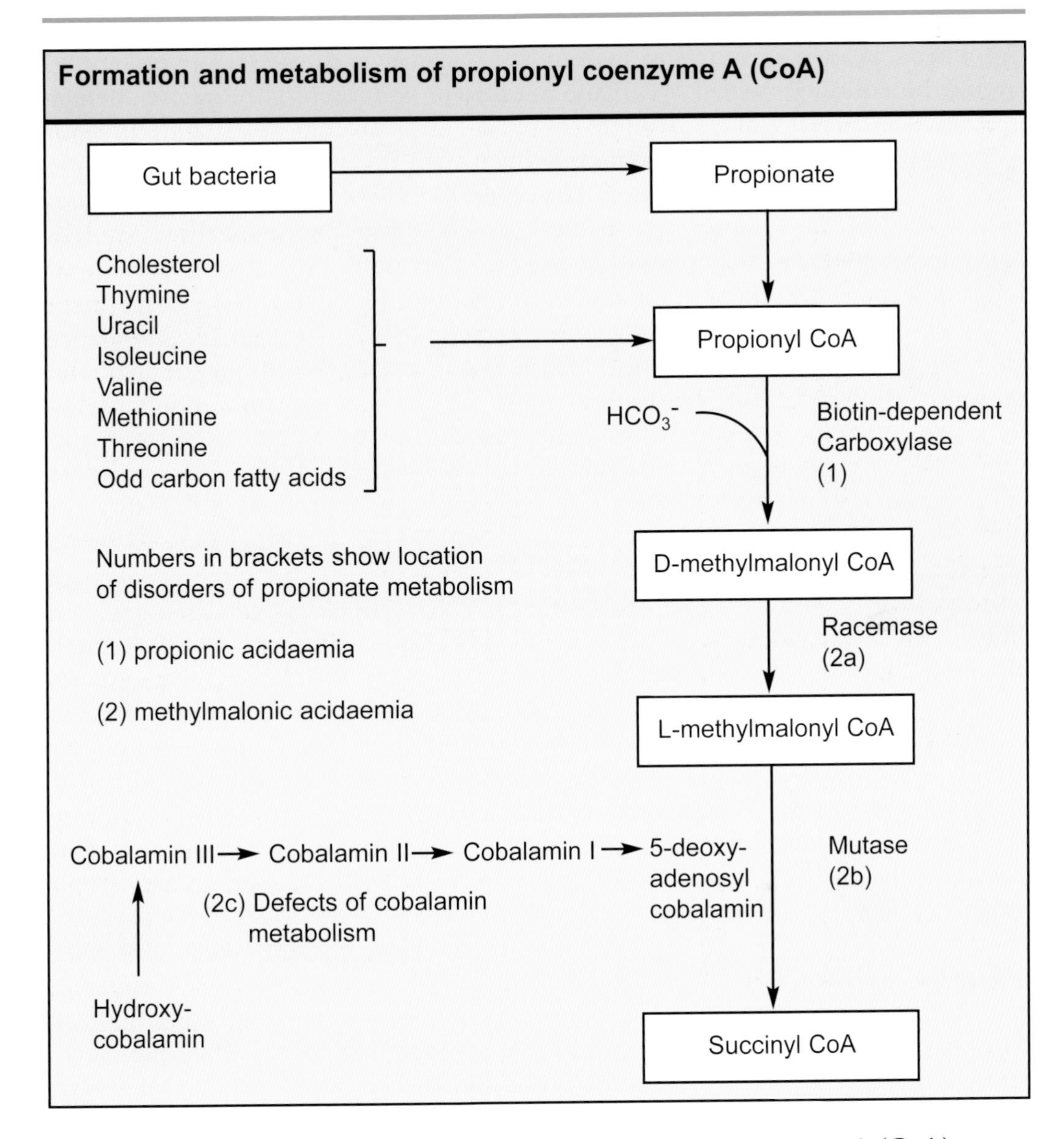

Figure 10.11 Formation and metabolism of propionyl coenzyme A (CoA)

While awaiting results of investigations, dietary protein should be withdrawn. Diagnosis of these disorders requires detailed investigations of organic acids and their metabolites. The accumulated organic acids exist as conjugates with carnitine, e.g. propionylcarnitine, and can be detected by tandem mass spectrometry. Measurement of carnitine species in blood spots or plasma is now the method of choice for rapid diagnosis. Urinary organic acid analysis by gas chromatography with mass spectrometry may also be required if the results of acyl carnitine measurements are equivocal.

Specimens, i.e. blood spot and heparinised plasma, and a *fresh* random urine, should be collected whilst the baby is acidotic and preferably before dietary protein is withdrawn. Treatment is by dietary protein restriction (0.8-1.5 g/kg/day) sometimes in combination with an artificial amino acid mixture. Some units treat with a vitamin cocktail. However, the basis for this is unproven as, although there are vitamin-responsive forms of these disorders, these are less likely to be the types that present acutely in a neonate. With the availability of rapid diagnosis, the use of vitamin cocktails should not be necessary.

Unfortunately, despite treatment, patients who have presented in the neonatal period continue to have intermittent crises of ketoacidosis and, generally, the long-term outcome is poor. A few patients with methylmalonic acidaemia and propionic acidaemias have undergone liver transplantation. Patients who have survived have some improvement, although mortality associated with the procedure has been high.

DISORDERS OF FATTY ACID TRANSPORT AND OXIDATION

Mitochondrial β-oxidation of fatty acids plays a major role in energy production, especially during periods of fasting. It is a complex process that involves uptake of fatty acids into the cell, activation to the acyl CoA and then transport into the mitochondria, which requires the carnitine transport cycle (see Figures 10.12 and 10.13). Within the mitochondria, the β-oxidation spiral requires a series of enzymes with carbon chain length specificity. There is a range of inherited disorders caused by defects in the carnitine cycle and the β-oxidation process. The defects of the β-oxidation process differ on the basis of the fatty acid chain length which is affected. The commonest disorder described is the defect of the medium chain acyl CoA dehydrogenase (MCAD) system, affecting fatty acids of carbon length C6 to C10.

Clinical severity varies widely in fatty acid oxidation disorders. They can cause sudden infant death but may also be present in asymptomatic adults. Many can lead to cardiac arrest, collapse or sudden infant death. Some of the disorders are candidates for prenatal diagnosis. Despite increasing knowledge of these disorders, many patients remain undiagnosed owing to the need to collect blood and urine specimens at an appropriate time in relation to illness.

The disorders characteristically present with hypoglycaemia. *Any neonate or infant with unexplained hypoglycaemia should have blood and urine collected for metabolic investigations at the time of presentation* (*see Chapter 7*). The hypoglycaemia is characteristically associated with inappropriately low concentrations of plasma and urine ketones, and an abnormally high ratio of plasma free fatty acids:3-hydroxy-

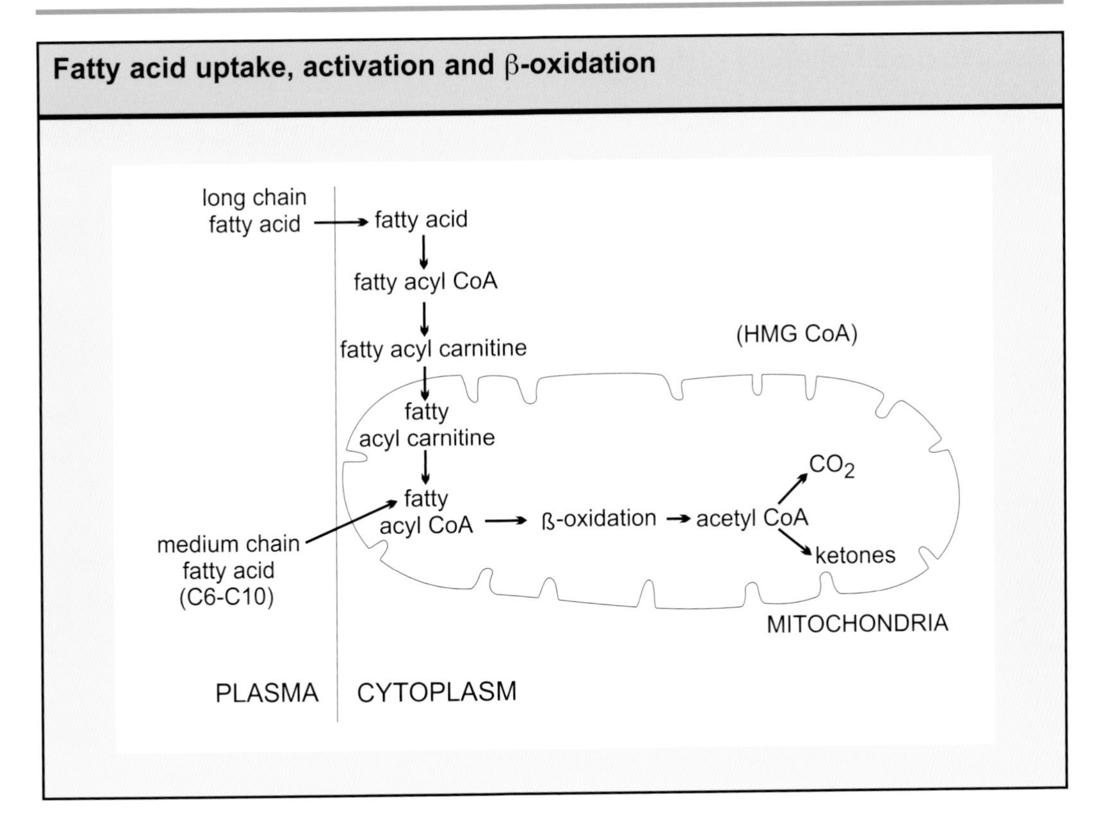

Figure 10.12 Fatty acid uptake, activation and β-oxidation

butyrate. During conditions of stress, e.g. fasting or catabolism, the fatty acid esters and corresponding dicarboxylic acids, e.g. sebacic, suberic and adipic acids accumulate (Figure 10.14).

The main features of presentation in the neonate are:

- malformations and facial dysmorphism
- cardiac
  - arrhythmias and conduction defects
  - cardiomyopathy
- neurological
  - lethargy, coma and hypotonia
- hypoketotic hypoglycaemia.

Metabolic acidosis may be a feature and hyperammonaemia is prominent in carnitine palmitoyl transferase II and translocase deficiencies.

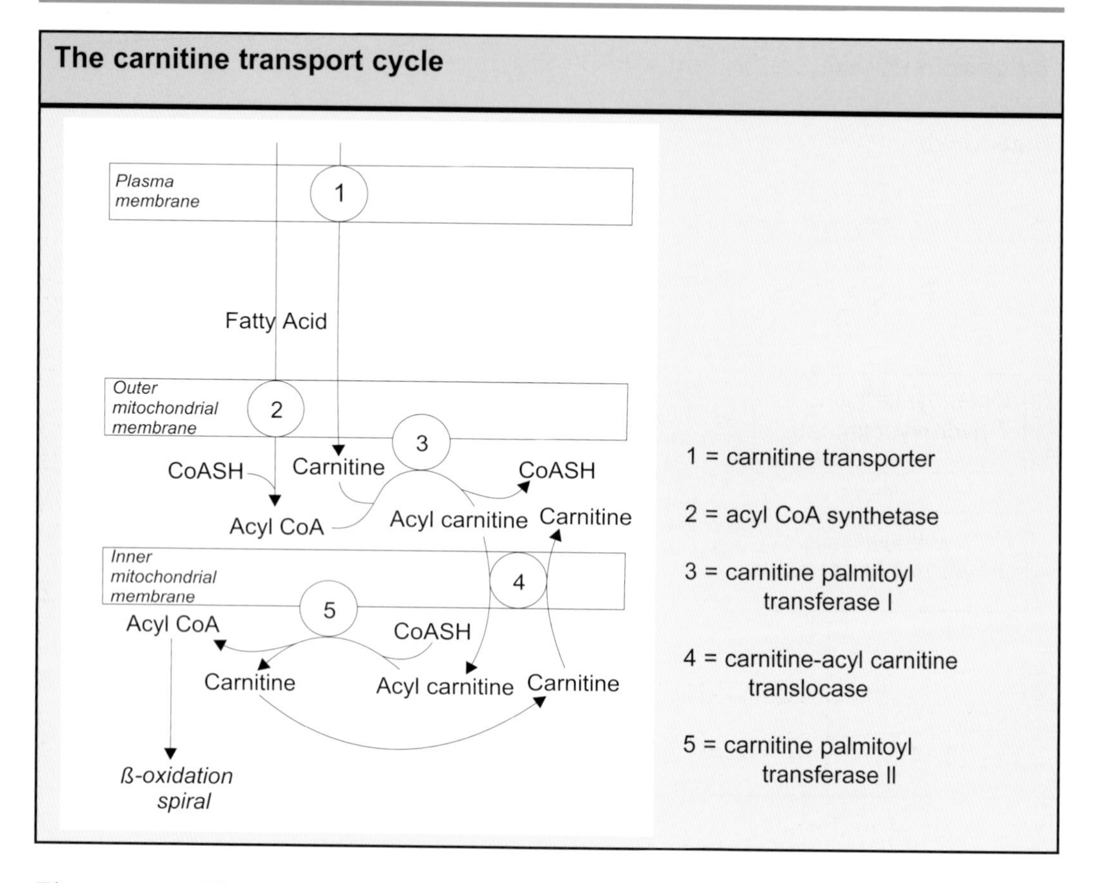

Figure 10.13 The carnitine transport cycle

Investigation is by analysis of acyl carnitine specimens in blood and organic acids in urine. It is important to investigate acyl carnitine species in plasma, as some defects may be less easy to diagnose from dried blood spots. For some disorders, e.g. MCAD, LCHAD, there are common mutations and specific DNA tests are available.

Diagnosis of these conditions can be very difficult, as the results of investigations may be completely normal when an affected infant is well, and abnormalities may only become evident when the infant is stressed by fasting. Undertaking a controlled (and extended) fast is potentially dangerous and should only be done if thorough investigation of acyl carnitines in plasma has revealed no clues to the diagnosis. It must only be undertaken under close medical supervision. It is particularly important to investigate newborn siblings of known patients by looking for characteristic metabolites in plasma (acyl carnitines) and urine (organic acids) that have been collected within the first 72 h of life, when the baby is stressed from the birth process.

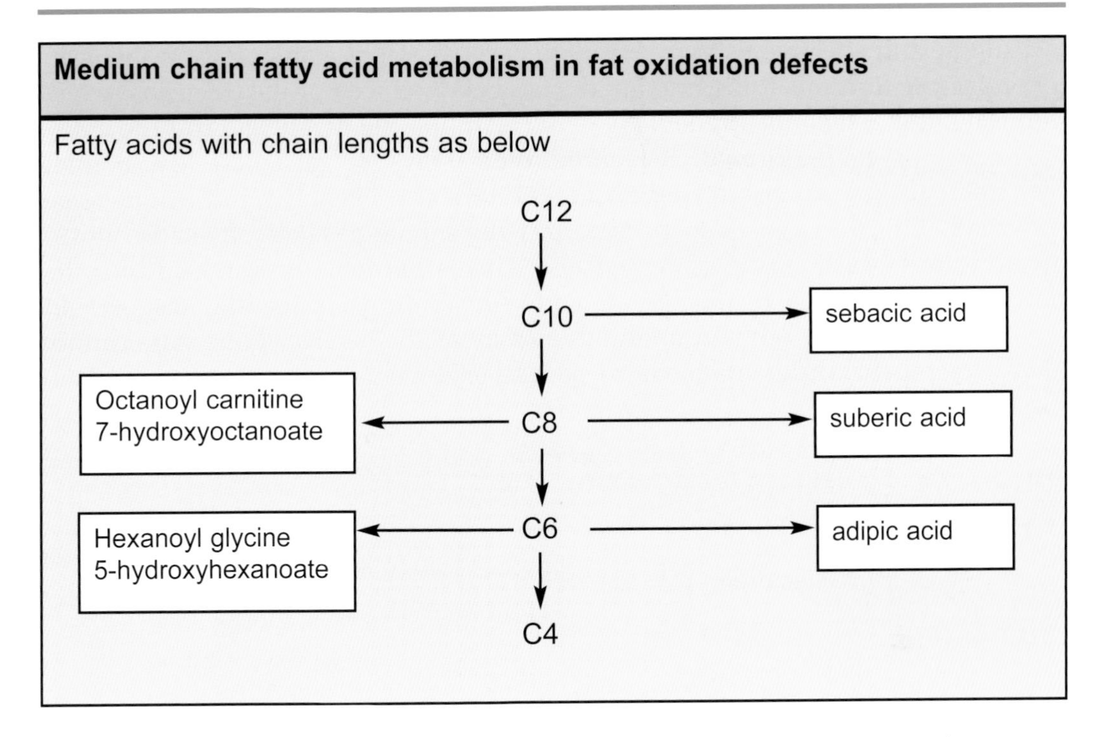

Figure 10.14 Medium chain fatty acid metabolism in fat oxidation defects

Syndromes of maternal illness during pregnancy, e.g. haemolysis, elevated liver enzymes and low platelets (HELLP) and acute fatty liver of pregnancy (AFLP), have been associated with a fetus being affected by some of these defects (in particular LCHAD).

CARBOHYDRATE DISORDERS

Galactosaemia

Classic galactosaemia, due to galactose 1-phosphate uridyl transferase deficiency (Figure 10.15), characteristically presents in the first week of life with failure to thrive, jaundice and hepatomegaly. The incidence in the UK is approximately 1 in 45,000. Some countries have neonatal screening programmes (*see p.146*). The severe illness is frequently associated with liver failure and septicaemia and, without treatment, death may ensue. In most of the UK and many other countries, there is no universal neonatal screening, and diagnosis relies on clinical acumen.

The diagnosis is supported by the finding of positive urinary reducing substances (Clinitest®), but the definitive test is measurement of galactose 1-phosphate uridyltransferase (gal 1-PUT) in erythrocytes. A negative test for urinary reducing substances, *provided that the baby is receiving lactose-containing milk formula,* is a simple and effective way of excluding classic galactosaemia. If the baby is on a non-lactose formula, if the milk intake has been reduced or the baby has severe vomiting, this test is not a reliable way of excluding the diagnosis, and the gal 1-PUT test must be performed. 'Screening' type assays for gal 1-PUT (e.g. Beutler test) are usually available in specialist laboratories and enable rapid results to be provided. If the diagnosis is suspected, the baby should be taken off lactose whilst awaiting the results of the screening test. This is particularly important for the newborn sibling of a confirmed patient. An abnormal screening test should always be confirmed with a quantitative assay as the heterozygous state cannot always be reliably differentiated; also, several enzyme variants (e.g. Duarte allele) exist.

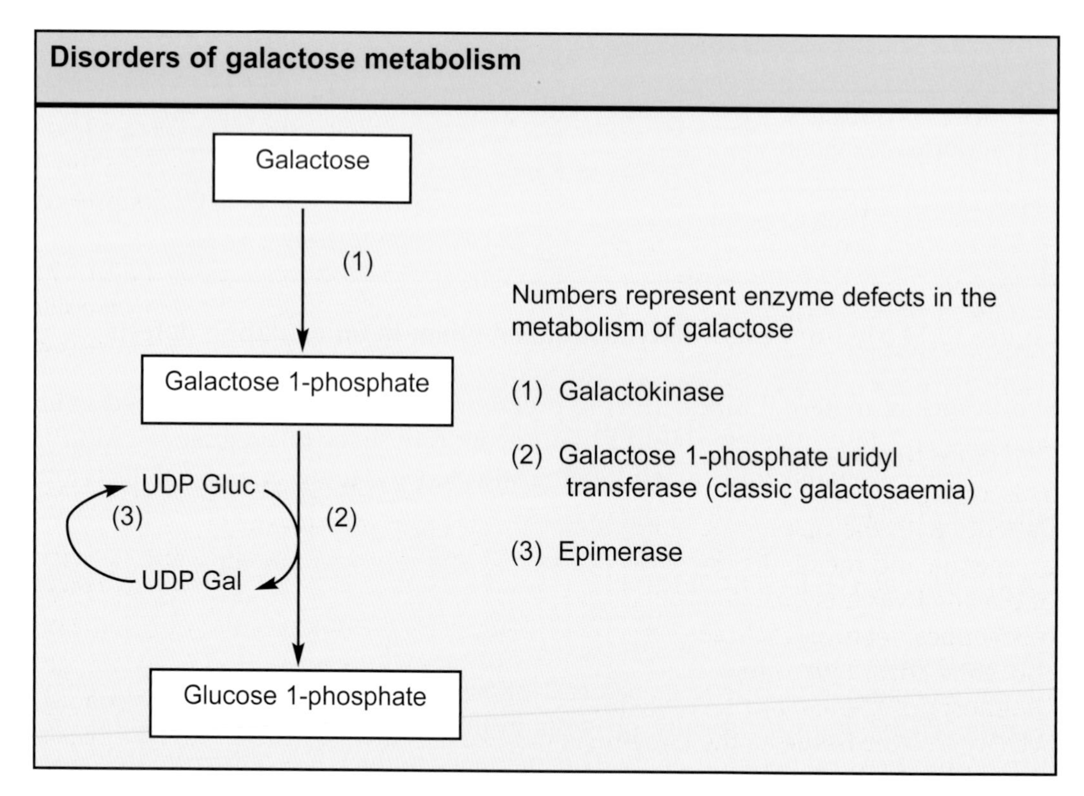

Figure 10.15 Disorders of galactose metabolism

Epimerase deficiency (Figure 10.15) has been described in a few cases and can present with a similar clinical picture to transferase deficiency; this deficiency should be considered if there is persistent galactosaemia and a normal gal 1-PUT. False positive Beutler screening tests can occur if the red cells are deficient in glucose 6-phosphate dehydrogenase. A high haemoglobin concentration can also interfere with the test, making interpretation of the results difficult and possibly giving rise to a false positive screening test. A false negative result may occur if the baby has recently had a blood transfusion and, therefore, the test is not valid if carried out within six weeks of a major transfusion. Persistent galactosuria in a baby must be taken seriously and a diagnosis pursued vigorously – the neonatologist and clinical biochemist should be aware of the possibility of a false negative screening result. If the baby has a classic galactosaemia picture with galactosuria, tyrosinaemia type I (*see p.166*) and hereditary fructose intolerance (*see p.182*) should be considered as part of the differential diagnosis.

Untreated babies with galactosaemia are susceptible to *E.coli* sepsis and galactosaemia should be considered when jaundice, hepatomegaly and sepsis occur in a neonate.

Patients with galactosaemia must have life-long treatment with a galactose-free diet. Recovery from the acute, life-threatening stage is usually rapid and complete. Dietary compliance should be monitored by measurement of erythrocyte galactose 1-phosphate. In spite of early and good compliance, the long-term outcome for some patients with treated galactosaemia is not good with some degree of neurological impairment and a high percentage of ovarian failure in females. Cognitive outcome appears to relate to genotype rather than metabolic control. Homozygosity for the Q188R mutation is invariably associated with a relatively poor outcome.

Glycogen storage disease (GSD) type I

This is a group of disorders caused by a deficiency of glucose 6-phosphatase. Patients with the disease can present within the first few days of life with hypoglycaemia and metabolic (lactic) acidosis. The liver may be enlarged and activity of plasma liver enzymes increased. Neutropenia is a feature of some types. Other biochemical features include increased plasma triglycerides, cholesterol and urate concentrations. Liver biopsy shows excess glycogen and associated fatty change. Diagnosis of the classic form requires measurement of glucose 6-phosphatase activity in liver tissue as the enzyme is not expressed in cultured skin fibroblasts or red blood cells. Further tests may be required to differentiate between the subtypes of GSD type I (A and non-A). Tolerance tests (e.g. using glucagon, galactose, glucose) are not appropriate in the young baby or infant and it is far better to proceed directly to histological investigation and specific enzyme measurements.

In some cases, the presentation is not so acute, and cases have been described where a baby has had unexplained hypoglycaemic episodes soon after birth, from which there was apparent full recovery until presentation several months later with unexplained hepatomegaly. Such cases stress the importance of adequately investigating hypoglycaemia (*see p.117*).

The main feature of GSD type I is repeated episodes of hypoglycaemia with elevated blood lactate. Treatment is aimed at preventing or minimising hypoglycaemia, and some patients manage with frequent feeds of a carbohydrate-rich diet. For others, continuous tube feeding is required. The use of corn starch as a carbohydrate source has improved management and, as the child gets older, the frequency of attacks usually declines. In the long term, impairment of renal and liver function can occur and follow up with relevant biochemical and clinical monitoring is required.

DISORDERS OF FRUCTOSE METABOLISM

Hereditary fructose intolerance (HFI) only presents after exposure to fructose (or sucrose) and is, therefore, very rare in neonates. The presentation is very similar to that of galactosaemia, and removal of the dietary sugar results in rapid clinical and biochemical improvement. Biochemical features include hypophosphataemia, hypoglycaemia and increased plasma lactate concentration. The diagnosis may be suspected from detailed nutritional history, clinical picture, the finding of a positive test for urinary reducing substances and amino aciduria.

Measurement of the enzyme fructose 1,6-bisphosphate aldolase activity in liver tissue is required for definitive diagnosis. Fructose tolerance tests, either oral or i.v, are not recommended in neonates or young infants. One specific mutation (A149P) is relatively common in north-western Europeans and may therefore provide a useful approach to diagnosis.

Fructose 1,6-bisphosphatase deficiency is less common. In contrast to HFI, dietary ingestion of fructose is not a prerequisite for clinical presentation. Presentation in the neonate is usually acute, within the first few days of life, as a life-threatening illness comprising hypoglycaemia, metabolic (lactic) acidosis, convulsions and hepatomegaly. Diagnosis requires measurement of the enzyme in leucocytes or liver.

LACTIC ACIDOSIS

There are several non-specific causes of lactic acidosis (Figure 10.16), the commonest being hypoxia/ischaemia. When considering metabolic causes of lactic acidosis, it is therefore important to ensure that the baby is well perfused and has an adequate blood volume and blood pressure. Poor peripheral circulation will occur following intraventricular haemorrhage and in the hypoplastic left heart syndrome. Concentrations of plasma lactate greater than 10 mmol/L can occur during hypoxia and excessive muscular activity, and concentrations may be even higher (up to 20 mmol/L) if there is severe respiratory failure. Lactate is usually measured in venous blood, although concentrations in free flowing capillary blood correlate well with venous blood measurement. Blood for lactate measurement is stable for at least three hours at room temperature if taken into fluoride-oxalate preservative; it is less stable in heparin.

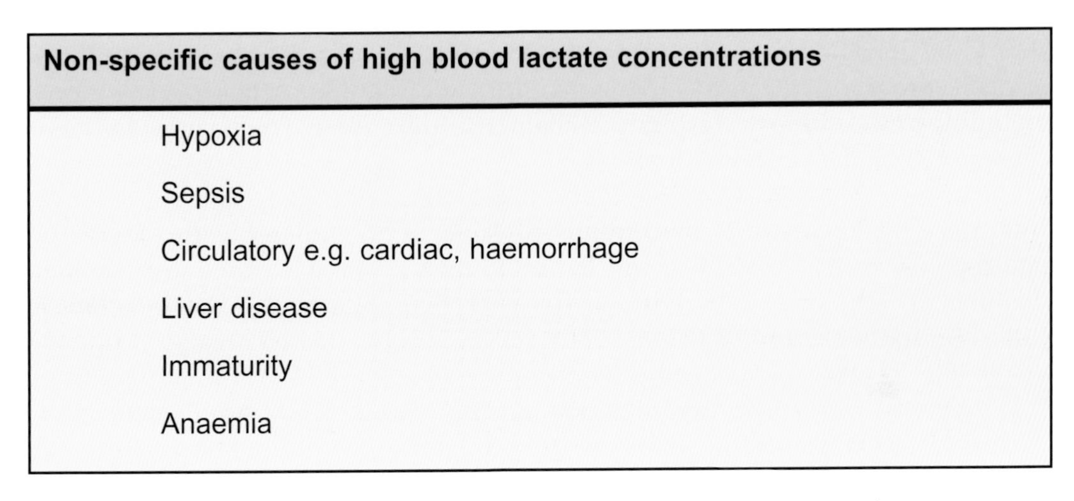

Non-specific causes of high blood lactate concentrations

Hypoxia

Sepsis

Circulatory e.g. cardiac, haemorrhage

Liver disease

Immaturity

Anaemia

Figure 10.16 Non-specific causes of high blood lactate concentrations

A moderately increased blood lactate concentration (2-4 mmol/L) may occur in infection or dehydration, or if there is liver dysfunction. Fitting can cause a significant increase in lactate in any infant, presumably as a result of hypoxia and excessive muscular activity.

If non-specific causes can be excluded, a persistently and significantly elevated lactate (i.e. $>$ 3 mmol/L) requires further investigation for the possibility of an IMD. This is particularly likely if associated with hypoglycaemia and/or hyperammonaemia. Differential diagnoses include:

- glycogen storage disorder type I
- organic acid disorders
- fatty acid oxidation defects
- disorders of pyruvate metabolism (pyruvate dehydrogenase deficiency)
- disorders of gluconeogenesis (phosphoenolpyruvate carboxykinase, pyruvate carboxylase, fructose 1,6-bisphosphatase deficiencies)
- electron transport chain defects/mitochondrial disorders.

Further tests will be directed by clinical history and should include consideration of blood spot or plasma acyl carnitines, urinary organic acids, plasma urate, plasma creatine kinase, plasma and urine amino acids, fasting blood glucose, plasma 3-hydroxybutyrate and free fatty acids, and liver enzymes. The results of these tests may be useful in establishing the significance of a mild or intermittent lactic acidosis and in guiding further investigations. It is important to measure CSF lactate if neurological features are present. Respiratory chain disorders should be considered in the differential diagnosis of a sick neonate with lactic acidosis, especially if there is hypotonia; this will require further investigations, including muscle biopsy. Respiratory chain disorders are one of the most frequent causes of neonatal cardiomyopathies.

Infants with Pearson's syndrome present with sideroblastic anaemia, neutropenia, watery diarrhoea and failure to thrive. There is exocrine pancreatic dysfunction and impaired redox status, which manifests as a lactic acidosis. Mitochondrial deletions or duplications are present in affected organs.

Investigations for urinary organic acids may not show an increased lactate if the plasma lactate concentration does not exceed 7 mmol/L. Normal urinary organic acids, therefore, do not preclude the possibility of a significantly increased plasma lactate.

PEROXISOMAL DISORDERS

Peroxisomes are subcellular organelles containing many enzyme systems. Their functions include the biosynthesis of plasmalogens (essential neuronal lipid compounds), catalase activity, oxidation of very long, long and medium chain fatty acids and phytanic acid, and metabolism of pipecolic acid (a metabolite of lysine oxidation). Several inherited metabolic disorders have been described that are caused by single or multiple defects in peroxisomal function.

The classic disorder of this group is Zellweger's syndrome. The major clinical features of this condition are dysmorphism, hypotonia, liver dysfunction, hepatomegaly and developmental delay. Presentation is at birth or shortly afterwards, often with seizures and severe hypotonia. The radiographic finding of calcific stippling of the epiphyses is an important clue. There are no simple biochemical tests for this condition; diagnosis requires measurement of plasma very long chain fatty acids (VLCFA).

PURINE AND PYRIMIDINE DISORDERS

Purine and pyrimidines are present in intracellular nucleotides involved in energy metabolism, e.g. ATP and GTP; nucleotides are the basic components of

DNA and RNA. Several inherited metabolic disorders of purine and pyrimidine metabolism have been described, affecting the functioning of the CNS, kidneys and immune system and having, therefore, a wide range of clinical presentations. The most severe disorder presenting in the neonatal period is xanthine oxidase/sulphite oxidase deficiency (molybdenum cofactor deficiency). Over 100 patients have been reported in a wide range of ethnic groups. The disorder presents with intractable seizures and can be suspected by the finding of a low plasma urate concentration and low urinary urate:creatinine ratio. In Lesch-Nyhan syndrome, plasma and urine urate concentrations are characteristically high; presentation in neonates is rare but may be suggested by the finding of an orange/red 'sand' in the nappy and/or haematuria. In a few instances, hypotonia has been recognised shortly after birth. Adenosine deaminase deficiency, associated with severe combined immune deficiency (SCID), manifests at birth with diarrhoea, failure to thrive and candidiasis.

LYSOSOMAL STORAGE DISORDERS

Lysosomes are subcellular oganelles that contain many enzymes required for the catabolism of large glycolipid molecules. Enzyme deficiencies result in storage of partly degraded, large, complex molecules, which subsequently damage tissues. Lysosomal disorders do not usually present in neonates, with the exception of those disorders that can present as hydrops (*see Appendix D*), or with dysmorphic features (Figure 10.17), cardiomyopathy (Pompe's disease) or cholestatic liver disease (Niemann-Pick type C). Hydrops is the most frequent neonatal presentation of lysosomal disorders.

DISORDERS OF CHOLESTEROL METABOLISM

Smith-Lemli-Opitz syndrome

Smith-Lemli-Opitz (SLO) syndrome is an inborn error of cholesterol metabolism caused by deficiency of 7-dehydrocholesterol reductase. It is relatively common, with estimates of incidence ranging from 1 in 20,000 to 1 in 40,000. In the severe form of SLO syndrome, patients have a distinctive facial appearance, with congenital microcephaly and ptosis. There are usually feeding problems and hypotonia. Other features may include syndactyly, and hypospadias and cryptorchidism in males. Some patients present with a severe, lethal form in the newborn period, from complications of visceral malformations. Biochemical diagnosis requires measurement of plasma 7-dehydrocholesterol. Cholesterol concentrations may be low or normal, but the ratio of 7-dehydrocholesterol:cholesterol is high. Dietary management with cholesterol replacement therapy has been used with reported benefits of improved behaviour and better growth in some patients.

Metabolic disorders with dysmorphic features

	Dysmorphic features	Other features	Specific investigation(s)
Maternal PKU	Microcephaly	Congenital heart disease	Plasma phenylalanine in the mother
Congenital lactic acidosis (pyruvate dehydrogenase deficiency)	Abnormal facies Microcephaly	Acidosis Hypotonia Seizures Abnormal brain (absence of corpus callosum)	Blood (& CSF) lactate Fibroblast studies Pyruvate oxidation DNA analysis
Zellweger's syndrome and related disorders	High forehead Shallow supra-orbital ridges Epicanthic folds Abnormal ear helices High arched palate Micrognathia Large fontanelle	Hypotonia Hepatomegaly Seizures Calcific stippling of epiphyses	Red cell membrane plasmalogens Platelet and fibroblast dihydroxyacetone phosphate acyl transferase Plasma C26:C24 fatty acid ratio
Glutaric aciduria type II (multiple acyl CoA dehydrogenase deficiency)	Macrocephaly Abnormal facies	Hypotonia Hypoglycaemia Polycystic kidneys	Urine organic acids Lymphocyte/fibroblast fatty acid oxidation Plasma acyl carnitines
Sulphite/xanthine oxidase deficiency (molybdenum cofactor deficiency)	Abnormal facies	Seizures Hypotonia	Urine sulphite Plasma urate Urine urate:creatinine ratio
Congenital adrenal hyperplasia	Ambiguous genitalia in females	Salt loss Recurrent vomiting Dehydration Hyponatraemia	Plasma 17-hydroxy-progesterone
Congenital hypothyroidism	Coarse facies	Jaundice	Plasma TSH and free T4
G_{M2} gangliosidosis	Frontal bossing Depressed nasal bridge Low set ears	Feeding difficulties Hypoactive Hypotonia Oedema	Urinary GAGs Leucocyte/fibroblast β-galactosidase
Mucolipidosis 2 (I cell disease)	Coarse facies Depressed nasal bridge Large tongue	Restricted joint movement Radiological changes	Plasma arylsulphatase A (I cell screen)

continued...

Metabolic disorders with dysmorphic features (cont.)

	Dysmorphic features	Other features	Specific investigation(s)
Mucolipidosis I (Sialidosis)	Coarse facies Depressed nasal bridge	Radiological changes Cherry red spot Myoclonus	Leucocyte/fibroblast neuraminidase Urine oligosaccharides
Mucopolysaccarid-osis VII (Sly's disease)	Coarse facies Depressed nasal bridge Large tongue	Hydrops fetalis Hepatomegaly	Leucocyte/fibroblast β-glucuronidase
Multiple sulphatase deficiency (Austin's variant)	Coarse facies Depressed nasal bridge Large tongue	Icthyosis Hepatomegaly Radiological changes	Leucocyte/fibroblast sulphatase (e.g. arylsulphatase A) Urine GAGs
Menke's disease	Abnormal facies	Hypothermia Fine hair Trichorrhexis nodosa Seizures	Plasma copper and caeruloplasmin
Carbohydrate deficient glyco-protein syndromes	Coarse facies Dysmorphism	Multisystem	Plasma transferrin isoforms
Cholesterol synthesis defects, e.g. Smith-Lemli-Opitz	Microcephaly Facial dysmorphism Syndactyly	Hypotonia	Plasma cholesterol Plasma 7-dehydrocholesterol Plasma steroids
Mevalonate kinase deficiency	Abnormal facies	Hepatospleno-megaly Anaemia Recurrent infections	Urine organic acids

GAGs = glycosaminoglycans

Figure 10.17 Some metabolic disorders that may present with dysmorphic features in the neonate

CARBOHYDRATE DEFICIENT GLYCOPROTEIN (CDG) SYNDROMES

These are a family of genetic disorders, with many sub-types, characterised by defective glycosylation of glycoproteins and other glycoconjugates.

The commonest type (type 1A) is caused by phosphomannomutase deficiency, and is a multisystem disease, presenting in neonates with dysmorphism, CNS dysfunction and involvement of several different organs, e.g. liver failure, pericardial effusion and nephrotic syndrome. Biochemical diagnosis requires the demonstration of a characteristically abnormal transferrin isoform pattern in plasma (though abnormal glycosylation may occur as a secondary phenomenon in other conditions, e.g. galactosaemia). Secondary abnormalities of several other plasma glycoproteins (e.g. coagulation factors and hormone-binding glycoproteins) can occur in type 1A CDG syndrome. The enzyme defect can be demonstrated in fibroblasts; many different mutations have been identified.

Patients with type 1B (caused by a defect in the microsomal glucose 6-phosphate transporter system) usually manifest with a gastroenterological presentation. No effective treatment is available for type 1A CDG syndrome; for type 1B, treatment with mannose may be effective.

THE DYSMORPHIC BABY AND INHERITED METABOLIC DISORDERS

Dysmorphic features in a newborn baby usually suggest an intrauterine insult, e.g. infection, drug exposure, chromosome abnormality, or a genetic syndrome without a known biochemical cause. In some cases, however, the malformation or dysmorphism can be associated with a biochemical disorder (Figure 10.17).

A neonate with dysmorphic features should have a careful and detailed examination to assess CNS function, and a sample should be taken for chromosome analysis. Neurological and/or radiological abnormalities may suggest particular biochemical defects and the need for more specific investigations. It is likely that an increasing number of syndromes will be found to have a biochemical basis and clinicians need to be aware of these possibilities and investigate accordingly.

NEONATAL SEIZURES AND INHERITED METABOLIC DISORDERS

There are numerous causes of seizures in neonates (Figure 10.18). Seizures are a feature of several inherited metabolic disorders (Figure 10.19). Clues that seizures may be metabolic in origin include:

- peculiar odour
- intractable seizures occurring after the first 72 hours
- normal prenatal and delivery history
- emergence of food intolerance
- increasing lethargy.

Neonatal seizures: non-metabolic causes
Hypoxic-ischaemic encephalopathy
Cerebrovascular accident/arterial or venous infarction
Intraparenchymal cerebral haemorrhage
Subdural haemorrhage
Subarachnoid haemorrhage
Infective encephalitis, e.g. Herpes
Meningitis, e.g. *E.coli* or Group B streptococcus
Congenital CNS malformations, e.g. lissencephaly, microgyria
Hydrocephalus (any cause)

Figure 10.18 Neonatal seizures: non-metabolic causes

Neonatal seizures: metabolic causes
Hypoglycaemia
Hypocalcaemia
Non-ketotic hyperglycinaemia
Urea cycle defects
Homocystinuria (remethylation defects)
Zellweger's syndrome
Molybdenum cofactor deficiency
Pyridoxine responsive seizures
Glucose transporter I deficiency
Familial neonatal seizures

Figure 10.19 Neonatal seizures: metabolic causes

Seizures may be the presenting feature in a primary disorder of the glucose transporter (GLUT) found primarily in the CNS, and responsible for glucose transfer across the blood brain barrier. Glucose transporter 1 deficiency usually presents in early infancy with seizures and developmental delay, and patients become progressively microcephalic. The characteristic abnormalities are a low concentration of glucose in CSF and a reduced CSF/blood glucose ratio. Seizures respond well to the institution of a ketogenic diet.

Benign familial neonatal convulsions is a dominant epilepsy syndrome presenting in the first week of life. The seizures usually remit within the first six months of life, although 10% of patients have seizures when older. It is caused by a mutation in one of the potassium channel genes.

Some neonatal seizures, which may start *in utero*, and are resistant to conventional anticonvulsants, are responsive to pyridoxine.

PREGNANCY AND INHERITED METABOLIC DISORDERS

It is now well established that there are complications associated with pregnancy in women with certain metabolic disorders. These may manifest as risks to the mother, detrimental effects on the fetus, or both. The best example of such a condition is phenylketonuria. If the mother is untreated there is a high incidence of spontaneous abortion, as well as the specific effects on the fetus of congenital heart disease and microcephaly (*see p.138*). It is now understood that there is a need for strict biochemical control at the time of conception and throughout pregnancy to ensure a good outcome. Although universal newborn screening programmes have been established since the early 1970s, there are still women with phenylketonuria/hyperphenylalaninaemia who are now of child bearing age who have either never been diagnosed or who have been lost to follow-up. Phenylketonuria (PKU) illustrates the need for careful and specific management of pregnancy in women with a metabolic disorder.

There are several other metabolic disorders in addition to PKU where adverse effects on the fetus or the mother clearly occur. Clinicians, particularly obstetricians, geneticists and biochemists, need to be aware of the potential for complications during pregnancy in this group of disorders.

FURTHER READING

Bennett MJ, Renaldo P, Strauss AW. Inborn errors of mitochondrial fatty acid oxidation. Crit Rev Clin Lab Sci 2000; **37:** 1-44.

Brown GK. Glucose transporters: Structure, function and consequences of deficiency. J Inher Metab Dis 2000; **23:** 237-46.

Chakrapani A, Cleary MA, Wraith JE. Detection of inborn errors of metabolism in the newborn. Arch Dis Child (Neonatal Ed) 2001; **84:** F205-210.

Cleary MA, Wraith JE. Antenatal diagnosis of inborn errors of metabolism. Arch Dis Child 1991; **66:** 816-22.

Fernandes J, Saudubray J-M, van den Berghe G. Inborn Metabolic Diseases: Diagnosis and treatment. New York: Springer, 2000.

Hoffman GF, Nyhan WL, Zchocke J, Kaher SG, Mayatepek E. Inherited metabolic disorders. Philadelphia: Lippincott, Williams & Wilkins, 2002.

Leonard JV, Morris AAM. Inborn errors of metabolism around the time of birth. Lancet 2000; **356:** 583-7.

Ogier de Baulny H. Management and emergency treatments of neonates with a suspicion of inborn errors of metabolism. Semin Neonatal 2002; **7:** 17-26.

Preece MA, Green A. Pregnancy and inherited metabolic disorders: maternal and fetal complications. Ann Clin Biochem 2002; **39:** 444-55.

Stacpoole PW, Bunch ST, Neuberger RE et al. The importance of cerebrospinal fluid lactate in the evaluation of congenital lactic acidosis. J Ped 1999; **134:** 99-102.

Van den Berghe G. Disorders of gluconeogenesis. J Inher Metab Dis 1996; **19:** 470-7.

Wraith JE. Inborn errors of metabolism in the neonate. Part 3. In: Textbook of Neonatology 3rd edn. Rennie JM, Roberton NRC. London: Churchill Livingstone, 1999, pp 986-1002.

Chapter 11

Haematological disorders

PHYSIOLOGY

FETAL HAEMOGLOBIN AND ERYTHROPOIESIS

Haematopoiesis begins in early embryonic development, taking place first in the yolk sac, then, between six weeks and six months gestation, in the liver. The main haemoglobins produced are fetal types, particularly HbF. From six months gestation onwards, the bone marrow becomes the main site of haematopoiesis. There is a gradual shift from fetal to adult type (HbA) haemoglobin production, starting at around 34 weeks gestation and continuing into infancy. At full term, about 20% of circulating haemoglobin is of the adult type: by six months of age fetal haemoglobin makes up less than 1% of the total.

Erythropoietin is an important stimulus in the fetus for bone marrow red cell production. After birth, erythropoietin production declines rapidly, and erythropoiesis virtually halts at the end of the first week, while the haemoglobin concentration and the haematocrit gradually decline. At six to eight weeks after birth, the haematocrit has usually fallen to about 30%; erythropoietin production by the kidney then increases, and erythropoiesis recommences. This early fall is exaggerated in the preterm infant.

Red cells transport oxygen to the tissues, bound reversibly to haemoglobin. This consists of four globin chains, each binding one molecule of haem. HbA (adult-type) has two α chains and two β chains; HbF (fetal-type) has two α chains and two γ chains. Fetal haemoglobin has a higher affinity for oxygen than HbA. This is thought to be advantageous to the fetus as it can achieve a higher oxygen content in its blood in the environment of a low partial pressure of oxygen from umbilical venous blood. After birth, when the PaO_2 rises, this is no longer an advantage.

The affinity with which haemoglobin binds to oxygen is affected by a number of factors as shown in the oxyhaemoglobin dissociation curve (*see p.76*). Factors that increase the affinity of haemoglobin for oxygen shift the curve to the left and potentially decrease the availability of oxygen to tissue. In term infants, 2,3-diphosphoglycerate in the erythrocytes increases in the first postnatal week, shifting the curve to the right and facilitating delivery of oxygen to tissues. This increase in delivery of oxygen to tissues more than compensates for the decreased oxygen carrying capacity associated with the physiological fall in haemoglobin concentration.

COAGULATION

Blood clotting systems have vascular, cellular and chemical components. Inappropriate activation of any part of the system can result in thrombosis and consumption of clotting factors. Deficiencies of elements of the system can result in bleeding.

The main processes involved in coagulation are summarised in Figure 11.1. Blood coagulation is initiated by tissue factor, which is released into the circulation as a result of tissue injury by trauma, inflammatory or allergic reactions, or malignancy. With factor VII, it forms tissue factor-factor VII complex. The activated complex (TF-VIIa) activates factor IX, which in turn activates factor X to produce factor Xa. Factor Xa, in the presence of Va, calcium and platelets, generates thrombin from prothrombin. Thrombin generation leads to the formation of fibrin and further activation of factor XI, which contributes to the activation of factor IX.

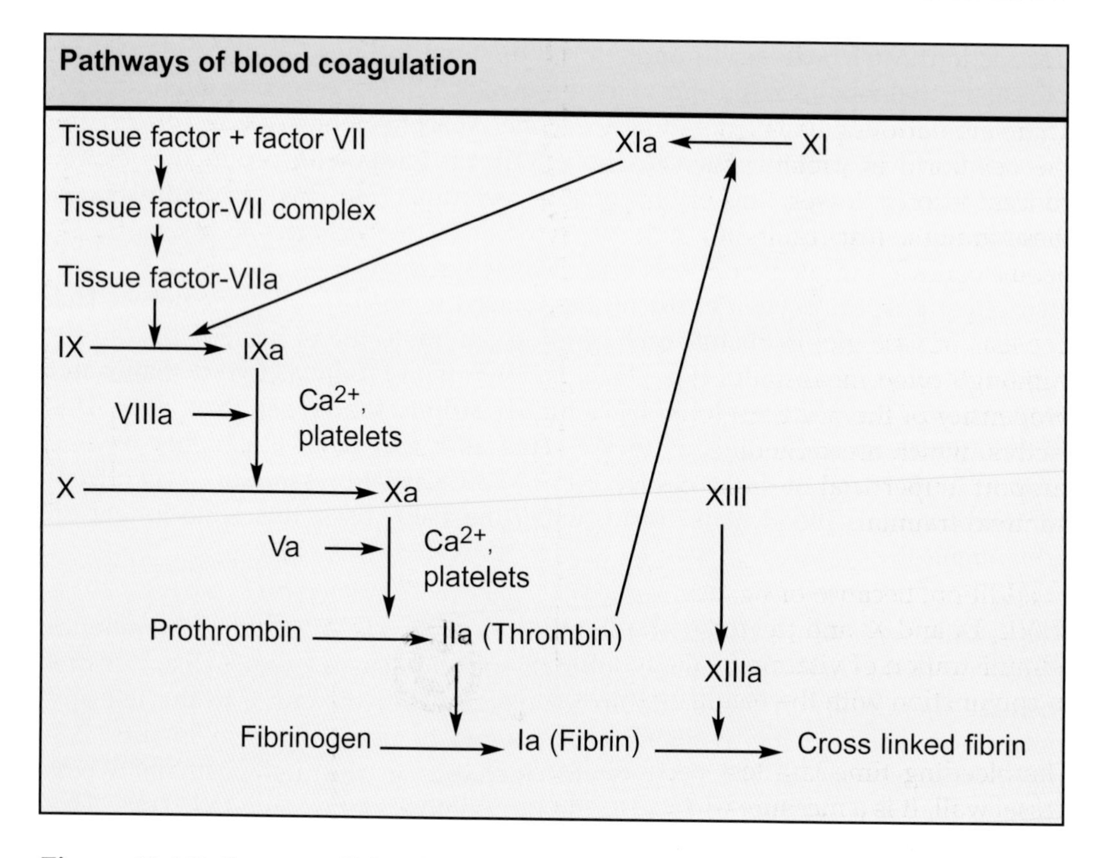

Figure 11.1 Pathways of blood coagulation

Factor XII's role in the coagulation pathway is not clearly understood. Patients with factor XII deficiency do not suffer from bleeding disorders and some of them are susceptible to thromboembolic disease.

Assessment of coagulation factor function involves two screening tests, prothrombin time (PT) and activated partial thromboplastin time (APTT), combined with inspection of a blood film, platelet count, and measurement of fibrinogen concentration. Prothrombin time measures the generation of thrombin after the addition of tissue factor *in vitro*. It is affected by vitamin K deficiency, as factors II, VII, IX and X are vitamin K dependent proteins. The APTT measures the time taken for thrombin generation after the addition of a contact activating factor through the factor IX pathway.

Reference ranges for coagulation indices

Reference ranges for individual coagulant proteins vary from fetal life through childhood. At term, plasma concentrations of the vitamin K dependent factors and contact factors are approximately equal to half adult values, while those of fibrinogen, factor VIII, factor V and von Willebrand factor are at similar concentrations to those found in adults.

There are various published reference ranges for the usual coagulation indices in the newborn. In preterm babies, the PT and APTT are longer and fibrinogen concentration is lower. Prenatal hypoxia and neonatal illnesses can further affect these indices. Test results for PT and APTT are always compared to a simultaneous 'control' sample using the same methodology.

Clinical significance of coagulation parameters

Although often measured, coagulation parameters do not themselves reflect the propensity of the newborn to bleed. This is determined by platelet and vascular factors, which are difficult to measure. Delicate immature skin and soft tissues support superficial vessels poorly and preterm babies bruise readily with minimal trauma.

In addition, because of hepatic immaturity, relatively poor production of factors II, VII, IX and X, and the relation of the timing of the sample to that of postnatal administration of vitamin K, the results of any one test should always be viewed in conjunction with the results of other investigations.

The bleeding time is a test performed to evaluate platelet interaction with the vessel wall. It is a measure of the duration of bleeding from a superficial skin incision. Difficulties in its interpretation arise from problems in standardising the method. In neonates, this involves using an automatic incision device to produce an incision on the volar aspect of the forearm, with a blood pressure cuff set to a standard pressure applied to the upper arm. This test is rarely used in clinical practice.

BLOOD GROUPS

Blood group incompatibility between a baby and its mother is clinically important only if the mother carries IgG antibodies (which cross the placenta freely) against a red cell or platelet antigen expressed by the fetus. Anti-A antibodies (carried by mothers of blood groups B or O) and anti-B antibodies (carried by mothers of blood groups A or O) are usually large IgM molecules, which do not cross the placenta. Some individuals carry IgG versions of these naturally occurring antibodies, called α and β haemolysins, which can affect the baby and cause haemolysis. Because this is unpredictable, these antibodies are not screened for routinely in pregnancy.

Other blood group antibodies that are IgG type can be acquired by the mother from previous blood transfusion, or from feto-maternal transfusion in a previous pregnancy. These will be detected at first booking with an antenatal clinic by a screen of maternal blood for irregular antibodies, and, if they are present, their titres should be monitored.

WHITE CELLS

There are several white cell growth factors active in the fetus, including the interleukins and other factors now becoming available for therapeutic use, such as G-CSF (granulocyte colony-stimulating factor) and GM-CSF (granulocyte-macrophage colony-stimulating factor).

Non-lymphoid and lymphoid cells are both necessary for many sorts of immune response. These functions are underdeveloped in preterm babies, who have defects in lymphocyte and phagocyte function, and reduced granulocyte production in response to bacterial infection. The total white cell count is high at birth, falling by about 25% in the first four weeks. The neutrophil count rises immediately after birth, peaking at 12 hours, then falling to a steady level from 60 hours onwards. Knowledge of postnatal age is therefore very important in interpreting white cell count, and especially neutrophil count, results.

NEONATAL HAEMATOLOGICAL DISORDERS

ANAEMIA

Anaemia at birth, usually defined as a haemoglobin concentration of < 12 g/dL , can arise in several different ways. Acute blood loss at, or prior to, delivery produces hypovolaemia as well as decreased oxygen carrying capacity, and requires emergency erythrocyte replacement. Group O negative blood, held in all delivery suites, can be used in an extreme emergency; partially packed cells compatible with the mother's blood group are preferable and should be as fresh as possible. Cell-free blood substitutes are not recommended in this situation.

Internal blood loss (placental loss to the maternal circulation) can be crudely estimated by performance of a Kleihauer test directly on maternal blood.

Preterm babies in neonatal units can lose proportionately huge volumes of blood in routine testing and monitoring, so care in sampling and use of micromethodology is vital. Many neonatal units (NNUs) electively replace sampling volumes after 10% of blood volume has been taken (average blood volume 90 mL/kg body weight, plasma volume 50 mL/kg) (*see p.10*).

Causes of anaemia in premature babies include excessive phlebotomy losses, somatic growth, resulting in a doubling or tripling of body weight and blood volume between birth and discharge, and prolongation of the normal postnatal suppression of erythropoietin release. Preterm babies develop a normochromic, normocytic anaemia, maximal at 3-12 weeks of age, which can be symptomatic. This may require correction by transfusion.

Indications for blood replacement in babies who become anaemic on neonatal units are consensus based, as measured haemoglobin concentration is likely to give only a poor representation of the oxygen carrying capacity of the blood when the blood volume is not known. The 'trigger' value at which an erythrocyte transfusion is ordered for an NNU patient varies according to the clinical situation. In seriously ill infants, the haemoglobin concentration is usually maintained at a higher level (> 13 g/dL) to ensure adequate oxygen carrying capacity, while in well babies, in order to minimise the hazards of transfusion and avoid marrow suppression, it can be allowed to fall to 8 g/dL as long as the baby is asymptomatic. Because it is not possible to infer the amount of oxygen available from the measured haemoglobin concentration or haematocrit in an individual baby, attention to clinical status is essential in deciding whether to transfuse. In all cases, samples for investigation of the anaemia must be taken prior to transfusion.

The product used for 'top up' transfusion in preterm babies is packed erythrocytes from CMV-negative donors, usually in a volume of 15 mL/kg body weight infused over 2-4 hours. Various published guidelines for red cell transfusions in this circumstance exist (*see* Further Reading).

Treatment of extremely premature babies with recombinant erythropoietin can stimulate red cell production if treatment is instituted early and sustained. This can reduce the need for postnatal replacement transfusion. Erythropoietin is administered at a dose of 250 units/kg body weight by subcutaneous injection three times a week for six weeks. Iron deficiency will reduce its efficacy, so iron supplementation should also be used. Cost effectiveness criteria have limited the use of erythropoietin in the UK, as attention to limiting phlebotomy losses may itself, together with a strict transfusion policy, reduce the need for transfusions. Erythropoietin has a place in the management of preterm babies whose parents have objections to blood transfusion.

Congenital anaemia

The cause of anaemia (Hb <12g/dL) at birth is usually clear from the history. Important causes of congenital anaemia include:

- feto-maternal haemorrhage some hours before delivery
- twin to twin transfusion
- accidental blood loss, e.g. from a placental vessel
- intrauterine haemolysis
- infection with parvovirus
- haemoglobinopathy
- thalassaemia
- neonatal blood loss, internal or external.

First line investigations of congenital anaemia should therefore be directed to exclude these diagnoses (see Figure 11.2).

If there has been postnatal bleeding, e.g. haematemesis, then Apt's test on the blood (acid elution test) will differentiate between maternal and neonatal blood. Maternal cells are haemolysed in the presence of an acid medium, while neonatal cells remain intact.

First line investigations in congenital anaemia
FBC, film, platelets
Reticulocyte count
Glucose 6-phosphate dehydrogenase (G6PD) screen
Group and direct antiglobulin test
Maternal blood group and antibody screen
Kleihauer test on maternal blood (to quantify any recent feto-maternal bleeding)
Congenital infection screen
Coagulation tests
Hb electrophoresis (if indicated)

Figure 11.2 First line investigations in congenital anaemia

Haemolytic disorders to consider include rhesus isoimmunisation; other blood group isoimmunisation, e.g. Duffy, Kell, ABO incompatibility with maternal α or β haemolysins (though the presence of these is not diagnostic as they can be inactive); G6PD deficiency, and rarer red cell abnormalities such as congenital spherocytosis or elliptocytosis.

Any longstanding cause of severe congenital anaemia may lead to heart failure and ascites, pleural or pericardial effusions, or hydrops, which may be detected and/or treated antenatally by fetal transfusion. The postnatal management of chronic anaemia should be by exchange transfusion rather than by a large volume 'top up'.

TRANSFUSION PRODUCTS

In the UK, special transfusion blood products are available for neonates. The standard product has a volume of about 230 mL, with a haematocrit of 55-75%, and is produced by removing plasma from donated blood. Donors are screened for known viruses, and all units are leucodepleted to reduce the risk of virus transmission. Additionally, blood that has been irradiated is indicated for *in utero* transfusions, and is currently recommended for post-delivery transfusion in these babies, or for babies with suspected immunodeficiency. Blood is tested for ABO,

RhD and compatibility with any irregular antibodies. In the authors' unit, maternal blood is used for cross matching, as long as ABO groups are compatible, as any neonatal IgG antibody will be derived from the mother.

Transfusion should be prescribed according to local protocols. The need for transfusion can be reduced by adherence to these and attention to volumes taken during blood sampling. Where possible, multiple satellite bags from single donors are used for serial transfusions to a single baby to minimise the potential risk from exposure to multiple donors. Units should be less than 35 days old for a 'top up' transfusion, and less than five days old for an exchange transfusion. In practice, the freshest blood available is used because of a lower potassium and acid load, and better oxygen carrying capacity.

The total volume of transfusion required for a given baby can be calculated as:

volume (mL of plasma reduced cells) = weight of baby (kg) x 3 x desired rise in Hb concentration (g/dL).

This is usually transfused over four hours. A single dose of diuretic can be administered at the beginning of the transfusion if the volume to be given is large (>15 mL/kg) or there is circulatory compromise, for instance as the result of a persistent patent ductus arteriosus.

POLYCYTHAEMIA

This is defined as a venous haematocrit of >65% in a newborn infant. Apparent polycythaemia from a capillary sample should always be confirmed on free flowing venous blood, as squeezing the baby's heel may produce a misleading result. Polycythaemia occurs in growth-restricted babies and infants of diabetic mothers owing to enhanced fetal erythropoietin production. It is also seen in pregnancy at high altitude and in trisomy 21.

Babies delivered at home, or babies who have had delayed cord clamping at delivery, may have received a transfusion of maternal blood at birth. Polycythaemia can also be part of twin-twin transfusion syndrome, although the major issue here is one of hyperperfusion in one twin, and haemoglobin concentrations at birth are not always elevated in the hyperperfused twin.

The underlying cause of polycythaemia is usually clear after taking a history and examining the baby, so further investigations are not usually necessary. Treatment depends on the absolute haematocrit or the presence of symptoms of hyperviscosity, which can include cardiac failure, respiratory distress or neurological signs of any sort. The baby appears plethoric, and is likely to develop jaundice. Complications can occur, such as necrotising enterocolitis, haematuria and proteinuria, or a pulmonary hypertension syndrome. It is very unusual for signs or symptoms to be present with a venous haematocrit below 70%. Many clinicians will treat an asymptomatic baby with a haematocrit between 70 and 75% with rehydration alone, but electively seek to reduce the haematocrit by dilutional exchange transfusion at values above this or if any symptoms of hyperviscosity are present. This involves exchanging 30 mL/kg of the baby's blood for 4.5% human albumin solution in 10 mL aliquots over about 20-30 minutes. Isotonic saline can be used safely in place of albumin.

HAEMOLYTIC DISORDERS

Conditions that lead to shortened red cell lifespan in the fetus or neonate may present as hydrops in the fetus, congenital anaemia or early (day 1) neonatal jaundice (*see Chapter 6*). Anaemia occurs if the rate of haemolysis exceeds the rate of red cell production.

The commonest neonatal haemolytic problems are caused by red cell membrane or enzyme abnormalities, or by blood group incompatibility between mother and baby where there is maternal IgG antibody production (haemolytic disease of the newborn). Intrinsic red cell membrane abnormalities frequently present as early jaundice. The commonest is congenital spherocytosis, an autosomal dominant condition, suggested either by family history, or by the presence of numerous spherocytes in the neonatal blood film, and confirmed by testing for osmotic fragility after the neonatal period. Congenital elliptocytosis and pyropoikilocytosis present similarly.

Red cell enzyme abnormalities should be considered in babies with early jaundice. It is our practice, with a local multiethnic population, to screen all infants with first day jaundice, or with plasma bilirubin concentration exceeding the phototherapy threshold, for G6PD deficiency. This is an X-linked disorder, also associated with drug-induced haemolytic crises: affected infants' families should be supplied with a list of drugs to avoid. The disease is expressed in males and in homozygous females, with highest frequency in those of Mediterranean, African or Asian ethnic origin. Twenty to thirty per cent of affected infants develop neonatal jaundice.

Prenatal factors

Feto-maternal blood group incompatibility involving the rhesus system or the Kell or Duffy systems can lead to fetal and neonatal anaemia through a process of haemolysis of fetal red cells and fetal marrow suppression. This is termed haemolytic disease of the newborn. These conditions also produce neonatal jaundice presenting on the first day of life.

There are five distinct antigen types in the rhesus system. They are known as C, D, E, c and e. The term 'rhesus-positive' refers to a person who has at least one copy of the D antigen. If the mother is 'negative' for the D antigen, but becomes pregnant with a baby who has the antigen, leakage of fetal blood into the maternal circulation may provoke maternal IgG antibody production against the fetal cells. Such bleeding commonly occurs at delivery but may occur silently during pregnancy or at the time of a miscarriage. The first appearance of these antibodies rarely produces an affected baby, but subsequent pregnancies are at risk.

Maternal antibodies of this type are screened for in rhesus-negative women (15% of the population) at booking, and during pregnancy at 24, 28 and 34 weeks. If they are present in high or rising titres, they may affect the fetus: they cross the placenta freely and cause haemolysis of antigen-positive fetal cells.

All non-sensitised (antibody negative) rhesus-negative women are given specific anti-D gamma globulin routinely at 28 and 34 weeks, after any event or procedure in pregnancy that might provoke bleeding, and after delivery. 250 I.U. is given before 20 weeks and 500 I.U. After 20 weeks or if the estimated blood loss is 5 mL or more. The bleed volume is estimated by a Kleihauer test, which detects fetal cells in maternal blood.

If a rhesus-negative pregnant woman has an antibody titre of >1, she is already immunised and should not be given anti-D. If the titre is 1-4, it should be repeated monthly to 20 weeks, then fortnightly; fetal ultrasound should also be performed. If the titre is >4, then amniocentesis or cordocentesis is indicated at, or after, 22 weeks. Subsequent management of the pregnancy, which may include fetal transfusion with irradiated antigen-negative red cells, is guided by serial estimation of liquor optical density at 450 nm at amniocentesis and by regular fetal ultrasound scanning, looking for development of oedema or ascites. This may indicate developing fetal hydrops (*see Appendix D*).

Postnatal care

Affected babies may be electively delivered prematurely to allow immediate postnatal treatment. At delivery, cord blood is taken for haemoglobin, bilirubin, blood group and direct antiglobulin test. It should be noted that if the baby has been transfused before birth with rhesus-negative blood, the blood group at birth will appear to be that of the donor, so rhesus grouping and direct antiglobulin test will appear to be negative.

If the baby appears pink and well at birth, no immediate action is necessary. Provided that cord haemoglobin concentration exceeds 12 g/dL, the baby's main problem is likely to be jaundice. Serum bilirubin should be checked four-hourly and phototherapy started promptly. Exchange transfusion (using 160 mL/kg warmed, CMV-negative, rhesus-negative blood less than five days old) may be needed if the bilirubin concentration rises above the exchange threshold for gestation (*see Chapter 6*). Multiple exchanges may be needed on successive days.

Follow-up after discharge includes monitoring for late anaemia for 12 weeks or until the haemoglobin starts to rise. This is particularly important if no exchange transfusion has been done, as the baby will have a full load of maternal antibodies and may require later 'top up' transfusion with rhesus-negative cells.

If the baby has received fetal transfusions and is pale at delivery but otherwise stable, a 'top up' transfusion may be appropriate instead of an exchange. Any baby who has had fetal transfusion and who requires blood postnatally – either as exchange or 'top up' – should receive irradiated cells, to prevent the possibility of graft versus host disease. If the baby is pale, hepatosplenomegaly should be looked for. This can result from extramedullary haemopoiesis *in utero*. There may be cardiomegaly, ascites or oedema, and the baby may need resuscitation and respiratory support. In these babies, the cord haemoglobin concentration will be <12 g/dL. Early exchange transfusion with 60 mL/kg of a high haematocrit blood preparation of partially packed cells (grouped prenatally against the mother's serum and less than five days old) within 3-4 hours is indicated. When the birth of a rhesus isoimmunised baby is anticipated, this blood product should be available on site so that it can be used for exchange transfusion immediately after delivery. Exchange transfusion can be performed through an umbilical vein, an umbilical artery, or a combination of a peripheral artery (e.g. radial) for the 'out' cycles, and a large vein (e.g. cephalic) for the transfusions into the baby. Close monitoring and 15 minute recording of heart rate, respiratory rate and blood pressure are needed. The procedure should be stopped briefly if the baby's condition deteriorates. If the baby is stable and there are no signs of hydrops, the 60 mL/kg exchange should be followed immediately by an 80 mL/kg exchange. The purpose of the first exchange is to give the baby red cells and thereby improve oxygen carriage to tissues; that of later exchanges is to remove antibody and also bilirubin.

Babies affected by any form of isoimmunisation are discharged home on oral folic acid supplements (1 mg daily). They should be monitored as outpatients for the development of late anaemia. If they have developed persistent conjugated hyperbilirubinaemia (sludging syndrome), they should be monitored until all signs of liver dysfunction have resolved. Treatment with oral ursodeoxycholic acid is sometimes given.

COAGULATION DISORDERS

Isolated deficiency of clotting factors may be suspected before birth because of a family history, and the risk of the fetus being affected may be defined by genetic testing. This is most commonly indicated in classic haemophilia, an X-linked recessive condition. If an affected baby is anticipated, delivery should be by elective caesarean section. The baby should not be given any intramuscular injections. Vitamin K should be given orally. Cord blood or baby's blood should be sent to the transfusion laboratory for elective quantitative clotting factor analysis by functional or immunological assay. If necessary, specific treatment can then be given. The low concentrations of coagulation factors in the neonate and reduced ability to generate thrombin cause vulnerability to internal bleeding.

Differential diagnosis of coagulation disorders

A relevant family history may be available (e.g. coagulation factor deficiencies, von Willebrand's disease). The mother may have a history of thrombocytopenia or antinuclear antibodies, or, in the obstetric history, there may have been a suspicion of fetal congenital infection. On examination of the baby, the presence of petechiae suggests a platelet deficiency or dysfunction, or a vascular problem, while bleeding from organs suggests a more generalised clotting failure. If the baby is generally unwell, this will suggest that the coagulation disorder is secondary to systemic disease.

Figure 8.3 summarises the use of laboratory screening tests in the differential diagnosis of coagulation disorders.

Haemorrhagic disease of the newborn

This group of conditions is caused by vitamin K deficiency. Haemorrhagic disease of the newborn was first described as self-limiting bleeding occurring between the first and fifth day of life associated with low plasma concentrations of prothrombin. This condition affected up to 1% of babies before routine postnatal vitamin K supplementation was established. Subsequently, the condition was attributed to deficiency of vitamin K, which is synthesised by intestinal flora. Concentrations are low at birth, because the gastrointestinal tract is sterile until feeding has become established. Breast milk is a poor source of the vitamin, so unfed or breast-fed infants, or those with underlying hepatic pathology and reduced ability to manufacture coagulation proteins, are particularly at risk of this condition.

Laboratory test results in the bleeding infant

Healthy infants

Platelets	Prothrombin time	Partial thromboplastin time	Likely diagnosis
Normal	Normal	Normal	Local factors (trauma, anatomical abnormality), qualitative platelet abnormality, factor XIII deficiency
Normal	Normal	Increased	Hereditary clotting factor deficiencies
Normal	Increased	Increased	Vitamin K deficiency
Decreased	Normal	Normal	Immune (auto- or allo-) thrombocytopenia, occult infection or thrombosis, marrow hypoplasia

Sick infants

Platelets	Prothrombin time	Partial thromboplastin time	Likely diagnosis
Normal	Normal	Normal	Compromised vascular integrity (hypoxia, prematurity, acidosis hyperosmolality)
Normal	Increased	Increased	Liver disease
Decreased	Normal	Normal	Platelet consumption (infection, necrotising enterocolitis, renal vein thrombosis)
Decreased	Increased	Increased	Disseminated intravascular coagulation

Figure 11.3 Laboratory test results in the bleeding infant

Early haemorrhagic disease may present in the first 24 hours, particularly if there is maternal intake of anticonvulsant drugs. Bleeding is rare but can be serious, including intracranial bleeds. Classic haemorrhagic disease occurs between 1 and 7 days and is characterised by cord or post circumcision oozing in a baby who has not received vitamin K at birth. 'Late' disease occurs at 1 to 3 months of age, in exclusively breast-fed infants or those with underlying malabsorption or liver problems such as cystic fibrosis or α_1-antitrypsin deficiency. PT and PTT are greatly prolonged and concentrations of vitamin K dependent factors are low, but are corrected by administration of 1 mg of parenteral vitamin K_1, with a rise in concentration within two hours and complete correction within 24 hours. Fresh frozen plasma (10-20 mL/kg) should be given immediately if there is active bleeding. Clotting factor concentrations can be measured when the diagnosis is suspected.

In the UK, all babies are given vitamin K_1 at birth (with parental consent) either 1 mg Konakion® intramuscularly, or, in well term babies, there is the option of 2 mg oral Konakion (Konakion MM Paediatric) followed by further oral doses for as long as exclusive breast feeding continues. Infants on prolonged total parenteral nutrition or who have chronic malabsorption should receive weekly parenteral Konakion (1-2 mg).

Disseminated intravascular coagulation (DIC)

This is a phenomenon resulting from activation and dysregulation of haemostatic systems, with generation of products of haemostasis and haemolysis, and consumption of haemostatic components. In the neonate, the usual presentation is with bleeding rather than thrombosis. DIC can be initiated by vascular injury, trauma, hypoxia, or sepsis, especially with Gram-negative organisms. The underlying common feature is thought to be exposure of blood to tissue factors, from which it is usually protected. Diagnosis depends on clinical features and laboratory tests: reduced platelet count (invariably), prolonged PT and APTT, low fibrinogen concentration (factor I) and elevated fibrin split products.

Treatment depends on managing the underlying condition; most babies with DIC will survive. Active bleeding should be treated with haemostatic agents. In milder cases, a combination of fresh frozen plasma (10 mL/kg) followed by cryoprecipitate (10 mL/kg) or factor VIII will significantly improve measured parameters. Platelet transfusion may also be required if the platelet count is less than 50 x 10^9/L. In sicker or preterm infants, exchange transfusion with group-compatible blood (as fresh as possible) is likely to be better tolerated.

In the premature population, much research has gone into judging when treatment with blood products should be given to prevent haemorrhagic complications. Preterm infants with intraventricular haemorrhages have been found to have clotting abnormalities prior to diagnosis, with prolongation of PT and APTT. It is now thought that this represents an indicator of risk rather than being the cause. Trials of prophylactic administration of fresh frozen plasma have given conflicting results, in general producing improvement in measured clotting parameters but no improvement in survival, and, in some series, reduced incidence of intraventricular haemorrhage. It is thought that at least some of the beneficial effect may be a result of stabilisation of the circulation and thus prevention of rapid changes in blood pressure, rather than a direct effect on coagulation. This notion is supported by other evidence suggesting that preterm babies are often hypovolaemic at birth.

THROMBOTIC DISORDERS

Homozygous deficiency of protein C or protein S, which are dominantly inherited anticoagulant proteins, can cause serious thrombotic events in the postnatal period, and should be investigated for in purpura fulminans, unexplained DIC, or suspected arterial or venous cerebral infarction. The parents will be heterozygous for the affected protein but are likely to be asymptomatic. Primary treatment is with fresh frozen plasma (10 to 15 mL/kg 8-hourly) or with protein C concentrate. Other rare inherited abnormalities of fibrinolysis also exist.

Acquired defects of thrombosis can follow vascular injury, altered blood flow or endothelial activation. Infants at risk are those with indwelling umbilical arterial or umbilical venous catheters, polycythaemia and hyperviscosity, hypoxia or dehydration. Treatment is usually supportive. Sometimes thrombi must be surgically removed. Anticoagulant treatment is usually contraindicated in infants below 34 weeks gestation because of the risk of cerebral haemorrhage.

PLATELET DISORDERS

Fetal platelet counts increase with gestation to a mean of $274 \times 10^9/L$ at 40 weeks. The normal range is generally taken to be the same for preterm and term infants as for adults ($150\text{-}450 \times 10^9/L$). However, many apparently healthy neonates have platelet counts of $100\text{-}150 \times 10^9/L$. If such a value is found, the measurement is usually simply repeated, and the infant monitored. Thrombocytopenia of some degree has been reported in up to 35% of infants admitted to NNUs. Sick neonates are highly susceptible to thrombocytopenia, probably because of a limited ability to increase platelet production in response to increased consumption. Thrombocytopenia can therefore be a useful non-specific warning of sepsis or inflammation. Some causes of thrombocytopenia are given in Figure 11.4.

Immune thrombocytopenias

Mild maternal thrombocytopenia due to shortened platelet survival in pregnancy is common and benign. Maternal immune thrombocytopenia is commonly due to IgG anti-platelet antibodies. These can cross the placenta, producing neonatal thrombocytopenia. This is seldom severe. The neonatal platelet count is low at birth and falls further for 72 hours before resolving within a week. Babies should be kept under observation until the platelet count starts to rise, and be treated with platelet transfusion if the count falls below 20 x 10^9/L or there is spontaneous bleeding. Alloimmune thrombocytopenia is much rarer: in this condition, maternal antibodies are directed against an antigen that is present in the baby's platelets but not the mother's. The maternal platelet count is therefore normal. Diagnosis is made on previous obstetric history or on investigation of a symptomatic thrombocytopenic baby. The usual antigen is PLA-1: the mother will be PLA-1 negative and the baby positive. Fetal steroid treatment or transfusion with IgG or PLA-I negative platelets have been employed to reduce the risk of fetal intracranial haemorrhage, and integrated fetal-neonatal care is important. Affected neonates, who are often severely thrombocytopenic (platelets < 50 x 10^9/L), should be given PLA-1 negative platelets or washed, irradiated maternal platelets and intravenous IgG (e.g. Sandoglobulin® 1 mg/kg/day for two days). Further details should be obtained from the local blood transfusion service.

Apparent thrombocytopenia should be confirmed on a free-flowing venous sample. Other indices of coagulation should be checked. Isolated thrombocytopenia causes bruises, petechiae or cephalhaematoma. Treatment is not usually needed if the platelet count is greater than 20 x 10^9/L in a term infant unless there is active bleeding or evidence suggesting DIC, in which case the platelet count should be kept above 50 x 10^9/L, and other coagulation abnormalities also corrected using appropriate factor concentrates.

NEUTROPENIA

In high risk neonates, neutropenia is usually caused by reduced production of granulocytes. The commonest association (40% of neutropenic infants) is infection. An increase in immature forms (myelocytes, band cells) is very suggestive of an infective cause. Other conditions associated with neutropenia are maternal pregnancy-induced hypertension, intrauterine growth retardation, and (rarely) neonatal alloimmune neutropenia, when the mother will also have a low neutrophil count. Some bone marrow disorders also produce neonatal neutropenia. These include the following conditions:

- severe congenital neutropenia (autosomal recessive)
- familial benign neutropenia
- cyclic neutropenia
- cartilage/hair dysplasia syndrome
- reticular dysgenesis
- humoral immunodeficiency.

Causes of neonatal thrombocytopenia

Aetiology	Disorder	Supporting features
Immune mediated	Alloimmune thrombocytopenia Maternal idiopathic thrombocytopenic purpura	Previous affected child Baby otherwise healthy
Infectious	Accompanies systemic infection - bacterial, candidal, congenital CMV, other viral infections	Accompanying signs of sepsis Neutropenia
Genetic	Thrombocytopenia-absent radius syndrome Fanconi anaemia Congenital thrombocytopenic syndromes Trisomy 13, 18, 21 Turner syndrome Wiskott-Aldrich syndrome Noonan syndrome Alport syndrome Some inherited metabolic diseases (*see Chapter 10*)	Other features of relevant genetic syndrome
Drug related	Maternal ingestion of quinine, hydralazine, tolbutamide, thiazide	Antibody against drug/hapten complex cross-reacts with platelet antigen Mother also thrombocytopenic
Part of disseminated intravascular coagulation (DIC)	Complicates severe neonatal illness	Prolonged PT and APTT Increased fibrin degradation products Increased D-dimers Decreased fibrinogen
Other	Secondary to thrombosis Necrotising enterocolitis Intrauterine growth retardation Maternal pregnancy induced hypertension Perinatal asphyxia	Renal vein thrombosis, sagittal sinus thrombosis, intravascular (catheter associated) thrombus, 80-90% of necrotising enterocolitis

Figure 11.4 Causes of neonatal thrombocytopenia

In neutropenic neonates with proven bacterial sepsis, recombinant growth factors (G-CSF and GM-CSF) are currently being evaluated for use in treatment.

HAEMOGLOBINOPATHIES AND THALASSAEMIAS

The commonly occurring haemoglobinopathies are caused by a mutation in the β chain of the haemoglobin molecule. In fetal life, the predominant haemoglobin is HbF, with two α chains and two γ chains. At birth, therefore, these conditions are clinically silent, presenting during infancy as the switch from γ to β chain synthesis occurs. In the common β thalassaemias, the production of β chains is reduced, so the presentation is similar to that of a haemoglobinopathy.

Screening tests (haemoglobin separation by HPLC or isoelectric focusing) on neonatal or cord blood, should detect sickle cell disease or homozygous thalassaemia by the absence of haemoglobin A (*see Chapter 9*).

FURTHER READING

Andrew M, Paes B, Milner R, Johnson M, Mitchell L et al. Development of the coagulation system in the full term neonate. Blood 1987; **70:** 165-72.

Andrew M, Massicote MP. Haemostasis. In: Pediatrics and Perinatology: the Scientific Basis 2nd edn. Gluckman PD, Heymann MA (Eds). London: Arnold, 1996, pp 877-89.

Bowman JM. RhD haemolytic disease of the newborn. N Engl J Med 1998; **339:** 1775-7

Canadian Pediatric Society. Guidelines for transfusion of erythrocytes to neonates and premature infants. Can Med Assoc J 1992; **147:** 1781-6

Franz AR, Pohlandt F. Red blood transfusions in very and extremely low birth-weight infants under restrictive transfusion guidelines: is exogenous erythropoietin necessary? Arch Dis Child 2001; **84:** F96-F100.

Ohls RK. The use of erythropoietin in neonates. Clin Perinatol 2000; **27:** 681-96.

Ouwehand WH, Smith G, Ranasinghe E. Management of severe alloimmune thrombocytopenia in the newborn Arch Dis Child 2000; **82:** F173-5.

Sola MC, Del Vecchio A, Rimsza LM. Evaluation and treatment of thrombocytopenia in the neonatal intensive care unit. Clin Perinatol 2000: **27:** 655-79.

Wee LY, Fisle HM. The twin-twin transfusion syndrome. Semin Neonatol 2002; **7:** 187-202.

Chapter 12

Neonatal infections

INTRODUCTION

Throughout pregnancy, until the membranes rupture, the fetal environment is usually sterile. Congenital infections are infections that are present before or at the time of birth. They can be acquired through transplacental spread of systemic maternal infections or from the genital tract, especially if there has been prolonged rupture of the membranes. These infections are relatively uncommon, but potentially very serious. After rupture of the membranes, the infant is exposed to the many different microorganisms present in the vagina, some of which are potentially pathogenic. Following delivery, the neonate continues to be exposed to a wide range of microorganisms originating from its mother, health care staff, family and visitors, and the hospital and home environments. There is considerable overlap between important pathogens that are acquired before, during and after birth (Figure 12.1). Serious infections in normal term infants in developed countries are relatively uncommon. Most of the microorganisms encountered are of low pathogenicity, the infant may be protected by passive immunity of maternal origin, and specific precautions (including maternal screening, see Figure 12.2) are routinely taken to protect against certain common and/or serious pathogens. Serious infections are a much more common problem in preterm neonates. These infants have much greater susceptibility to infection because of immaturity of both the immune system and non-specific defences such as the skin, and because there is likely to have been less transfer of passive immunity. They are also at risk of hospital-acquired infections associated with neonatal intensive care.

INFECTIONS THAT ARE TRANSMITTED TRANSPLACENTALLY

The effects on the fetus of infections that are transmitted transplacentally depend on the microorganism and the stage of pregnancy when infection occurs. The most common outcome, especially after the first trimester, is that the fetus is unaffected. Any serious maternal infection may result in loss of the pregnancy or onset of premature labour. Some infections have specific effects on the fetus (Figure 12.3). Some infections mimic the pattern of infection in other age groups, but the fetus is more severely affected because of its immunological or physiological immaturity. A small number of infections may cause developmental abnormalities of the fetus. These include the TORCH organisms: *Toxoplasma gondii*, rubella virus and cytomegalovirus. Herpes simplex virus is sometimes also considered as a TORCH organism, although congenital infection is extremely rare.

Mother to infant transmission of important pathogens

Bacteria	Antenatal	Perinatal	Postnatal
Group B streptococcus	-	+++	+
Staphylococcus aureus	-	+	+++
Listeria monocytogenes	+++	+	+
Escherichia coli	-	+++	++
Treponema pallidum	+++	-	-
Neisseria gonorrhoeae	-	+++	+
Chlamydia trachomatis	-	+++	-
Ureaplasma urealyticum	-	+++	-
Coagulase-negative staphylococci	-	-	+++
Viruses			
Cytomegalovirus	+++	+	+
Herpes simplex virus	+	+++	++
Varicella zoster virus	+	+	+++
Hepatitis B virus	+	+++	+
Hepatitis C virus	±	+	±
HIV	+	+++	+
Rubella virus	+++	-	-
Enteroviruses	-	-	+
Parasites			
Toxoplasma gondii	+++	-	-

Key

-	no significant risk of transmission of the agent at this stage
±	transmission of the agent occasionally occurs at this stage
+	small but measurable risk of transmission of the agent at this stage
++	significant risk of transmission of the agent at this stage
+++	most infections with the agent are transmitted at this stage

Note that this table does not provide a quantitative comparison of the risks of mother to infant transmission of different agents

Figure 12.1 Timing of mother to infant transmission of important fetal and neonatal pathogens

Infection screening during pregnancy		
Infection	**Screening method**	**Rationale/action**
Infections for which screening is routinely offered in the UK		
Rubella	Antibody detection	Non-immune women offered immunisation after delivery (since rubella vaccine is a live vaccine it is contraindicated in pregnancy)
Syphilis	Antibody detection	Antimicrobial therapy given, where evidence of active infection to prevent congenital syphilis
Hepatitis B	Detection of viral surface antigen (HbsAg)	Immunisation of neonate to prevent mother to baby transmission
HIV	Antibody detection	Preventative measures before, during and after delivery greatly reduce risk of mother to baby transmission
Infections for which screening is routinely offered in some countries other than the UK		
Toxoplasmosis	Repeated testing of sero-negative women	Antimicrobial therapy given to women who seroconvert during pregnancy may prevent or limit fetal damage
Group B streptococcus	Culture of vaginal and/or rectal swabs	Intrapartum antimicrobial prophylaxis given to carriers

Figure 12.2 Infection screening during pregnancy

GENERAL PRINCIPLES OF DIAGNOSIS OF CONGENITAL INFECTIONS

Early *in utero* diagnosis of these infections can facilitate optimal management. However, this is dependent on first identifying maternal infection, which in many cases is either asymptomatic or causes only mild non-specific symptoms. For this reason, screening during pregnancy is routinely offered for a number of infections (see Figure 12.2). Occasionally, fetal infections are identified as a result of investigations of maternal illness. However, many fetal infections are only diagnosed after abnormalities are detected in antenatal scans or after birth.

Possible effects of transplacental fetal infections	
Infection	**Possible effects on the fetus**
Toxoplasmosis (*Toxoplasma gondii*)	Developmental abnormalities
Rubella	Developmental abnormalities
Cytomegalovirus	Developmental abnormalities
Human parvovirus B19	Hydrops fetalis
Listeriosis (*Listeria monocytogenes*)	Septicaemia, meningitis
Syphilis (*Treponema pallidum*)	Developmental abnormalities

Figure 12.3 Possible effects of transplacental fetal infections

Infections may be diagnosed by the direct detection of the infectious agent or by demonstration of an antibody response. The former depends on the infecting organism still being present at the time when diagnostic specimens are collected, and is also limited by the fact that many of the agents that cause fetal infection are difficult or impossible to culture *in vitro*. Serological techniques must be able to demonstrate that antibodies detected relate to acute infection, and not to past infection or immunisation.

Samples from the mother, the fetus and the infant during the first few months of life may be helpful in diagnosing intrauterine infections. It is generally technically straightforward to diagnose acute maternal infection. Serodiagnosis is usually based on detection of specific IgM or demonstration of seroconversion. Many laboratories retain sera collected from women at their booking antenatal appointment; retrieving these samples for testing in parallel with sera collected later in pregnancy is often helpful in demonstrating seroconversion. However, demonstration of maternal infection does not necessarily mean that the infection has been transmitted to the fetus.

Fetal blood sampling is the mainstay of investigation of fetal infection *in utero*, although other samples such as amniotic fluid and placental biopsy are occasionally helpful. Samples from the fetus or infant may be used for antibody testing or for direct detection of the organism. Serodiagnosis using fetal or infant blood depends on distinguishing between antibodies that have been produced by the baby and passively acquired antibodies of maternal origin. This may be done by:

- detection of IgM antibodies, which do not cross the placenta or occur in breast milk
- demonstration of a rising antibody titre in the infant after birth
- demonstration of the persistence of antibody beyond the age when passively acquired antibodies would be expected to have been lost. Traditionally, antibodies persisting beyond six months of age were considered diagnostic of fetal infection. However, with highly sensitive techniques, such as enzyme immunoassay for anti-HIV antibodies, passive antibody may be detectable for a year or more.

TOXOPLASMOSIS

Toxoplasma gondii is a protozoan parasite whose definitive host is the cat. Oocysts excreted in cat faeces sporulate to form infectious sporocysts that are ingested by secondary hosts (virtually any animal or bird, including farm livestock) in which parasitaemia and tissue invasion occurs. The life cycle is completed when a cat predates secondary hosts such as rodents or birds. Humans may acquire infection by:

- contact with or consumption of raw or undercooked meat, especially lamb
- direct or indirect (for example eating raw vegetables) contact with cat faeces
- contact with sheep at lambing
- mother to fetus transmission *in utero*. Very rarely, toxoplasmosis may also be transmitted by blood transfusion or organ transplantation. However, person to person transmission of toxoplasmosis cannot occur by any other route.

In the UK, seroprevalence rates rise from 20% at age 20 years, to 50-60% by age 60, with a risk of infection during pregnancy of 0.5% to 0.7%. In some other countries, such as France, toxoplasmosis is more common and occurs at an earlier age, such that as many as 80% of pregnant women are sero-positive. Possession of antibodies is normally indicative of immunity.

Toxoplasmosis in humans usually causes no, or only subclinical, illness. When a pregnant woman acquires toxoplasmosis, the risk of transmission to the fetus increases from 25% in the first trimester to 65% in the third. However, the risk of serious effects decreases from 75% to 5% between the first and third trimesters.

Severe congenital infection is characterised by hydrocephalus, cerebral calcification, hepatitis and myocarditis. It is estimated that in England and Wales, around 50 infants are born each year with overt congenital infection. Another 400 infected babies are born each year who are asymptomatic at birth. Many of these will develop chorioretinitis in later life, with a peak incidence in the second or third decades.

Diagnosis

Detection of IgM antibodies to *T. gondii* is usually the first indicator of possible maternal infection. However, this is not diagnostic of acute toxoplasmosis having occurred during pregnancy, because IgM usually remains detectable for many months after acute infection. Infection during pregnancy may be confirmed by demonstration of seroconversion, or by IgG avidity studies.

Fetal infection may be diagnosed by detection of IgM antibodies in fetal blood or by detection of *T. gondii* in amniotic fluid, usually by polymerase chain reaction (PCR).

The presence of IgM antibodies in neonatal blood is diagnostic of congenital infection, but only around one third of congenitally infected neonates produce a detectable IgM response. Detection of *T. gondii* in neonatal blood by PCR may be helpful, but sometimes the diagnosis can only be confirmed or excluded by serological follow-up until at least one year of age when maternal antibodies will normally have disappeared.

Treatment

A number of drugs are active against *T. gondii*, and treatment is indicated during pregnancy to try to prevent the parasite from invading the fetus, or at least to limit fetal damage. Treatment is continued for the newborn during the first year of life. Combination therapy with pyrimethamine and sulphadiazine is believed to be the most active regimen, but is potentially toxic. It is, therefore, usually given in three week courses alternating with spiramycin (which is much less toxic).

RUBELLA

Rubella is a highly infectious viral illness that is spread by the respiratory route. After an incubation period of 14-23 days, rubella presents with mild constitutional upset, a skin rash, lymphadenopathy and occasionally arthropathy. Patients may be infectious for up to seven days before, and seven days after, onset of the rash. Childhood immunisation has led to rubella becoming an uncommon illness, whilst ensuring that around 95% of pregnant women are immune.

When rubella is contracted by a woman during the first 12 weeks of pregnancy, the fetus is virtually always severely affected. Thereafter, the risk decreases rapidly, from 17% between 13 and 16 weeks to nil by 20 weeks. The classic triad of manifestations of congenital rubella is cataracts, heart disease and deafness. Natural infection and immunisation are both usually followed by long-lasting immunity to rubella. However, reinfections can occur even in the presence of detectable antibody, and these can damage the fetus.

Diagnosis

Maternal infection is diagnosed by serology, either by demonstration of specific IgM or a rising antibody titre by haemagglutination inhibition. There is rarely any place for *in utero* diagnosis of fetal infection with rubella. After birth, congenital rubella can be confirmed by demonstration of specific IgM, or by culture of the virus in urine or upper respiratory tract specimens.

Treatment

There is no specific anti-viral therapy for rubella. Termination of the pregnancy is usually offered to women who acquire rubella during the first twelve weeks of pregnancy. The risk of congenital defects declines rapidly during the subsequent 4-6 weeks, and careful counselling is required to help women infected at this stage to decide whether to continue with their pregnancies.

CYTOMEGALOVIRUS

Cytomegalovirus (CMV) is a member of the herpes group of viruses. CMV is not very infectious, and is usually only spread by prolonged close contact with infected body fluids, such as saliva, semen, blood and urine. In the UK, around 40% of individuals have detectable antibody by the age of 20 years, and around 1% of susceptible pregnant women acquire primary infection with CMV (that is 5 to 7 infections per thousand pregnancies). In developing countries, CMV infections are more common in childhood, and adult seroprevalence rates are consequently higher.

Most infections in healthy individuals outside the neonatal period are asymptomatic, or cause mild non-specific and self-limiting illness. Occasionally, CMV causes more severe symptoms, such as a glandular fever-like illness or hepatitis. When a pregnant woman experiences a primary infection with CMV, the risk of transmission to the fetus is around 40%. At least 85% of infected babies will have no adverse effects. Around 5% will be symptomatic at birth: clinical manifestations include hepatosplenomegaly, thrombocytopenia, prolonged neonatal jaundice, pneumonitis, growth retardation, microcephaly and cerebral calcification. A further 5-10%, although asymptomatic at birth, will develop long-term sequelae (usually cognitive, motor, visual or hearing defects). It is estimated that each year in England and Wales, around 120 infants have defects at birth, and a further 175 will develop defects during the first year of life as a consequence of CMV infection. Like other herpes viruses, CMV may persist in the body after infection, and reactivate months or years after the original infection. Reinfections with different strains of CMV can also occur. There is a small and unquantified risk that the fetus may be affected when a woman experiences a reactivation or reinfection during pregnancy.

DIAGNOSIS

Maternal CMV infection is usually diagnosed by detection of IgM antibodies in a single blood sample. Seroconversion in the period between two blood samples is also diagnostic.

Fetal infection can be diagnosed by detection of IgM antibodies in fetal blood, or by detection of CMV in amniotic fluid by culture or polymerase chain reaction.

Congenital infection in neonates can be diagnosed by detection of IgM antibodies or detection of virus in a throat swab or urine by culture or PCR. Since CMV infection may also be acquired at birth or during the first few days of life, congenital infection can only be diagnosed with certainty on samples collected within the first three weeks of life.

TREATMENT

Drugs that are active against CMV, such as ganciclovir, are toxic, and have largely been used for treating serious CMV infections in immunocompromised patients. However, they are increasingly being used to treat congenital CMV infections, where they may limit damage to hearing and vision.

HUMAN PARVOVIRUS B19

Human parvovirus B19 (HPV B19) is a small, single-stranded DNA virus that replicates in, and is cytotoxic for, erythroid progenitors. Transmission is via the respiratory route, but HPV B19 is much less infectious than many other respiratory viruses. Epidemics of infection occur every five to six years, and primarily affect children aged 6-10 years; 40% of the adult population is non-immune. After an incubation period of 6-15 days, the early symptoms of HPV B19 infection are non-specific, and indistinguishable from those of other respiratory viruses. In around half of cases, the illness is biphasic, the initial viraemic phase being followed by a skin rash (characteristically giving the appearance of slapped cheeks) and/or arthropathy.

When HPV B19 infection occurs during the first 20 weeks of pregnancy, there is a 10% risk of fetal loss, and between 9 and 20 weeks a further 3% risk of hydrops fetalis. Infections after 20 weeks of gestation do not cause serious morbidity, but are occasionally associated with transient anaemia in the mother or newborn. Note that there is no evidence of HPV B19 being associated with teratogenicity or developmental abnormalities.

DIAGNOSIS

Detection of IgM antibodies in maternal blood is diagnostic of recent infection, but because the window of IgM seropositivity is short (typically six weeks) IgM antibodies may have disappeared by the time fetal HPV B19 infection is suspected. Detection of IgM antibodies in the antenatal booking blood sample or demonstration of seroconversion since that sample was collected are also diagnostic.

Detection of IgM antibodies in fetal or neonatal blood is diagnostic of intrauterine infection, but is positive in fewer than 50% of cases. In IgM antibody negative cases where maternal infection has not been excluded, the fetal or neonatal blood should be tested for the presence of viral genome by polymerase chain reaction.

TREATMENT

There is no specific anti-viral therapy for HPV B19. Hydrops fetalis can usually be managed successfully by intrauterine transfusion. The prognosis after delivery is excellent.

LISTERIOSIS

Listeria monocytogenes is a Gram-positive bacillus that is ubiquitous in nature and thrives over a wide temperature range (including refrigeration temperatures). It is usually transmitted to man via food such as soft cheeses, pâtés, salads and poultry, but person to person transmission has been described in neonatal units. Only 30 to 40 pregnancy-associated cases of listeriosis are reported each year in the UK. Although still a rare condition, the incidence of listeriosis is higher in countries such as France and Belgium, where there is greater consumption of high risk foods.

Infection can occur at any time during pregnancy, but is most common in the third trimester. In most cases, the infant is infected by transplacental transmission following maternal bacteraemia, although transvaginal spread can probably also occur. Nosocomial spread of *L. monocytogenes* between infants can also occur. Pregnant women usually experience only a mild febrile illness. Neonatal listeriosis usually causes severe generalised sepsis, often with meningitis. The risk of severe morbidity or mortality may be as high as 60%. Occasionally, localised cutaneous or ocular infections are seen; these generally have a favourable outcome.

Diagnosis

Blood cultures collected from the mother and/or neonate are the mainstay of diagnosis of listeriosis. Other neonatal samples from which *L. monocytogenes* may be isolated include cerebrospinal fluid and skin swabs. Culture of other sites in the mother is rarely revealing. Serology is unhelpful in diagnosing listeriosis.

Treatment

L. monocytogenes is usually sensitive to a wide range of antibiotics, including amoxicillin, gentamicin and chloramphenicol, but importantly is resistant to cephalosporins. Amoxicillin, given together with gentamicin in order to obtain a synergistic bactericidal effect, is the treatment of choice for confirmed listeriosis.

CONGENITAL SYPHILIS

Syphilis is a sexually transmitted infection caused by the highly delicate spiral bacterium (spirochaete), *Treponema pallidum*. The incidence of syphilis in developed countries declined dramatically during the twentieth century. In England and Wales only 100-200 new cases are now diagnosed each year, whereas in the early 1900s 10% of adults had serological evidence of syphilis. However, syphilis remains common in many developing countries.

Without treatment, syphilis in adults runs a course over many years that is divided into a number of stages. A mother with untreated syphilis can infect her fetus. The risk of vertical transmission during the first year after infection is 80-90%, and diminishes rapidly thereafter until after four years transmission is rare. Without interventions, up to 50% of babies with congenital syphilis die *in utero* or post-natally. Symptomatic congenital syphilis in survivors is classified into early and late stages. Early congenital syphilis is a generalised infection that usually presents between 2 and 12 weeks of age with features such as rhinitis, skin rash and hepatosplenomegaly. Late congenital syphilis usually presents at age 6 to 14 years and is associated with local infection, affecting sites such as eyes, ears, bones and central nervous system. Lesions of early and late congenital syphilis heal to leave characteristic stigmata such as nasal, dental and bony deformities, blindness and deafness.

Diagnosis

Congenital syphilis may be diagnosed either by microscopic demonstration of spirochaetes in material from mucous membrane and skin lesions, or by serology. *T. pallidum* cannot be cultured *in vitro*. Maternal infection is usually diagnosed by serology because most pregnant women with untreated syphilis do not have clinical lesions. Dark ground or fluorescence microscopy is used to detect *T. pallidum*, because the bacteria are too slender to be visualised by light microscopy, even after staining.

There are two types of serological test. Non-treponemal tests (e.g. Venereal Disease Research Laboratory (VDRL), rapid plasma reagin (RPR)) measure antibody against a cardiolipin antigen that is not specific for *T. pallidum*. These tests are useful because the results tend to correlate with disease activity. Treponemal tests (e.g. *T. pallidum* haemagglutination assay (TPHA), fluorescent treponemal antibody absorbed test (FTA-ABS) and most enzyme immunoassays (EIAs)) measure specific anti-treponemal antibodies, but tend to remain positive for life. Some treponemal tests can be used to detect specific IgM. Newer EIAs are more reliable than the previous FTA-ABS IgM, and can be especially helpful in early confirmation of congenital syphilis. However, a single negative IgM result around the time of delivery does not exclude congenital infection; serological follow-up with standard non-treponemal and treponemal antibody tests, as well as repeat IgM testing, is always required.

TREATMENT

T. pallidum remains highly sensitive to penicillin, which is the treatment of choice for all types of syphilis. Treatment during the first and second trimesters of pregnancy is highly effective in preventing congenital syphilis, but it is less effective in later pregnancy. Unless it is certain that mothers with active syphilis have been adequately treated, their infants should be treated at birth. Treatment of infants of mothers who were treated before or during pregnancy is only indicated if serological or clinical evidence of infection is detected during follow-up.

INFECTIONS THAT ARE USUALLY ACQUIRED DURING OR AFTER DELIVERY

Potential neonatal pathogens that may be acquired from the mother at the time of delivery include both microorganisms that are regarded as commensals (e.g. group B streptococci and *E. coli*) and pathogens of the female genital tract (e.g. *Neisseria gonorrhoeae* and *Chlamydia trachomatis*). Vaginal delivery is also the time of highest risk of transmission of blood-borne viruses such as hepatitis B and HIV from mother to baby, although these infections can also be transmitted transplacentally and via breast milk. After delivery, neonates are at risk of infection with a wide variety of microorganisms that may be acquired inside or outside hospital.

Because neonatal infections rarely present with clinical features that are pathognomic of the causative microorganism, they are considered here both in terms of the infectious syndromes they may cause, and on an individual microorganism basis.

INFECTIOUS SYNDROMES IN NEONATES

EYE INFECTIONS

Sticky eyes are a common problem in neonates, and are not always caused by infection. *Staphylococcus aureus* is the most common cause of infective conjunctivitis in the newborn. Other bacteria, such as *Streptococcus pneumoniae* and *Haemophilus influenzae,* occasionally cause eye infections. Although uncommon, the sexually-transmitted pathogens *N. gonorrhoeae* and *C. trachomatis* are important causes of severe conjunctivitis, ophthalmia neonatorum. Gonococcal ophthalmia almost always develops within a week (usually 1-4 days) of delivery. Chlamydial ophthalmia usually has a longer incubation period, and may present at any time from 2-30 days after delivery. Occasionally, conjunctivitis during the neonatal period may be of viral origin.

INVESTIGATIONS

Mild conjunctivitis is usually self-limiting, and investigation is often not necessary. Swabs are recommended in all cases where antibiotic therapy is prescribed. Local laboratories will advise on procedures for investigating suspected gonococcal, chlamydial and viral infections. Bacteria seen in Gram stained preparations can be presumptively identified on the basis of their morphological appearance. Demonstration of inflammatory cells in the absence of bacteria is suggestive of a chlamydial or viral aetiology. Most bacteria that cause conjunctivitis can be cultured from clinical samples within 24 hours. The availability of results of testing for *C. trachomatis* will depend on individual laboratories' testing protocols. Viral cultures are usually maintained for at least three weeks.

TREATMENT

Mild conjunctivitis usually resolves without antimicrobial therapy. Topical treatment with chloramphenicol or gentamicin drops suffices for most cases of purulent conjunctivitis. Systemic antibiotic therapy is indicated for ophthalmia neonatorum (*see p.234*).

UMBILICAL CORD AND SKIN INFECTIONS

Infections of the umbilical cord stump occur quite frequently. *S. aureus* is the most common cause. Mixed infections with coliforms and anaerobic bacteria are also common, but usually respond to conservative management. The presence of flare or cellulitis around the umbilicus is suggestive of streptococcal infection.

Cutaneous infections are also common in neonates; *S. aureus* is again the main cause. The most common presentation is the appearance of small septic spots with little or no systemic upset. However, more invasive cutaneous infections such as cellulitis can also occur. Some strains of *S. aureus* are able to produce an exfoliative exotoxin that causes staphylococcal scalded skin syndrome (SSSS). This begins abruptly with fever and a scarlatiniform rash, and progresses rapidly to bullae, which slough off to leave red, raw skin. Outbreaks of SSSS in neonatal nurseries are now uncommon, but do still occur from time to time.

Candidiasis is often associated with napkin rash, and should be suspected where the rash is florid and confluent, involving the skin flexures.

INVESTIGATIONS

Swabs should be collected from the infected areas. If the skin is dry, the swab should be moistened first with sterile water or saline to enhance bacterial survival during transport to the laboratory. Gram staining of skin swabs is not usually helpful, because it is often impossible to distinguish between commensal and pathogenic bacteria, but may be of use in investigating suspected candidiasis. A preliminary culture result is usually available within 24 hours.

TREATMENT

Most infections are successfully treated topically. Antiseptics such as hexachlorophene and chlorhexidine are highly active against staphylococci. Topical nystatin or miconazole are recommended for candidiasis. Indications for systemic antibiotic therapy include widespread infection, cellulitis, and evidence of systemic upset. Flucloxacillin will suffice in most situations. Benzylpenicillin should be considered in addition if cellulitis is present (to improve cover against streptococci), or gentamicin if the patient is seriously unwell.

GASTROINTESTINAL TRACT INFECTIONS

These are now rare in neonates in developed countries. However, epidemic infantile diarrhoea due to enteropathogenic *E. coli* (EPEC) used to be a problem in neonatal nurseries, with a mortality rate of up to 50%. It remains a major cause of neonatal death in some developing countries. Nowadays, outbreaks of diarrhoea on neonatal units are more likely to be due to viruses, especially rotavirus. Infections with other gastrointestinal pathogens such as campylobacter, salmonella or shigella are rare, and virtually never occur in an outbreak setting.

INVESTIGATIONS

Microscopy is generally of little use in the investigation of diarrhoea in neonates. Stool samples should be cultured on a non-selective medium that supports growth of *E. coli*, as well as the usual selective media for salmonella, shigella and campylobacter. Samples should be tested routinely for rotavirus, usually by antigen detection. Electron microscopy may be helpful, especially if other causes of viral gastroenteritis are suspected.

TREATMENT

Fluid replacement is the mainstay of management of gastrointestinal tract infections. For most infections, antimicrobial therapy is either not available or of limited value. However, neonates with salmonellosis should always be treated, because they are at increased risk of invasive disease.

NECROTISING ENTEROCOLITIS

Necrotising enterocolitis (NEC) is a major cause of morbidity and mortality in low birth weight infants in neonatal units. The cause of NEC is unknown, but a number of factors may be important in causing the initial mucosal damage that culminates in necrosis of the bowel wall, including inadequate tissue oxygenation, enteral feeding, immaturity and bacterial overgrowth. Epidemics of NEC can occur in neonatal units, supporting the aetiological role of infection. Various pathogens have been associated with outbreaks of NEC. Usually these have been Enterobacteriaceae, although both *S. aureus* and coagulase-negative staphylococci have also been implicated. However, it is unclear whether there is a direct aetiological relationship, or whether abnormal bacterial gastrointestinal colonisation is a consequence of an already abnormal gastrointestinal tract. Whether or not bacteria are involved in the primary aetiological process, systemic bacterial infection as a result of translocation of bacteria across the abnormal bowel wall is common. Broad spectrum antibiotic therapy (such as penicillin, gentamicin and metronidazole) is routinely given to patients with NEC.

SERIOUS SYSTEMIC SEPSIS

Most serious systemic infections in term neonates without underlying disease present within the first few days of life, and are usually acquired from the maternal genital tract after the membranes have ruptured. Neonates receiving intensive care are susceptible to the same infections as any other neonate, and the spectrum of infections seen in the two groups during the first few days of life is similar. However, the longer the preterm neonate is in hospital, and the higher the level of intensive care, the more likely it is that it will become infected with hospital-acquired pathogens. Thus, the spectrum of microorganisms causing infection changes with increasing age, until after seven days almost all infections are nosocomial in origin. On this basis, infections in the preterm neonate undergoing intensive care are usually categorised as very early onset (within 24 hours of birth), early onset (1-7 days after birth), and late onset (more than seven days after birth) (Figure 12.4).

Bacterial and fungal infections in neonatal intensive care

Species	Typical species distribution (%) where the onset of infection is:		
	Very early (<24 hours)	Early (1-7 days)	Late (>7 days)
Group B streptococcus	30-50	10-15	5
E. coli	10-30	10-30	10-15
Streptococcus pneumoniae	5-10	0-5	0-5
Haemophilus influenzae	5-10	0-5	0-5
Staphylococcus aureus	5-10	0-5	-
Listeria monocytogenes	5	10-20	10-15
Enterococci	0-5	5-10	5-10
Enterobacter	-	-	5-10
Klebsiella	-	0-5	10-25
Coagulase-negative staphylococci	0-5	5-25	15-50
Candida	-	0-5	10-15

Figure 12.4 Pattern of bacterial and fungal infections in neonatal intensive care units

Early onset systemic infections usually present with signs of generalised sepsis (Figure 12.5), accompanied by septicaemia. Although patients may have an associated focus of infection, such as meningitis or pneumonia, localising signs are rarely seen because of the rapidly progressive nature of the illness.

Intravascular devices are an increasingly important source of late onset sepsis in neonatal units. Occasionally, these infections become disseminated, leading to infective endocarditis, or osteomyelitis in bone near the insertion site. Other possible foci of infection include the urinary tract, skin and gastrointestinal tract (especially associated with NEC). Late onset pneumonia is usually associated with mechanical ventilation and endotracheal tube colonisation, and is rarely accompanied by bacteraemia. Occasionally, late onset pneumonia is caused by congenitally acquired pathogens that have a long incubation period, especially *C. trachomatis.*

Clinical signs of systemic neonatal sepsis	
Decreased activity	Temperature instability
Respiratory distress	Irritability
Poor feeding	Lethargy
Apnoea	Jaundice
Hepatomegaly	Thrombocytopenia

Figure 12.5 Clinical signs of systemic neonatal sepsis

INVESTIGATIONS

It is important to consider the possibility of infection in any unwell neonate, because the clinical presentation is often non-specific, and untreated infections in neonates can be rapidly progressive. In addition to microbiological investigations to demonstrate the aetiologic agent, a variety of other laboratory tests can provide circumstantial evidence of infection. These are important because results are available within minutes or hours, compared with a day or more for most microbiological investigations. They are also useful in assessing the possible significance of isolates from infants on neonatal units, where the microorganisms that are common pathogens (especially coagulase-negative staphylococci) are also commonly seen as commensals or contaminants. Neonatal infection can sometimes be the initial presentation of metabolic or haematological disorders. Investigations for these conditions should be considered where infection is of unusual severity and/or due to an uncommon pathogen (*see Chapters 10 and 11*).

Microbiological investigations

Blood cultures are mandatory in the investigation of any unwell neonate. Blood culture media specially formulated for paediatric use are recommended. These are designed to support the growth of common paediatric pathogens and to cope with relatively small blood volumes. Because anaerobic bacteraemia is very uncommon in infants, anaerobic blood cultures are rarely necessary. Although blood cultures are usually maintained in the laboratory for 5-7 days, at least 90% of isolates are detected within the first 48 hours. Examination of CSF is desirable in all neonates with suspected systemic sepsis. However, it is now common practice to await the results of blood cultures, and perform lumbar puncture only on infants with bacteraemia. The interpretation of the results of CSF analyses can be difficult in neonates. During the first week of life the white cell count may be as high as 32 cells/mm^3, and it only gradually decreases thereafter. Both the normal CSF protein concentration and CSF:blood glucose ratio may also be considerably higher than in adults. Endotracheal tube aspirates from neonates who are ventilated should be collected for microscopy and culture. Nasopharyngeal aspirates (NPAs) are of limited value in investigating suspected bacterial or fungal infection, because the upper respiratory tract flora may not be representative of that in the lower respiratory tract. However, virological testing of NPAs is occasionally useful, especially during the winter months when respiratory viruses are most prevalent. Urinary tract infection is diagnosed by microscopic examination and culture of urine. Leucocytes may appear in neonates' urine in a number of other conditions, including hypoxia. Occasionally, the differential diagnosis of neonatal sepsis will include congenital infections such as CMV or toxoplasmosis (*see p.217 & 219*).

Some neonatal units undertake routine surveillance cultures in which samples are examined, usually at regular intervals, regardless of the clinical condition of the infant. Samples used in surveillance cultures include swabs from superficial sites (e.g. ear, nose, skin, rectum), gastric aspirates at the time of birth, and nasopharyngeal or endotracheal tube aspirates. The principle of surveillance cultures is that knowledge of the resident microbial flora of the infant can be used to direct the choice of antibiotic therapy in the event that systemic infection occurs; however, the value of this approach is uncertain. The use of antibiotic therapy to eradicate potential pathogens detected in surveillance cultures in order to prevent systemic infections is sometimes advocated, although this practice is controversial.

Other laboratory investigations

Non-specific changes may be found in various haematological and biochemical parameters (Figure 12.6). Measurement of early inflammatory mediators may provide more direct evidence that sepsis is present or absent. The most readily available is C-reactive protein (CRP). CRP measurement at the time of presentation is poorly predictive of infection, but two normal CRP concentrations (<10 mg/L) on samples taken 24 hours apart between 8 and 48 hours after presentation reliably excludes bacterial or fungal infection. Of the many other markers that have been studied, the two that appear to offer most promise are interleukin-6 (IL-6) and procalcitonin (PCT). Several studies suggest that both offer sensitivities and specificities of around 90% for the detection of sepsis, although, as with CRP, the best predictive values are obtained from serial measurements.

Laboratory parameters in neonates with systemic sepsis	
Haematological	Neutropenia or neutrophilia Increased immature:total neutrophil ratio Thrombocytopenia Deranged clotting
Biochemical	Hyperglycaemia or hypoglycaemia Congenital hyperbilirubinaemia Deranged liver function tests Elevated C-reactive protein

Figure 12.6 Changes in haematological and biochemical parameters in neonates with systemic sepsis

TREATMENT

The most widely used antibiotic therapy for early onset serious neonatal sepsis is penicillin, ampicillin or amoxicillin, together with an aminoglycoside such as gentamicin. Alternatively, ampicillin or amoxicillin may be combined with cefotaxime to provide similar cover without the risk of aminoglycoside toxicity. However, widespread use of cephalosporins on neonatal units may lead to the emergence and spread of *Enterobacter* and similar cephalosporinase-producing bacteria as troublesome pathogens.

The choice of antibiotics for late onset neonatal sepsis should take account of local antibiotic resistance patterns and the individual patient's previous microbiology results and antibiotic therapy. Broad-spectrum cover is required, encompassing Gram-negative bacteria, streptococci and *Staphylococcus aureus*. Cefuroxime or cefotaxime together with an aminoglycoside are commonly used antibiotic choices that provide better activity against Gram-negative bacteria than the regimens recommended for early onset sepsis. Giving an aminoglycoside along with the cephalosporin also minimises the risk of selection of resistant bacteria.

In all cases of serious neonatal sepsis, empirical antibiotic therapy should be reviewed once the results of microbiological investigations become available. When cultures are positive, treatment may need to be altered because of unexpected antibiotic resistance, or to optimise antibiotic delivery to the site of infection. When cultures are negative, cessation of antibiotic therapy should be considered.

BACTERIAL AND FUNGAL PATHOGENS OF NEONATES

GROUP B STREPTOCOCCUS (*STREPTOCOCCUS AGALACTIAE*)

Group B streptococci (GBS) are common commensals of the gastrointestinal and female genital tracts. Reported maternal colonisation rates range from 2% to 40%, with some of the highest incidences being reported from the USA and Australia. Carriage rates in the UK have usually been found to be 5% to 10%. Although GBS rarely cause clinically significant infections outside the neonatal period, they are the most common serious neonatal pathogen in most developed countries.

The risk of mother to baby transmission of GBS is around 50%. The vast majority of infants who acquire GBS are asymptomatically colonised, while a few develop mild infections of superficial sites such as the umbilical stump and conjunctivae. The risk of serious GBS sepsis in an infant born to a mother who is a GBS carrier is 1%. Neonatal GBS sepsis is classified as early onset (within the first six days after delivery) or late onset (seven or more days after delivery). Most early cases present within 24 hours of delivery with overwhelming generalised sepsis, sometimes accompanied by meningitis. Late onset disease is uncommon and is more often focal, meningitis being the most common manifestation.

GBS infections require aggressive antimicrobial therapy. GBS remain universally sensitive to penicillins, and penicillin, ampicillin or amoxicillin, combined with an aminoglycoside such as gentamicin in order to achieve a synergistic effect, remains the treatment of choice on many units. GBS are also sensitive to cephalosporins, such as cefotaxime, and to chloramphenicol.

STAPHYLOCOCCUS AUREUS

S. aureus is carried by 20-40% of the general adult population, and by up to 70% of health care workers. Carriage sites include the skin, nose and upper respiratory tract. Many neonates become colonised in the first few days of life from their mothers, health care staff or other infants in hospital. Colonisation is often asymptomatic, but infections (usually mild) of the umbilicus, skin and eyes are also common. *S. aureus* is one of the most important causes of bacteraemia in neonatal units. Bacteraemia is almost always related to a primary focus of infection, such as an intravascular device, pneumonia, osteomyelitis or infective endocarditis. Without aggressive and prolonged treatment, infections can become disseminated and/or recur.

Although almost all *S. aureus* are now penicillin-resistant, most strains remain sensitive to a wide range of other antibiotics, including flucloxacillin, gentamicin, erythromycin, vancomycin, and cephalosporins such as cefuroxime and cefotaxime. Fusidic acid is useful for treating deep-seated *S. aureus* infections because of its excellent penetration into bone and pus. However, it must always be given along with another antibiotic to prevent the emergence of resistance during therapy. MRSA (methicillin-resistant *S. aureus*) are strains of *S. aureus* that are resistant to methicillin and other β-lactam antibiotics, including flucloxacillin, and often to several other classes of antibiotics. However, they do remain sensitive to some antibiotics, most reliably the glycopeptides vancomycin and teicoplanin.

COAGULASE-NEGATIVE STAPHYLOCOCCI

Coagulase-negative staphylococci (CNS) comprise a number of *Staphylococcus* species that are easily distinguished from *S. aureus* by the absence of a coagulase enzyme. CNS are highly ubiquitous, and generally of low virulence. However, they are important opportunistic pathogens in neonatal intensive care units. Infections are particularly associated with prosthetic devices such as intravascular catheters, endotracheal tubes and CSF shunts; some strains produce an extracellular mucoid substance (glycocalyx) that promotes adherence of bacteria to synthetic polymers. It can be difficult to distinguish between true infection and colonisation because CNS often constitute the predominant surface flora of neonates.

CNS causing hospital-acquired infections are usually multiply antibiotic-resistant, and treatment often necessitates use of a glycopeptide antibiotic such as vancomycin or teicoplanin.

ENTEROCOCCI

Enterococci are another increasingly important cause of opportunistic infections. Their ability to survive for prolonged periods in the environment and their resistance to many commonly used antibiotics (including flucloxacillin and the cephalosporins) contribute to their success as nosocomial pathogens. Early onset neonatal sepsis is occasionally seen, where the infection is acquired from the maternal genital tract. However, enterococci are more important as a cause of hospital-acquired late onset neonatal sepsis, usually against a background of recent or current antibiotic exposure. Enterococcal infections can be treated with amoxicillin or ampicillin, or with a glycopeptide antibiotic such as vancomycin. An aminoglycoside antibiotic such as gentamicin is sometimes added in order to obtain a synergistic effect. Up to 50% of enterococci are resistant to amoxicillin and ampicillin. Enterococci that are also resistant to vancomycin have emerged as important pathogens in some hospitals (although not usually in neonatal intensive care units). Infections with vancomycin-resistant enterococci are difficult to treat, and rigorous infection control measures are required to prevent spread.

ENTEROBACTERIACEAE (*E. COLI, KLEBSIELLA, ENTEROBACTER*)

The Enterobacteriaceae are a large family of Gram-negative bacteria often referred to in the UK as coliforms, because the gastrointestinal tracts of humans and animals are the normal habitats of many species. However, coliforms also survive well in moist environments. *Escherichia coli* is the most common species found in humans. It is the second commonest cause of early onset serious neonatal sepsis after GBS, and is the most common cause of urinary tract infection. Enteropathogenic *E. coli* (EPEC) are strains that possess a unique virulence factor that causes diarrhoea in infants. In western countries, serious outbreaks of infection with these strains in neonatal nurseries are now rare, but they remain an important cause of morbidity and mortality in developing countries. *E. coli* is also an important cause of late onset hospital-acquired neonatal sepsis such as bacteraemia and ventilator-associated pneumonia. Other coliforms, such as *Enterobacter* and *Klebsiella*, are mainly hospital-acquired pathogens.

All coliforms are now frequently resistant to commonly used antibiotics such as amoxicillin and trimethoprim. *E. coli* and *Klebsiella* are usually sensitive to cephalosporins such as cefuroxime or cefotaxime, and aminoglycosides such as gentamicin or netilmicin. *Enterobacter* species commonly produce broad-spectrum β-lactamases (cephalosporinases) that hydrolyse cephalosporins as well as penicillins such as amoxicillin. It is important to note that these enzymes may not be detected by routine antibiotic susceptibility testing, so that strains may falsely appear to be cephalosporin-sensitive. Strains of *Klebsiella* and even *E. coli* that possess similar enzymes are also now emerging. There have been many reports of large-scale use of cephalosporins as monotherapy in neonatal units being followed by outbreaks of infection with cephalosporinase-producing coliforms, most notoriously *Enterobacter* species.

PSEUDOMONAS AERUGINOSA

P. aeruginosa is resistant to many commonly used antibiotics and disinfectants and is commonly found in moist environments. Infections range from mild to severe, and antibiotic choices are often severely restricted. Antipseudomonal antibiotics include aminoglycosides (such as gentamicin), ceftazidime, imipenem and ciprofloxacin (not licensed for general use in children). Although sporadic pseudomonas infections may occur in neonatal units, the main importance of *P. aeruginosa* is as a cause of outbreaks of infection. In such situations, an environmental source should be sought, although health care workers' hands have been implicated in some outbreaks.

NEISSERIA GONORRHOEAE

Gonorrhoea is a sexually transmitted infection of adults. In women, gonorrhoea causes cervicitis; however, at least 50% of infections are asymptomatic. Conjunctivitis (ophthalmia neonatorum) is the most common manifestation of neonatal gonococcal infection. The conjunctivitis is often severe and, without treatment, can lead to blindness owing to corneal ulceration and scarring. Infections of other sites, including septicaemia, pneumonia and arthritis, are very uncommon in neonates.

Because *N. gonorrhoeae* is highly susceptible to drying and cooling, swabs should ideally be plated directly onto culture media. Where this is impractical a non-nutritive transport medium such as Stuart's or Amie's should be used. For isolation of *N. gonorrhoeae,* specialised culture media are required that are both highly enriched and contain selective agents to suppress the growth of competing flora. It is important that the identity of presumptive *N. gonorrhoeae* is confirmed, usually by biochemical testing.

An injectable cephalosporin such as cefuroxime or cefotaxime is the usual empiric therapy for neonatal infections, because significant numbers of strains of *N. gonorrhoeae* are now penicillin-resistant.

CHLAMYDIA TRACHOMATIS

Chlamydiae are Gram-negative bacteria that are obligate intracellular pathogens. *C. trachomatis* survives poorly outside the body, so that exacting specimen transport and storage conditions are required to ensure the viability of organisms in clinical samples. The organism can only be cultured *in vitro* in cell culture, a technique that is not widely available.

C. trachomatis is now much the most common bacterial sexually transmitted disease in most developed countries. Like gonorrhoea, chlamydial genital tract infection in women is frequently asymptomatic. Purulent conjunctivitis is the most common presentation of *C. trachomatis* infection in neonates. Untreated chlamydial ophthalmia does not appear to cause permanent ocular damage, but symptoms can persist for many months. *C. trachomatis* can also cause an interstitial pneumonia. This usually presents at 4 to 6 weeks of age, with gradual onset dyspnoea, but usually no fever and little or no cough. Up to half of patients with untreated chlamydial ophthalmia may subsequently develop pneumonia, but pneumonia is not always preceded by conjunctivitis.

Culture of *C. trachomatis* has largely been superseded by diagnostic techniques that are not dependent on maintaining the viability of the bacteria. Originally, methods based on detection of chlamydial antigens were used, including direct immunofluorescence and enzyme-linked immunosorbent assay (ELISA). These in turn are now being replaced by molecular techniques such as polymerase chain reaction (PCR) or ligase chain reaction (LCR).

Neonatal chlamydial infection should always be treated with a systemic antibiotic such as erythromycin. In ophthalmia neonatorum, topical tetracycline can be given in conjunction.

MYCOPLASMA AND UREAPLASMA

Mycoplasmas are small, highly fastidious, cell wall deficient bacteria that can only be cultured using specialised techniques. In humans, mycoplasmas are found in the respiratory and genital tracts. Genital tract mycoplasmas include *Ureaplasma urealyticum* as well as various *Mycoplasma* species. *U. urealyticum* is the species most commonly implicated in neonatal infections. It may be carried by up to 80% of women, and transient surface colonisation of neonates is, therefore, common. Respiratory tract colonisation is increased in infants with a gestational age of less than 36 weeks, and is probably acquired *in utero* rather than at the time of delivery. There is evidence that congenital pneumonia due to *U. urealyticum* is a risk factor for chronic lung disease in low birth weight neonates that is independent of gestational age. There is some evidence that early treatment with erythromycin may prevent the development of chronic lung disease.

FUNGAL INFECTIONS

Candida infections of flexures are not uncommon in infants. Neonates receiving intensive care are at risk of systemic fungal infections. Infection rates of up to 5% have been reported in very low birth weight babies in some centres. The most important risk factors are prior broad-spectrum antibiotic therapy, hyperglycaemia, parenteral nutrition and the presence of indwelling devices. Yeasts, especially *Candida* species, account for almost all systemic fungal infections in neonates. Neonates with systemic fungal infections have a high mortality rate, but systemic fungal infection is often simply the final event in a progressive clinical deterioration.

Culture of fungi from blood cultures or other specimens from deep tissues and organs provides definitive evidence of systemic fungal infection. However, fungi are often difficult or impossible to isolate from clinical material, so that infections are often diagnosed late. Sometimes anti-fungal therapy has to be started empirically for patients who have risk factors for invasive fungal infection and evidence of sepsis that has not responded to anti-bacterial therapy.

Superficial candidiasis can usually be treated with topical agents. There is an increasing number of anti-fungal drugs for systemic fungal infections, and microbiological advice on treatment should always be sought. Initial treatment is usually with intravenous fluconazole or amphotericin. Fluconazole is less toxic and easier to administer than even liposome-based preparations of amphotericin. In infections with fungi that are sensitive to both agents they appear to have comparable efficacy. However, fluconazole has a narrower spectrum of activity than amphotericin; it is inactive against some yeasts, and has no useful activity against many other groups of fungi, including *Aspergillus* species.

VIRAL INFECTIONS OF NEONATES

HERPES SIMPLEX VIRUSES

Two types of herpes simplex virus (HSV) cause mucocutaneous herpes in humans. HSV-I is mainly associated with orolabial herpes and HSV-II with genital herpes, although this demarcation is not absolute. After primary infection with HSV the infection usually becomes latent, and may later reactivate.

HSV are transmitted by close contact. Infections in neonates are usually acquired perinatally from the maternal genital tract. Occasionally, infections may be transmitted postnatally from orolabial herpes in the mother or another person. Intrauterine infections are very rare, but may cause fetal death.

The risk of serious neonatal infection is greatest if the mother has active lesions of a primary herpes infection at the time of vaginal delivery. Where the mother has had a previous primary infection the baby will be protected by passive immunity; serious infections in these neonates are uncommon, even if the mother has active recurrent disease at the time of delivery. The most serious form of neonatal HSV infection is disseminated disease, where the virus is found in many organs, including the brain, liver and skin. Infants may also present with localised neurological or mucocutaneous disease.

Recurrent genital herpes can usually be diagnosed clinically, without recourse to laboratory tests. Culture of HSV is easier than for many other viruses, but results may take several days, and low numbers of viruses present in samples such as CSF may not be detected. Rapid techniques for direct detection of HSV in clinical material, such as immunofluorescence or electron microscopy, may be useful for examination of samples from skin lesions and other tissues that are likely to contain a large number of virus particles. Amplification of viral genome by PCR may be the most sensitive method of detecting HSV in CSF.

Aciclovir is the drug most commonly used to treat infections with HSV. However, even with treatment, serious neonatal herpes infection is associated with a high rate of major morbidity and mortality.

VARICELLA ZOSTER VIRUS

Chickenpox is the result of primary infection with varicella zoster virus (VZV). Like other herpes viruses, VZV may persist in the body after recovery from chickenpox, and reactivate as shingles months or years after the original infection. Chickenpox is highly transmissible by both the respiratory route and direct contact with the rash; patients are infectious from 48 hours before the rash appears. Shingles is much less infectious than chickenpox, and is generally transmitted only by direct contact with the rash. In western countries, chickenpox is very common in children, and around 90% of adults are immune. Neonates whose mothers have previously had chickenpox will normally be protected by passive immunity unless they are very premature.

Chickenpox tends to be more severe in adults than in children, and as with any other serious systemic infection, there is a risk that a pregnancy may be lost when a woman develops chickenpox. Chickenpox during the first trimester also carries a small risk (less than 3%) of fetal malformation (congenital varicella syndrome). The other time of high risk to the baby from chickenpox is the immediate postnatal period. Neonates who develop chickenpox are highly vulnerable to severe disseminated infection, especially during the first week of life. A neonate may acquire chickenpox if the mother develops chickenpox (but not shingles) around the time of delivery (when there will be no opportunity for transfer of passive immunity), or if it has significant exposure to another person with chickenpox or shingles and has no passive immunity.

It is often easy to diagnosis chickenpox and shingles on clinical grounds alone. In cases of doubt, the virus may be detected in vesicle fluid by immunofluorescence or electron microscopy for rapid confirmation, or by culture. Serological diagnosis is of little help in diagnosing chickenpox, because of the unreliability of methods for detection of IgM. The main role for serology is in determining whether or not contacts of a case of chickenpox are immune.

Because of the high morbidity and mortality associated with chickenpox during pregnancy and in the neonatal period, passive immunisation with varicella zoster specific immunoglobulin (VZIG) should be offered to non-immune pregnant women and neonates who have had significant contact with chickenpox or shingles. VZIG is most effective at modifying or preventing disease when it is given within 72 hours of exposure. However, it may attenuate an attack even when given up to ten days after exposure. The recommended dose of VZIG for neonates is 250 mg (one vial) administered by intramuscular injection.

Neonates who develop chickenpox should be treated with aciclovir as soon as possible.

HEPATITIS B

Hepatitis B virus has three important antigens, HbsAg, HbcAg and HBeAg. HbsAg and HBeAg, together with the antibodies formed against the three main antigens, are used, along with detection of viral DNA, as markers of the various stages of hepatitis B infection (Figure 12.7).

Significance of serological markers of hepatitis B	
Marker	**Significance**
HbsAg	Acute or chronic hepatitis B
Anti-HBs	Immunity to hepatitis B
Anti-HBc (total)	Past or current hepatitis B
Anti-HBc (IgM)	High titre: acute infection Low titre: chronic infection
HbeAg	Active viral replication High infectivity
Anti-Hbe	Low infectivity
HBV DNA polymerase	Active viral replication
HBV DNA	Active viral replication Infectivity depends on viral load

Figure 12.7 Significance of serological markers of hepatitis B

Following infection, a significant proportion of individuals fail to eliminate the virus and so become carriers. Not only do carriers represent an infectious risk to others, but they are at risk of developing serious long-term sequelae, including chronic hepatitis, cirrhosis and hepatocellular carcinoma.

Hepatitis B is hyperendemic in south-east Asia and parts of Africa, where up to 90% of the population is infected. Vertical transmission from carrier mothers to their infants is the major route of infection in these areas. In areas of low endemnicity (including northern Europe and North America), less than 10% of the population has been exposed to infection, and fewer than 1% are carriers. The most common routes of infection in these countries are sexual contact or drug abuse. However, carriage rates in immigrant women tend to parallel rates in their countries of origin.

Without interventions, the risk of vertical transmission from a mother who is a hepatitis B carrier depends on her HBeAg and anti-HBe status. Where the mother is HBeAg positive, the risk is greater than 90%, compared with around 10% where she is negative for both HBeAg and antibody to HBeAg (anti-Hbe), and less than 5% when the mother possesses anti-HBe. Most neonatal infections are perinatally acquired, with intrauterine infections accounting for fewer than 5% of cases. Whereas the majority of infected neonates become HbsAg positive without developing clinical hepatitis, up to 90% may become chronic carriers.

In the UK, all pregnant women are screened for hepatitis B infection by testing for HbsAg. Reactive sera then undergo further testing (including HBeAg and anti-HBe) in order to ascertain the infectivity of the woman. Babies born to HBsAg-positive mothers are protected by immunisation. In addition, those whose mothers have high infectivity (that is those who are HBeAg positive, HBsAg positive without e markers, or who have had acute hepatitis B during pregnancy) are given hepatitis B immunoglobulin (HBIG) at birth (Figure 12.8). Mothers infected with hepatitis B may breast feed, provided that their babies have been appropriately immunised. Although immunisation gives over 95% protection, infants should be tested for serological evidence of hepatitis B infection at intervals during at least the first year of life.

Immunisation policy for newborns of HBsAg-positive mothers
1st dose vaccine: at birth (+ HBIG 200 IU* if indicated)
2nd dose: at 1 month
3rd dose: at 2 months
4th dose: at 1 year
*Note that this is a higher dose than is recommended in some other countries

Figure 12.8 Recommended immunisation policy for newborns of HBsAg-positive mothers in the UK

HEPATITIS C

Hepatitis C is another blood-borne viral hepatitis. The seroprevalence in the general UK population is around 0.01%, but is higher in some southern European countries. Acute infection is usually a subclinical illness, but up to 80% of patients progress to chronic liver disease. Mother to infant transmission of hepatitis C occurs relatively infrequently (well under 10% in most studies), but high maternal viral load and co-infection with HIV are important risk factors. No interventions are routinely employed to prevent vertical transmission of hepatitis C. Infants born to mothers infected with hepatitis C require serological follow-up; persistence of anti-hepatitis C antibodies and/or detection of viral genome by PCR are diagnostic of infection.

HIV

Mother to infant transmission now accounts for almost all paediatric HIV infection. The prevalence of HIV infection in pregnant women in most of the UK remains at around 0.01%, but is significantly higher in London. Because fewer than half of HIV-infected pregnant women have been previously diagnosed, antenatal HIV screening is now offered to all women. Interventions reduce the risk of mother to infant transmission from 30-50% to 2-3% or less. The most important preventative measure is anti-retroviral treatment for the mother and neonate. The mother should receive highly active anti-retroviral therapy (HAART) with the aim of suppressing her plasma viral load to undetectable levels. Neonates born to HIV-positive mothers should receive anti-retroviral therapy (usually with zidovudine). Delivery by caesarean section reduces the vertical transmission rate, but may not be necessary where the maternal viral load is undetectable. HIV-positive mothers in developed countries should not breast feed, but in developing countries the benefits of breast feeding probably outweigh the risk of HIV transmission.

HIV-infected infants tend to have high viral loads and progress rapidly to symptomatic disease. They may then present with non-specific symptoms and signs such as failure to thrive, diarrhoea, anaemia, lymphadenopathy and hepatosplenomegaly. Alternatively, they may present with an unusually severe episode of infection with a recognised neonatal pathogen such as candida, cytomegalovirus or herpes simplex virus, or with an opportunistic infection such as *Pneumocystis carinii* pneumonia.

Maternal infection is diagnosed by detection of anti-HIV antibodies, with appropriate confirmatory testing. Monitoring of viral load in sero-positive individuals is used to optimise therapy. Antibody tests are of limited value in diagnosing HIV infection in infants because passively transferred anti-HIV antibodies remain detectable for up to 18 months. Infected infants usually mount an antibody response after 3-4 months, when IgA (and sometimes IgM) anti-HIV may be detected. However, infants whose HIV infection is rapidly progressive may never produce detectable antibodies. Because of the limitations of serology, early diagnosis of HIV infection depends heavily on direct detection of HIV components (p24 antigen, or viral nucleic acid) in the infant's blood. Testing schedules, and results interpretation, are shown in Figures 12.9 and 12.10.

Testing schedule for infants born to HIV-positive mothers	
Timing of sample	**Rationale**
Around the time of birth (*not* cord blood)	May permit detection of infections that have been acquired *in utero*
1 month	Many perinatally acquired infections are diagnosable by this stage
3 months	Most infections are diagnosable by this stage
6 months	If tests remain negative at this stage HIV infection is very unlikely
12 months	Anti-HIV reactivity should be reduced or absent in the uninfected child
18 months	Most uninfected children will have lost anti-HIV by this stage
≥ 2 years	To exclude possibility of delayed HIV infection (e.g. due to breast feeding)

Figure 12.9 Recommended testing schedule for infants born to HIV-positive mothers

HIV diagnostic criteria
HIV infected
In *two* specimens collected on different dates, detection of *two or more* of:
HIV proviral DNA
HIV viral RNA
HIV p24 Ag
Anti-HIV Abs at >18 months of age
HIV uninfected
Absence of reactivity in any tests for HIV infection in at least *two* specimens collected at least one month apart, the former at age ≥ 3 months, and the latter at age ≥ 6 months.
HIV indeterminate
Failure to fulfil either of the above criteria

Figure 12.10 HIV diagnostic criteria

ENTEROVIRUSES

Enteroviruses are small RNA viruses that include polio viruses and hepatitis A virus. In neonates, other enteroviruses, coxsackie B and echoviruses can cause infections that range in severity from mild subclinical illness to fatal overwhelming infections. Mother to infant transmission can occur, but the main hazard is nosocomial transmission leading to outbreaks in neonatal nurseries. Manifestations include rapid onset circulatory collapse, fulminant liver failure and meningitis or meningoencephalitis.

FURTHER READING

British HIV Association. http://www.bhiva.org.

Crowcroft NS, Roth CE, Cohen BJ, Miller E. Guidance for control of parvovirus B19 infection in healthcare settings and the community. J Public Health Med 1999; **21:** 439-46.

Jenson HB, Baltimore RS (Eds). Pediatric infectious diseases. Principles and practice, 2nd edn. Philadelphia: WB Saunders, 2002.

McCartney AC. Prevention of early onset neonatal group B streptococcal infection. J Med Screen 2001; **8:** 170-2.

Remington JS, Klein JO (Eds). Infectious diseases of the fetus and newborn infant, 5th edn. Philadelphia: WB Saunders, 2001.

Shaw IM. Viral infections of the fetus and neonate. London: Jones-Sands, 1998.

Chapter 13

Infection control

INTRODUCTION

The neonatal unit (NNU) presents many challenges for infection control. Not only do the patients share all the risk factors for infection of any other group of patients receiving intensive care, but they are also uniquely microbiologically and immunologically naïve. Before admission to the NNU, a neonate will only have been exposed to a few different microorganisms, mostly from the mother's genital tract. By definition, any microorganism that a neonate acquires after delivery must be hospital-acquired. Almost all infections acquired at the time of delivery present in the first few days of life, with the proportion that are hospital-acquired increasing with age (*see Chapter 12*). On this basis, infections are categorised as very early onset (within 24 hours of birth, and always of maternal origin), early onset (1-7 days after birth), and late onset (more than 7 days after birth, and almost always hospital-acquired). Microorganisms may be acquired on the delivery suite or NNU from the environment, other patients, staff, family and other visitors.

ORGANISATION OF INFECTION CONTROL

In the UK, all hospitals are required to have an Infection Control Team (ICT), which is responsible for day to day management of infection control. The members of the ICT are consultant microbiologists (one of whom is designated the Infection Control Doctor), and Infection Control Nurses. Many NNUs have identified one or more Infection Control Link Nurses, who act as a resource and role model for colleagues alongside their regular nursing duties on the unit. There should be close liaison between NNU staff and the ICT, which is best achieved by regular visits to the unit by members of the Team. As well as providing advice on good practice, and monitoring compliance with policies and procedures, the ICT should undertake infection surveillance, so that trends in infection can be identified and acted upon if necessary. The most widely used system is laboratory-based surveillance of clinically important neonatal pathogens that may cause outbreaks of infection, such as *Staphylococcus aureus* and Gram-negative bacteria.

BASIC REQUIREMENTS FOR INFECTION CONTROL

High standards of infection control are dependent on certain basic requirements in the design and operation of the NNU. These include:

- induction and update training for all staff in infection control
- adequate hand-washing facilities
- adequate space between cots
- adequate isolation facilities for infected patients; cubicles that are mechanically ventilated should be under negative air pressure
- clinical areas designed to be easy to clean
- schedule of regular and thorough cleaning
- medical equipment and consumables kept at the cot side restricted to the minimum required for that patient
- no reuse of medical equipment intended for single use only
- reusable medical equipment decontaminated according to manufacturers' recommendations
- restrictions on visitors with transmissible infections
- policies for microbiological screening and/or isolation of patients readmitted from the community or transferred from other hospitals.

MANAGEMENT OF INFECTIOUS CASES

The infectious case may be a patient, a member of staff, a family member, or another visitor. There are two broad management considerations:

- infection control precautions are required to prevent spread of infection from the case. These should be based on an understanding of the risks and routes of transmission of the infection (Figure 13.1)
- there must be recognition that individuals who were contacts of the case before infection control precautions were implemented may be at risk of infection.

RECOMMENDED INFECTION CONTROL PRECAUTIONS FOR IMPORTANT NEONATAL INFECTIONS

STAPHYLOCOCCUS AUREUS

S. aureus is the most common hospital-acquired neonatal pathogen. For this reason, many centres routinely apply antiseptic dusting powder prophylactically to sites such as the cord stump and skin flexures that are common sites of colonisation. Two preparations are available: hexachlorophene, which has proved to be dependable over many years, despite the theoretical risk of toxicity due to systemic absorption, and chlorhexidine, with which there is much less experience.

Controversy surrounds the efficacy and cost-effectiveness of routine anti-staphylococcal prophylaxis; however, in our experience, prophylaxis reduces the incidence of clinical infections with *S. aureus* by around 50%.

Prevention of spread of infection from an infected patient

Measure	Required for	May not be required for
Isolation of patients(s) in a single room*	Infections that may be spread by the airborne route, are associated with environmental contamination, or are highly transmissible by other routes	Infections that are only transmitted by direct contact with blood or other body fluids
Enhanced hand washing	Frequent and thorough hand washing is required for all infections. Consider using antiseptics instead of soap and water for infections where hand contamination is likely, and during outbreaks of infection	
Wearing of protective clothing (gloves, aprons) whenever entering cubicle	Infections that are associated with environmental contamination	Infections that are transmitted only by close contact
Wearing of protective clothing for direct contact with patient	Infections that are transmitted only by close contact	
Use of dedicated equipment for infected patients	All infections, where practicable: especially important for infections associated with environmental contamination, and for equipment that is difficult to clean	
Enhanced daily cleaning of the patient's bedspace	All infections: especially important for infections that are associated with environmental contamination	
Thorough final cleaning of the vacated bedspace	All infections: especially important for infections that are associated with environmental contamination	

*Where more than one patient has the same infection it may be more convenient to isolate them as a cohort

Figure 13.1 Measures used to prevent spread of infection from an infected patient

Some strains of *S. aureus* have particular properties that justify additional infection control precautions. The two most important are methicillin-resistant *S. aureus* (MRSA) and *S. aureus* that produce toxins that are the cause of staphylococcal scalded skin syndrome. Without infection control measures, such strains can spread rapidly from patient to patient.

MRSA

Routes of nosocomial transmission Directly from person to person, or indirectly via contaminated equipment or the environment. Individuals encountering MRSA may develop infection, or may become asymptomatically colonised at sites such as the nose, throat and skin. Anyone carrying MRSA, whether colonised or infected, may be the source of spread of the bacterium. In units with a high prevalence of MRSA, colonised or infected patients are the main reservoirs of the bacterium, whereas in units where MRSA is not endemic, colonised staff members are more important. For this reason, all staff on our NNU are screened for MRSA on commencement of employment.
Incubation period Variable.
Period of infectivity Carriers are considered to be infectious until three sets of negative swabs at least one week apart, and whilst off all antimicrobial treatment, have been obtained.
Control measures (infected or colonised patient) Isolation in a single cubicle. Gloves and apron on entering cubicle. Topical therapy to eradicate carriage.
Control measures (infected or colonised healthcare worker) Topical therapy to eradicate carriage. Consider excluding from work until MRSA-negative.
Control measures (infected or colonised visitor) Discourage MRSA-positive individuals, who are not close family members, from visiting. Isolate neonates if an MRSA-positive family member is visiting (high risk that the neonate will become colonised). MRSA-positive visitors must go directly to and from the infant's isolation cubicle.
Control measures (contacts of a case) Consider screening patient contacts. Investigation of other contacts not usually required.

Staphylococcal scalded skin syndrome

Routes of nosocomial transmission Directly from person to person, or indirectly via contaminated equipment or the environment. Source individual may be symptomatic, or an asymptomatic carrier.
Incubation period Variable, usually 2-7 days.
Period of infectivity Until carriage has been eliminated.
Control measures (infected or colonised patient) Isolation in a single cubicle. Gloves and apron on entering cubicle. Antibiotic therapy also reduces infectivity.
Control measures (infected or colonised healthcare worker) Often not identified,

but if so give topical therapy to eradicate carriage. Consider excluding from work.
Control measures (infected or colonised visitor) Not usually identified.
Control measures (contacts of a case) Measures not usually required.

HERPES SIMPLEX VIRUSES

Routes of nosocomial transmission Direct spread from person to person. Type I virus is usually spread by contact with saliva or orolabial lesions. Transmission of type II virus usually occurs at the time of delivery through exposure to maternal genital tract lesions. However, both virus types can affect either or both sites.
Incubation period 2-12 days.
Period of infectivity Individuals are most infectious when lesions are present. Asymptomatic virus shedding also occurs.
Control measures (infected patient) Isolation in a single cubicle. Gloves and aprons if direct patient contact likely.
Control measures (infected healthcare worker) Staff with orolabial herpes should be offered treatment with topical aciclovir, and should avoid direct contact with neonates until lesion has crusted.
Control measures (infected visitor) Mothers with active orolabial herpes normally pose little risk to their babies, because of passive transfer of antibody. Other individuals may represent a greater risk, because the baby may have no passive immunity. Offer treatment with topical aciclovir, and advice on careful hand washing and avoiding holding the baby close to the face.
Control measures (contacts of a case) Prophylactic aciclovir may be effective in accidental inoculation injuries with material from a herpetic lesion.

LISTERIOSIS

Routes of nosocomial transmission Patient to patient spread uncommon: may occur via health care workers' hands or environmental contamination.
Incubation period Variable; usually less than one week.
Period of infectivity Uncertain, but reasonable to assume potentially infectious until clinical recovery.
Control measures (infected patient) Isolation in a single cubicle. Gloves and apron for direct patient contact.
Control measures (infected visitor) Restrict mothers whose infant has neonatal listeriosis from direct contact with other babies.
Control measures (contacts of a case) None necessary.

OPHTHALMIA NEONATORUM (GONOCOCCAL OR CHLAMYDIAL)

Routes of nosocomial transmission Person to person spread uncommon, and almost always occurs via hands.
Incubation period Gonococcal ophthalmia 1-4 days; chlamydial ophthalmia 5-10

days.
Period of infectivity Until after 48 hours antibiotic therapy.
Control measures (infected patient) Isolation in a single cubicle not usually necessary. Gloves and apron for direct patient contact.
Control measures (infected visitor) Encourage parents to attend a GU Medicine Clinic for assessment and treatment.
Control measures (contacts of a case) None necessary.

CYTOMEGALOVIRUS

Routes of nosocomial transmission Close contact with body fluids, especially urine and respiratory secretions.
Incubation period 3-12 weeks.
Period of infectivity Children with congenital CMV infection may remain infectious for years.
Control measures (infected patient) Isolation in a single cubicle. Gloves and apron for contact with body fluids. Pregnant staff should, if possible, avoid contact with body fluids, although the risk is low.
Control measures (infected visitor) CMV rarely diagnosed in older children and adults.
Control measures (contacts of a case) None necessary.

ENTEROVIRUSES

Routes of nosocomial transmission Airborne spread, direct or indirect contact with respiratory secretions, skin rashes and faeces.
Incubation period 3-5 days.
Period of infectivity Virus can persist in faeces for several weeks, but infectivity highest during symptomatic illness.
Control measures (infected patient) Isolation in a single cubicle. Gloves and apron for direct patient contact.
Control measures (infected healthcare worker) Exclude from work until asymptomatic. Advice on careful hand washing on return to work.
Control measures (infected visitor) If possible, exclude while symptomatic.
Control measures (contacts of a case) Consider isolating contacts of a case for five days.

CHICKENPOX AND SHINGLES

Routes of nosocomial transmission Chickenpox via respiratory secretions and vesicle fluid; shingles via vesicle fluid only.
Incubation period Chickenpox 10-21 days; shingles is due to reactivation of latent virus.
Period of infectivity Chickenpox, from two days before onset of the rash until

vesicles have all crusted. Shingles, while vesicles are present.
Control measures (infected patient) Isolation in a single cubicle. Gloves and apron for contact with patient. Non-immune staff should avoid contact.
Control measures (infected healthcare worker) Chickenpox, exclude from work. Shingles, exclude from patient contact but may undertake administrative work if rash is on a non-exposed part of the body.
Control measures (infected visitor) Chickenpox, exclude from visiting. Shingles, visitors must go directly to and from the infant's isolation cubicle.
Control measures (contacts of a case) Assess immunity and indications for passive immunisation with VZIG (*see p.237*). Isolate patients and exclude staff/visitors from contact with vulnerable patients during potentially infectious period (8-21 days after contact).

INFANTS BORN TO MOTHERS WITH BLOOD-BORNE VIRUS INFECTIONS (HEPATITIS B, HEPATITIS C, HIV)

Routes of nosocomial transmission Risk of transmission through mucous membrane or percutaneous exposure to blood and body fluids (inoculation injury).
Incubation periods Variable, usually 2-3 months.
Period of infectivity Regard as potentially infectious until mother to infant infection can be excluded (usually at least six months). Infected individuals are infectious indefinitely.
Control measures (infected patient) Isolation in a single cubicle not usually necessary, unless there is uncontrolled bleeding. Gloves and apron for contact with blood and body fluids. Eye protection and mask where risk of spattering with blood or body fluids
Control measures (infected healthcare worker) Healthcare workers who know or suspect that they have one of these infections must contact their Occupational Health Service immediately.
Control measures (infected visitor) HIV-positive mothers are advised not to breast feed.
Control measures (contacts of a case) Follow local policy in the event of an inoculation injury.

ANTIBIOTIC-RESISTANT GRAM-NEGATIVE BACTERIA (E.G. SERRATIA, PSEUDOMONAS, ACINETOBACTER)

Routes of nosocomial transmission Direct or indirect patient to patient spread. Environmental colonisation can become widespread.
Incubation period Variable.
Period of infectivity Until cessation of colonisation.
Control measures (infected patient) Isolation in a single cubicle. Gloves and apron

on entering cubicle or for direct patient contact only, depending on the likelihood of environmental contamination.
Control measures (contacts of a case) None usually necessary.

Tuberculosis
Routes of nosocomial transmission Children with primary tuberculosis are not usually infectious. Risk is of adult to infant transmission by the airborne route.
Incubation period 4-12 weeks.
Period of infectivity Until a patient with smear-positive tuberculosis has been treated for two weeks.
Control measures (infected patient) Isolate in a single cubicle (because the source of the infection may be one of the visitors).
Control measures (infected healthcare worker) Exclude from work until treated for two weeks.
Control measures (infected visitor) Exclude until treated for two weeks.
Control measures (contacts of a case) Contacts require assessment; infants and young children who are significant contacts require chemoprophylaxis. Involve local public health/chest clinic personnel in contact-tracing.

Necrotising enterocolitis
Routes of nosocomial transmission Epidemiological evidence that some cases of NEC are infective in aetiology. Routes of transmission unclear, but direct and indirect patient to patient transmission likely.
Incubation period Unknown.
Period of infectivity Unknown; usually considered to be until complete clinical recovery.
Control measures (infected patient) Isolation in a single cubicle. Gloves and apron for patient contact.
Control measures (contacts of a case) None necessary.

MANAGEMENT OF OUTBREAKS OF INFECTION

Even with the best infection control precautions in place, outbreaks of infection inevitably occur from time to time. An outbreak is defined as the occurrence of an unexpectedly high number of cases of an infection. The occurrence of a single case of an uncommon and serious infection may therefore constitute an outbreak, but more usually the term relates to two or more cases of infection that are linked. An outbreak of infection may be suspected as a result of:

- routine surveillance of microbiology results showing an unexpectedly high rate of detection of a single species
- medical or nursing staff on a ward noticing an increased incidence of a specific infection

- the Occupational Health Department noticing an increased incidence of a specific infection amongst staff members.

Suspected outbreaks of infection must be reported *immediately* to the ICT. Where there is evidence that there is, or may be, an outbreak, the ICT will immediately institute appropriate infection control procedures, and assess the current and potential severity of the outbreak. Many outbreaks are small and can be controlled by the ICT without causing significant disruption to the operation of the unit. For more serious outbreaks, an Outbreak Control Group may have to be convened to direct the management of the incident. The core membership of an OCG comprises the ICT, the local Consultant for Communicable Disease Control (CCDC), senior medical, nursing and other staff from affected areas of the hospital and the Chief Executive. Depending on the circumstances of the outbreak, other individuals may be required on the OCG, e.g. occupational health, facilities or estates staff. There is no clear definition of when an outbreak becomes serious enough to require a control group. Considerations include the number of cases, the severity of the infection, the effect on the routine operation of the hospital, and the possible impact of the outbreak on other NNUs or on the community.

FURTHER READING

Damani NN. Manual of infection control procedures, 2nd edn. London: Greenwich Medical Media, 2002.

Hospital Infection Working Group of the Department of Health and Public Health Laboratory Service. Hospital Infection Control. Guidance on the control of infections in hospitals. London: Department of Health, 1995.

Sohn AH, Garrett DO, Sinkowitz-Cochran RL, Grobskopf LA, Levine GL *et al.* Prevalence of nosocomial infections in neonatal intensive care unit patients: results from the first national point-prevalence study. J Pediatr 2001; **139:** 821-7.

Wilson J. Infection control in clinical practices, 2nd edn. London: Balliere Tindall, 2001.

Chapter 14

Breast feeding

INTRODUCTION

Breast milk has many advantages that determine that it is the preferred nutrition, not only for healthy term babies, but usually also for babies who are separated from their mothers on neonatal units. Breast milk is nutritionally complete, protects against infection and necrotising enterocolitis, and promotes neurological development. Allergies in later infancy may be less common in babies fed with breast milk. The mother's own fresh milk is optimal in terms of nutritional availability and biological activity. However, where a supply of fresh milk cannot be maintained for infants who are hospitalised, stored mother's milk or milk from an unrelated donor (the former being preferred) may be used.

Most problems with breast feeding relate to establishing and maintaining feeding, and are outside the remit of this book. However, there are also some uncommon but important biochemical and microbiological issues, including breast milk jaundice and the risk of transmission of infection via breast milk. In addition, breast milk may be contraindicated for some babies with, or at risk of, rare inherited metabolic disorders (*see Chapter 10*); potentially harmful drugs that are secreted in breast milk are discussed in Chapter 16.

BREAST MILK JAUNDICE

This is a benign problem that usually presents at 14-21 days of age with persistent unconjugated hyperbilirubinaemia of greater than 170 µmol/L in an infant who is otherwise entirely well. The jaundice may persist for as long as four months, but will resolve within a week of cessation of breast feeding, although it is not necessary to curtail feeding to make the diagnosis if other causes of jaundice can be excluded (*see Chapter 6*). The aetiology of breast milk jaundice is not fully understood, but there is evidence for the role of extrinsic factors, such as 3α, 20β-pregnanediol and free fatty acids in breast milk, in conjunction with a background of inherited susceptibility. Mutations of the uridine diphosphoglucuronate glucuronosyltransferase gene, similar or identical to those associated with Gilbert's syndrome, have been found in a large proportion of infants with breast milk jaundice.

BREAST FEEDING BY VEGAN MOTHERS

Animal products are the main source of vitamin B12. Vegans, therefore, have low body stores of B12, and babies who are exclusively breast-fed by vegan mothers are at risk of B12 deficiency. Clinical problems usually only occur in infants who have been breast-fed for at least six months, when they may present with anaemia or neurological signs. Investigations will reveal macrocytic anaemia, methylmalonic aciduria and low serum B12 concentrations. Treatment is with B12 injections, and full recovery can be expected.

VIRAL INFECTIONS

A number of viruses can be found in breast milk, including hepatitis B & C, HTLV-I & II, HIV 1 & 2 and CMV. Although on a global scale breast feeding is an important route of transmission of some of these agents, breast milk is often not a very efficient means of transmission of infection, and the risk to the individual breast-fed baby is often quite small. Especially in developing countries, this risk may be outweighed by the nutritional and anti-infective benefits to the infant from breast feeding. Important determinants of the risk of transmission include the stage of maternal infection, and the duration of breast feeding.

HEPATITIS B

Most hepatitis B infections in infants are perinatally acquired, and breast feeding does not appear to be a major means of transmission of hepatitis B whether or not the infant has been immunised. In the UK, and other countries that undertake routine antenatal screening for hepatitis B, babies born to mothers infected with hepatitis B are given additional protection through immunisation at birth. Babies who have been immunised can be safely breast-fed by mothers who are hepatitis B carriers, even if they are HBeAg positive (and therefore of high infectivity).

HEPATITIS C

Hepatitis C virus has been found in the breast milk of infected mothers. Most studies have not found an increased risk of mother to infant transmission in infants who are breast-fed compared with those who are not. However, these studies have not been large enough to detect a small increased risk, nor have they taken into account the possible influence of factors such as viral maternal load. Until more information is available, all that can be advised is that there is currently no basis for strongly advising a mother against breast feeding, but equally, there is no basis for reassurance that breast feeding carries no risk.

HUMAN IMMUNODEFICIENCY VIRUSES (HIV)

Breast feeding may more than double the risk of mother to infant transmission of HIV. The risk of infection is increased if the mother has a high viral load, for example if she becomes newly infected during the breast feeding period. In the UK and other developed countries, bottle feeding poses less risk to the health of the baby of a mother infected with HIV than the risk of HIV transmission. Breast feeding is therefore not recommended, even by mothers whose viral load has been rendered undetectable by highly active anti-retroviral therapy. If a mother insists on breast feeding (for example for religious reasons), then she should be encouraged to do so for as short a period as possible, and given advice on how to avoid inflammatory breast conditions that may increase the risk of HIV transmission.

CYTOMEGALOVIRUS (CMV)

There is a high incidence of post-partum transmission of CMV to infants of seropositive mothers, for which breast feeding probably accounts for one third of cases. Most infections are asymptomatic, but there is a theoretical risk to preterm babies who are especially susceptible to severe disseminated CMV infections. That such infections are rarely seen is probably because the neonate will usually also be protected by passive immunity from its own mother. There is a low risk of transmission of CMV via donated milk because the virus is largely inactivated by freezing.

HUMAN T-CELL LEUKAEMIA VIRUS TYPE I (HTLV-I)

HTLV-I is a retrovirus that is endemic in areas such as southern Japan, the Caribbean and West Africa. In the UK, HTLV-I is uncommon, and occurs mainly amongst immigrants from endemic areas. The vast majority of carriers develop no related disease, but HTLV-I is recognised as the cause of two serious conditions: an aggressive T-cell malignancy, adult T-cell leukaemia/lymphoma (ATLL), and a progressive demyelinating disease, tropical spastic paraparesis (TSP).

Breast feeding appears to be the major route of transmission of HTLV-I. At least 25% of infants breast-fed by seropositive mothers will become infected during the first year of life. In Japan, antenatal screening is used to identify seropositive mothers, who are then discouraged from breast feeding. The prevalence of infection in the UK, even in areas with a high Afro-Caribbean population, is low, and there is no programme for either routine screening or selective testing of antenatal patients. When a mother is known to be infected with HTLV-I, breast feeding is not advised.

BREAST FEEDING AND IMMUNISATION

Both inactivated and live vaccines can be safely administered to breast feeding mothers. Attenuated virus may be found in breast milk after administration of live vaccines such as rubella, but this almost never leads to infection in the infant. Note that immunisation of the mother does not usually confer sufficient passive immunity to protect the baby against the infection. This is an important consideration with travel vaccines such as yellow fever and meningococcal meningitis.

EXPRESSED BREAST MILK

Mothers who are separated from their babies should be encouraged to express milk for feeding to their babies. Mothers who have too much milk may also be asked to donate the surplus. Feeding of expressed breast milk (EBM) entails considerably more handling of the milk than direct breast feeding, creating opportunities to introduce microbial contamination and also to adversely affect the nutritional and anti-infective properties of the milk. Moreover, some precautions that can reduce microbial contamination, such as freezing and pasteurisation, may themselves have a deleterious effect on other properties of the milk. Therefore, wherever possible, babies should receive fresh EBM from their own mothers.

EXPRESSED BREAST MILK FOR THE MOTHER'S OWN BABY

Guidelines on the administration of the mother's EBM to her own baby are available in many countries, including the UK. Measures to optimise the collection, storage and handling of EBM are outlined in Figure 14.1. UK guidelines suggest that by following these precautions, the need for either pasteurisation of mother's milk or any routine microbiological testing is obviated. However, there are many reports of serious, sometimes fatal, bacterial sepsis being transmitted via EBM, and some centres (including the authors') continue to undertake routine microbiological testing of EBM. Milk expressed at home should be regarded as particularly hazardous, because the cleanliness of the home environment cannot be guaranteed, and the conditions during transport from home to hospital may not be ideal. The procedures followed in the authors' hospital for milk expressed at home and in hospital are outlined in Figure 14.2.

DONOR BREAST MILK

Microbiological safety is a key consideration in the use of donor breast milk. As well as the risk of microbial contamination during collection, handling and storage, there is the potential risk of transmission of viral infections from the donor. As a minimum, donors must be screened for antibodies to HIV 1 & 2 and hepatitis C virus, and for hepatitis B surface antigen (HBsAg). Screening for antibodies to HTLV I is also undertaken in some countries, including the UK, where routine testing was introduced in 2002. There is generally no need to test donors for antibodies to CMV, because the virus does not survive freezing.

Procedures for handling and microbiological testing of donated milk should be more stringent than for EBM fed to a mother's own baby. The procedure used in the author's hospital is outlined in Figure 14.3.

Collection, storage and administration of expressed breast milk	
MEASURE	**RATIONALE**
Collection	
Encourage good hygiene in the mother	Minimises risk of contamination with bacteria from maternal skin
Ensure collecting kit is cleaned and disinfected or sterilised after use, and stored dry	Minimises risk of contamination with bacteria of maternal or environmental origin
Collect milk in volumes as close as possible to required feed size, but not less than 15-20 mL	Excess volumes result in waste Very small volumes contain higher bacterial counts
Use suitable containers	Considerations include ease of cleaning (if not disposable); suitability for freezing; minimisation of immunoglobulin loss
Refrigerate milk as soon as possible	Inhibits bacterial multiplication after collection
Ensure that samples are clearly labelled	Ensures milk is given to the correct infant and within the defined shelf life
Storage	
Milk that is to be used within 48 hours may be stored refrigerated	Microbial multiplication is minimal during this time
Milk that is to be stored for over 48 hours should be frozen	Prevents microbial multiplication during prolonged storage
Administration	
Care to ensure that the infant receives the correct milk	Maternal viral infections can be transmitted via breast milk. Accidental administration of breast milk to the wrong infant should be managed as an inoculation injury
Where possible frozen milk should be thawed in the refrigerator	Low temperature minimises microbial multiplication
Unused frozen milk that has been thawed must be disposed of after 12 hours	Microbial counts in frozen milk may be higher, giving risk of rapid multiplication after thawing

Figure 14.1 Recommended measures to optimise the collection, storage and administration of expressed breast milk

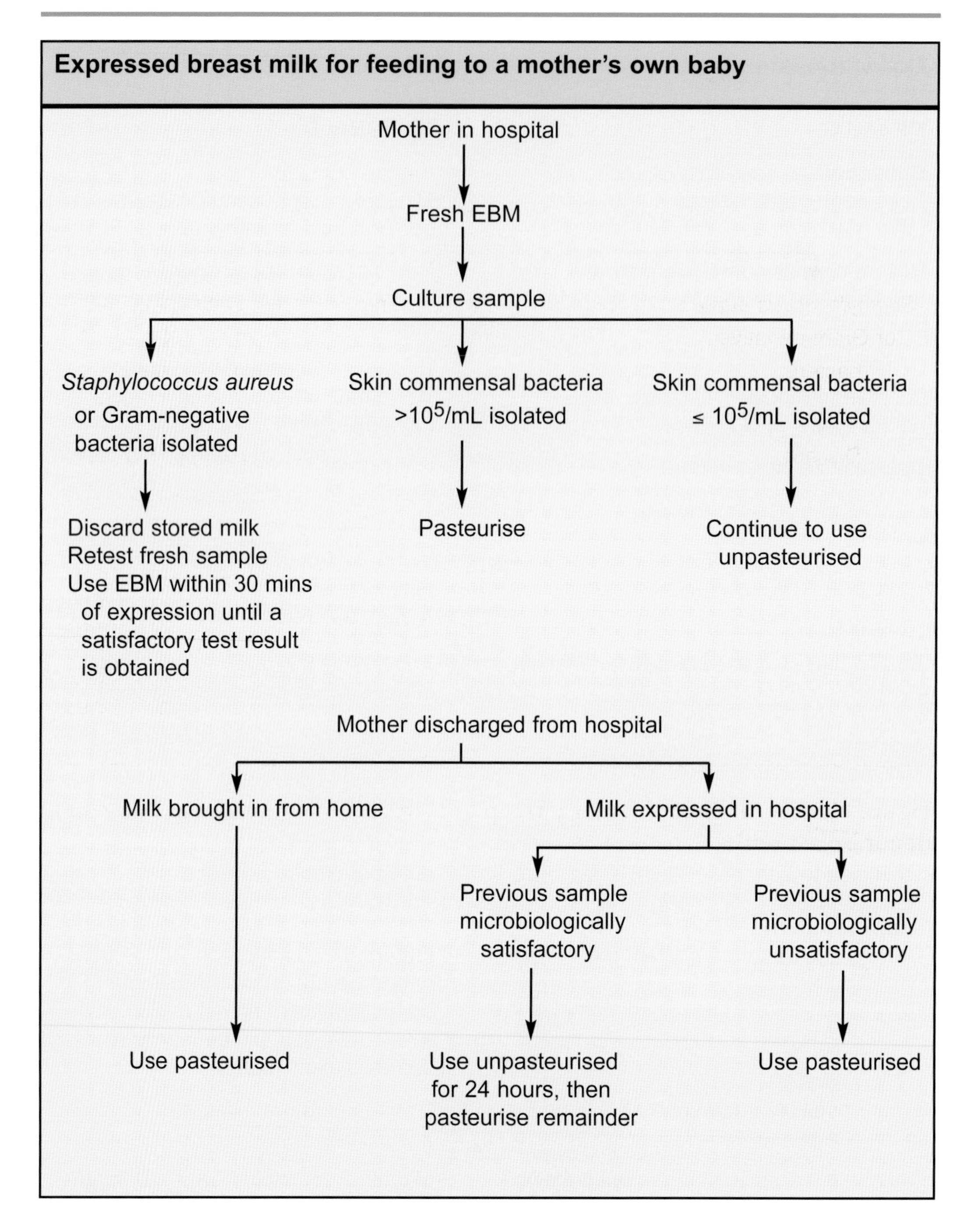

Figure 14.2 Birmingham Women's Hospitals procedure for handling and testing expressed breast milk for feeding to a mother's own baby

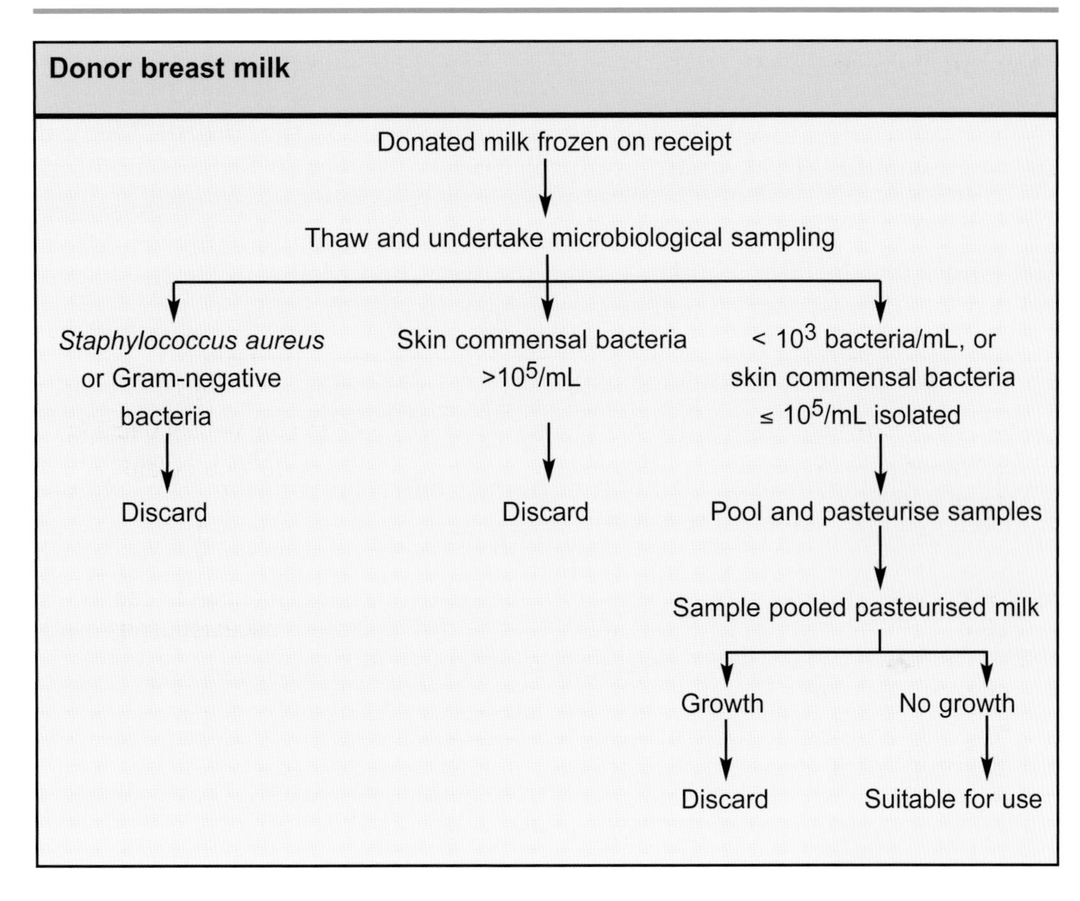

Figure 14.3 Birmingham Women's Hospitals procedure for handling and testing donor breast milk

FURTHER READING

British National Formulary. Published biannually by the British Medical Association and Royal Pharmaceutical Society of Great Britain, London. http://BNF.org.

HIV and infant feeding. Guidance from the UK Chief Medical Officers' Expert Advisory Group on AIDS. London: Department of Health, 2001.

Human Milk Banking Association of North America. http://www.hmbana.org

Standing Committee of Nutrition of the British Paediatric Association. Guidelines for the establishment and operation of human milk banks in the UK. London: British Paediatric Association, 1994.

Chapter 15

Parenteral nutrition

INTRODUCTION

Parenteral feeding is an important component of the management of both preterm infants and low birth weight infants born at term, as well as term infants with compromised gastrointestinal function (e.g. protracted diarrhoea, short bowel syndrome, etc.).

There is wide variation in practice and no agreed position on when premature infants should receive parenteral nutrition (PN) because of immaturity alone. The extent of the contribution of PN in improving outcome in premature neonates is unclear, as it is impossible to consider it separately from the other support received in the neonatal intensive care environment. However, it is common practice to provide PN if the birth weight is less than 1.5 kg and almost universal practice if birth weight is less than 1 kg.

Minimal enteral feeding is often used as an adjunct to PN, as it has the advantages of providing protection against sepsis, reducing the risk of cholestasis, promoting faster growth and reducing the time required to establish full enteral feeding. It may also protect the intestinal mucosa from the degeneration that can occur with prolonged fasting. Minimal enteral feeding takes the form of 0.5-1 mL/kg/h of expressed breast milk feed, given nasogastrically.

Parenteral nutrition is a skilled procedure, expensive and not without risks. It should, therefore, only be undertaken by experienced medical and nursing staff, with specialist support provided by a multidisciplinary team including a clinician, dietitian, pharmacist, nurse, biochemist and microbiologist. Most infants receive PN for no more than 2-3 weeks. However, in a minority of surgical patients, PN extends well beyond the post-operative phase of intestinal failure. Home parenteral nutrition is now well established for those patients requiring long-term support.

INDICATIONS FOR PARENTERAL NUTRITION

Whenever possible, nutrition should be maintained enterally, e.g. by the nasogastric route. If the gastrointestinal tract is compromised and it is judged that the neonate will be unable to absorb sufficient nutrients to prevent catabolism, then parenteral feeding should be considered. Absolute indications include intestinal failure, bowel obstruction and necrotising enterocolitis. Neonates who have had gut resection (e.g. for volvulus or ileal atresia) and have a short bowel (loss of more than 50% of small intestine) are particular candidates for parenteral nutrition.

Preterm infants have very little stored energy resources (i.e. glycogen and fat): at 28 weeks gestation virtually all of the carbohydrate, fat and protein is structural. Failure to supply adequate nutrition to low birth weight babies will result in a catabolic state and tissue breakdown will ensue rapidly. It may be impossible to ensure adequate nutrient intake enterally without the risk of overloading the gut and consequent diarrhoea, or regurgitation and aspiration pneumonia. The decision to start PN in this situation is therefore based on how much enteral feed the baby can tolerate and whether there are any additional stress factors, e.g. sepsis, respiratory difficulties or severe intrauterine growth retardation.

REQUIREMENTS

There is a general trend to start PN earlier than was previously the practice, usually by 24 hours in a baby weighing less than 1 kg; the volume and nutrient content of the feed are increased gradually, usually over about 3-4 days, particularly with regard to the amino acid and lipid content. For details of intravenous regimens and practicality of administration, the reader is referred to the texts mentioned at the end of this section.

In term infants, an intake of at least 110 kcal/kg body weight /24h is required to promote anabolism. Recommended 24 hourly intakes are: amino acids 2.5 g/kg, fat 3 g/kg, and carbohydrate 14 g/kg. In preterm infants, growth may be possible on a significantly lower caloric intake than this, for example, with an average energy intake of 80 kcal/kg/24h and approximately 3 g/kg/24h of amino acids.

The fluid requirement of extremely preterm infants nursed in maximally humidified incubators is 60-80 mL/kg/24h, increasing to 100-120 mL/kg/24h in week two. If measures to reduce transcutaneous water loss are not taken, fluid requirements for extremely preterm infants can be greater than 150 mL/kg/24h.

ADMINISTRATION

Peripheral or central venous lines can be used. Central lines should be placed with the tip in the superior vena cava or inferior vena cava, not the right atrium, and will allow up to 20% glucose solution to be given. There should be a bacterial filter in the line before a Y connector. Lipid is not usually mixed with amino acid solutions in neonatal practice and is either not filtered or is passed through a 1.2 micron pore filter via the other limb of the connector. The high requirement for calcium and phosphate risks destabilising the lipid emulsion and precludes the use of a single bag system in neonates. Positioning central lines with the tip in the right atrium should be avoided because there have been case reports of fatal cardiac tamponade in neonates with lines in this position.

NUTRIENT SOURCES AND THE COMPOSITION OF INTRAVENOUS SOLUTIONS

Requirements for parenteral nutrition formulae are based on data from normal, enterally fed babies and regimens have been developed to take account of the differing needs of the term or pre-term baby. Commercial amino acid preparations suitable for neonates are available (e.g. Primene®, Vaminolact®) and can be used as the basis for the preparation of a nutritionally complete regimen. This needs to contain carbohydrate, lipid, amino acids, vitamins and minerals.

CARBOHYDRATE

Glucose is the carbohydrate of choice. Solutions more concentrated than 12.5% should not be given peripherally, but only via a central vein.

LIPID

Parenteral lipid emulsions (e.g. Intralipid®) are isotonic fluids that provide essential fatty acids and are energy rich. They are metabolised in the same way as chylomicrons. Olive oil based intravenous fat emulsions may be more suitable than the more widely used soya bean based emulsions. Parenteral lipid should be introduced gradually, particularly in babies who are preterm or small for gestational age, in those at risk from chronic lung disease or who have jaundice or liver dysfunction. A regimen of continuous fat infusion over a period of 20 or 24 hours (*see p.273*) is better than one involving intermittent infusion.

AMINO ACIDS

A balanced mixture of L-amino acids (including adequate essential amino acids) is required. Preterm infants require more amino acids, and in different proportions, than term infants. Formulae particularly suited for preterm babies are available. Cysteine, taurine, tyrosine and histidine are considered essential in low birth weight infants. Glutamine is probably essential in stressed infants, but currently is not routinely included in PN solutions.

VITAMINS

Water-soluble and fat-soluble preparations are given in doses appropriate to the baby's weight.

MINERALS

Only small amounts of sodium and potassium are provided in commercial amino acid solutions and supplements of sodium and potassium chloride are needed to meet the basic requirements (*see Chapter 4*).

Preterm infants require additional phosphate supplementation (*see Chapter 8*). The limited solubility of the inorganic salts of calcium and phosphate may make provision of the full requirements impossible, particularly in preterm infants. Recently, glucose 1-phosphate and calcium glycerophosphate, which have greater solubility, have been used to increase the calcium and phosphate concentrations of intravenous feeding solutions. Plasma phosphate concentration should generally be kept above 2.0 mmol/L in very low birth weight infants.

TRACE ELEMENTS

These are provided as a supplement based on body weight. Routine supplements may not supply enough trace elements for preterm infants on long-term PN (i.e. > 4 weeks), especially if there are abnormal losses of fluid from the gut.

INFECTION RISKS

Catheter-related blood stream infection (CRBSI) is a frequent complication of intravenous feeding, with reported incidences of 3-30 infections per thousand catheter days. Serious complications of CRBSI include disseminated infection and predisposition to PN-related liver disease. Most episodes of CRBSI are caused by cutaneous microorganisms (Figure 15.1), which may reach the catheter tip by migrating either along the catheter track from the skin or endoluminally from the hub. Enteric bacteria account for a greater proportion of cases of CRBSI in neonates than in older age groups. The cause is thought to be translocation of gastrointestinal bacteria into the blood stream.

CRBSI may present as a generalised infection or with signs localised to the catheter insertion site. It is vital that insertion sites are inspected daily, as local infection in neonates can rapidly extend into deeper tissues. Prevention is important to avoid morbidity and the costs of treatment (up to £5,000 per episode). The most important preventative measures are administration of PN through a dedicated line and scrupulous aseptic precautions during catheter insertion and accessing the hub. Diagnosis is usually based on isolation of microorganisms typically associated with CRBSI in blood cultures taken through the line, in the absence of another obvious focus of infection (*see Chapter 12*).

Microbial causes of parenteral nutrition related CRBSI in children aged less than 1 year	
Coagulase-negative staphylococci	58.4%
Coliforms (*E.coli, Enterobacter, Klebsiella*)	13.5%
Enterococci	12.4%
Candida	5.6%
Pseudomonas species	4.5%
Staphylococcus aureus	4.5%
Streptococcus bovis	1.1%

Figure 15.1 Microbial causes of parenteral nutrition related CRBSI in children aged less than 1 year at Birmingham Children's Hospital (Jan-Dec 2000)

METABOLIC COMPLICATIONS OF PARENTERAL NUTRITION

The metabolic complications of PN are summarised in Figure 15.2. Babies with compromised gastrointestinal function frequently have electrolyte abnormalities, e.g. hyponatraemia, hypokalaemia or hypocalcaemia, as a result of their primary disorder, whether or not they receive PN. Neonates with continuing abnormal fluid and electrolyte losses, e.g. diarrhoea, upper gastrointestinal fluid loss or renal losses, are particularly prone to electrolyte depletion and require regular monitoring of plasma sodium, potassium and calcium concentrations. If hypocalcaemia occurs, the plasma albumin concentration should be checked; plasma magnesium concentration should be measured if there is refractory hypocalcaemia. Measurement of urine sodium and potassium may be helpful to identify renal loss or conservation.

Hyperglycaemia and glycosuria (> 0.5% measured by dipstick) may occur in very low birth weight babies and 6-hourly blood glucose monitoring and urine testing for glucose is recommended. Hyperglycaemia is managed initially by reducing the carbohydrate concentration to avoid an osmotic diuresis. The neonate may subsequently require an insulin infusion to allow adequate energy intake, especially if of very low birth weight or if steroids are being given for lung disease.

Hyperglycaemia in term infants or previously stable infants is uncommon and, when it occurs, is suggestive of infection or other stress or accidental over-supply, or, in premature neonates, may be a complication of steroid therapy.

Metabolic complications of parenteral nutrition in neonates	
Frequent complications	**Less frequent complications**
Sodium depletion*	Hyperphenylalaninaemia (– hypertyrosinaemia)*
Potassium depletion*	Hyperlipidaemia (cholesterol ↑, triglycerides ↑)*
Hyperglycaemia/hypoglycaemia*	Zinc deficiency**
Glycosuria*	Copper deficiency**
Jaundice*	Selenium deficiency**
Hypophosphataemia*	Molybdenum deficiency**
Metabolic acidosis	Essential fatty acid deficiency
Calcium depletion	Hyperammonaemia
	Anaemia (associated with longer term PN or and/or excessive bleeding)
	Dysfunction of thrombocytes or neutrophils
	Carnitine deficiency

* particularly important in extreme preterm infants
** associated with longer term PN

Figure 15.2 Metabolic complications of parenteral nutrition in neonates

Hyperbilirubinaemia occurs in some neonates, particularly if on PN for more than 14 days. The cause of the jaundice is probably multifactorial, with enteral starvation being an important component. Free fatty acids in the blood displace bilirubin from albumin and may increase the risk of kernicterus. It is therefore recommended that lipid emulsions should not be given if plasma bilirubin concentration exceeds 170 μmol/L and the amount infused should be reduced at bilirubin concentrations between 100 and 170 μmol/L. Cholestasis with conjugated hyperbilirubinaemia occurs as a complication of prolonged parenteral nutrition. However, it is important not to assume that this is the cause, and other causes of prolonged jaundice, e.g. biliary atresia, sepsis and neonatal hepatitis should be considered and appropriate investigations undertaken (*see p.101*). Both a complete absence of any enteral feeding and systemic infection may increase the likelihood of cholestasis. In our experience, central venous catheter infections are an important factor that can precipitate cholestasis in infants receiving parenteral nutrition.

Hypophosphataemia is one of the commonest abnormalities arising from PN and regular measurement of plasma phosphate is essential. Increased phosphate provision may be required because of excessive losses from the gastrointestinal tract or because of bone disease in premature infants (*see Chapter 8*). Treatment with oral vitamin D, calcium and phosphate supplements should be provided in infants at risk of bone disease of prematurity when PN is discontinued.

Mild acid-base disturbances are common, particularly with increasing duration of PN. Such findings are rarely associated with any clinical symptoms and, unless the base deficit exceeds 5 mmol/L, are generally safely ignored. In very immature infants, it is common to see the base deficit exceed 10 mmol/L, presumably because of renal immaturity; this may require bicarbonate treatment.

Hypercholesterolaemia has been noted in some babies receiving Intralipid. The phospholipid present as an emulsifier has been implicated as the cause, and its intake can be reduced by giving the Intralipid as a 20% rather than a 10% emulsion, since the former preparation has a lower proportion of phospholipid. The significance of this hypercholesterolaemia is not known but it is probably best avoided. Hypercholesterolaemia may not be a complication when Lipofundin®, a lipid source with 50% long chain triglycerides and 50% medium chain triglycerides, is used. Hypertriglyceridaemia should not occur if the rate of lipid infusion is controlled appropriately. Essential fatty acid deficiency should not occur if lipid emulsion is being given but is a risk if, for any reason, it is not.

Amino acid imbalances have been observed over many years with the use of products formulated primarily for administration to adult patients. With the advent of newer products (e.g. Vaminolact), whose formulae are based on breast milk and hence specifically tailored for the premature/low birth weight baby, there is now much less of a problem. Taurine deficiency has been associated with a reversible abnormality in the electroretinogram in patients on long-term therapy and is a cause for concern. There have been several reports of hyperphenylalaninaemia in babies receiving Vamin (an amino acid solution widely used in adult

PN). Vamin contains more than twice as much phenylalanine as breast milk, whereas the specially designed infant formulae, Vaminolact, has a considerably reduced phenylalanine concentration.

Hyperammonaemia is a rare complication with the currently available nitrogen sources and if liver function is normal. If, however, the baby becomes lethargic or develops fits, plasma ammonia concentration should be measured.

Carnitine plays an essential role in the oxidation of fatty acids (*see p.176*). Preterm infants, fed parenterally with carnitine-free solutions, develop low blood and tissue carnitine concentrations because of limited carnitine storage and biosynthesis. If PN is required for more than one month, consideration should be given to adding carnitine to the regimen.

Deficiencies of both zinc and (less frequently) selenium can occur during long term PN. A falling plasma alkaline phosphatase activity, or a value lower than that often seen in premature babies, may be an indicator of zinc deficiency. If PN is prolonged, i.e. for more than three weeks, then plasma zinc, copper and selenium should be measured. Zinc and selenium are both negative acute phase reactants and their concentrations tend to fall during an inflammatory response, whereas copper concentrations increase; assessment of trace metal status should therefore be interpreted in conjunction with CRP concentration as a measure of the acute phase response. Plasma selenium concentration is an indicator of recent intake, whereas erythrocyte glutathione peroxidase activity or whole blood selenium are better markers of overall selenium status. If PN is supplemental or required for only two weeks, only zinc needs to be added to the infusion. If PN continues for longer than a month, other trace metals need to be added. The risk of zinc deficiency is increased with excessive gastrointestinal loss. Chromium may be added to the regimen for long-term PN but, as it has been implicated as a cause of renal impairment, it is not current practice to use it routinely. Molybdenum and fluoride supplements are recommended with long-term (3-6 months) PN. In practice, Peditrace® is used as a trace metal supplement. This contains zinc, copper, manganese, selenium, fluoride and iodide. Copper and manganese supplements should be withheld when cholestasis is present, by omission of Peditrace and provision of the other trace elements on an individual basis.

Selenium deficiency, presenting as a myopathy, has been described as a complication of long-term PN and selenium is now included in routine supplements. The recommended manganese intake has been reduced following reports of accumulation associated with basal ganglia damage in children with cholestasis. Clinical effects of trace element deficiencies are shown in Figure 15.3.

Clinical effects of trace element abnormalities	
Zinc	Dermatitis (symmetrical periorificial) Diarrhoea Alopecia
Copper	Hypochromic anaemia Neutropenia
Selenium	Cardiomyopathy Skeletal myopathy

Figure 15.3 Clinical effects of trace element abnormalities

Some elements may unintentionally be given in excess of requirements as contaminants, particularly of amino acid solutions. Aluminium accumulation can occur in preterm infants after prolonged IV feeding and is associated with impaired neurological development and metabolic bone disease. In very long-term PN, consideration should be given to measurement of aluminium.

LABORATORY MONITORING OF PARENTERAL NUTRITION

There are numerous guidelines for biochemical monitoring, most of them based on little hard scientific data. With increasing experience, and availability of more appropriate products for neonates, concerns about potential biochemical complications have been reduced and reported complications are now uncommon.

Unnecessary blood sampling is traumatic to the baby and creates an added risk of infection and anaemia. Our experience suggests that for those infants who are being monitored *solely* because they are receiving parenteral nutrition, a conservative approach to monitoring can be recommended (Figure 15.4). However, in an infant who is clinically unstable, has major organ failure or has unusual fluid losses, more frequent or extensive monitoring may be needed. It may also be needed in premature infants, though in practice what can be achieved may be limited by the low blood volume and the consequently small specimen sizes.

POINTS TO NOTE

- Preterm infants will require additional monitoring, particularly plasma phosphate and glucose, and urine glucose.
- More frequent phosphate monitoring will be required if plasma phosphate

concentration is low.

- 'Apparently' low glucose results by a 'stix' method (i.e. < 2 mmol/L) must be confirmed with a laboratory result.
- The frequency of glucose monitoring can be reduced after first week, unless glucose intake is being increased or baby is preterm.
- With refractory hypoglycaemia, consider administration problems (e.g. leak, disconnected catheter), hypopituitarism and hyperinsulinism.
- Vitamin K should be given weekly during long-term PN.

Biochemical and haematological monitoring of term neonates on PN

Timing	Body fluid	Tests
Pre-PN	Blood	Sodium, potassium, bilirubin, phosphate
	Urine	Sodium, potassium
Throughout PN	Blood	Sodium, potassium: twice weekly Phosphate, ALT, bilirubin (total and conjugated): once weekly Glucose: daily first week or more frequently if unstable or preterm. Haemoglobin, haemotocrit, WBC and differential, platelets: weekly Triglycerides: weekly
	Urine	Sodium, potassium: as required
Additional tests after two weeks PN	Blood	Calcium, alkaline phosphatase: weekly
Additional tests after three weeks PN	Blood	Selenium, zinc, copper, manganese: three weekly
Long-term PN		Aluminium, chromium (molybdenum, ferritin) : after six months

Figure 15.4 Protocol for routine biochemical and haematological monitoring of term neonates on PN

In some units, the timing of blood collections is standardised so that blood is collected after the lipid infusion has been turned off for four hours. Blood taken during, or soon after stopping, the lipid infusion may be artefactually lipaemic and can produce spurious results, depending on the methodology in use in the laboratory. If the methods in use present no problem, then continuous 24 hour infusion is given with no break for blood samples. If there is particular concern about lipid clearance, e.g. due to liver dysfunction, plasma triglyceride and free fatty acid concentrations should be measured; visual lipaemia provides an insensitive assessment and does not correlate well with quantitative measurements. Triglycerides should be measured and if the concentration exceeds 3.0 mmol/L, the lipid intake should be reduced. In babies with no particular susceptibility to acid-base disturbances, routine hydrogen ion and blood gas measurements are not indicated. Osmolality measurements are not included in our protocol as, in our experience, they add little if anything to management. It is usually more informative to measure individual analytes.

FURTHER READING

Aspen Board of Directors and the Clinical Guidelines Task Force. Guidelines for the use of parenteral and enteral nutrition in adult and paediatric patients. JPEN, 2001; **26 (suppl 1):** 1SA-138SA.

Ball, PA, Booth IW, Holden CE, Puntis JWL. Paediatric Parenteral Nutrition 3rd edn. Runcorn: Fresenius Kabi, 1998.

Hay WW Jr (Ed). Neonatal Nutrition and Metabolism. St Louis: Mosby Year Book, 1991.

Heird WD. Parenteral feeding. In: Effective care of the newborn infant. Sinclair JC, Bracken MB (Eds). Oxford: Oxford Medical Publications, 1992, pp. 141-60.

Puntis JWL. Parenteral nutrition in infants. In: Nutrition in the infant: problems and practical procedures. Grimble GK, Preedy VR, Watson RR (Eds). London: Greenwich Medical Media, 2001, pp 93-102.

Puntis JWL. Paediatric parenteral nutrition. In: Artificial Nutrition Support in Clinical Practice 2nd edn. Payne-James J, Grimble G, Silk DRW (Eds). London: Greenwich Medical Media, 2001, pp 461-84.

Yu VYH. Parenteral nutrition. In: Textbook of Neonatology, 3rd edn. Rennie JM, Robertson NRC. London: Churchill Livingstone 1999, pp. 349-59.

Chapter 16

Drugs and the neonate

Neonates are very different from older children and adults in their handling of, and response to, drugs. However, only a relatively small number of drugs are regularly prescribed for neonates, and suitable dosing and monitoring regimens for these agents are relatively well-defined. The laboratory often has an important role in monitoring for direct or indirect evidence of both the efficacy and potential toxicity of these agents. For drugs that are prescribed infrequently, there is often little information to guide the prescriber. These agents have to be administered particularly cautiously, with close monitoring during therapy.

As well as drugs that are administered directly, the neonate may be exposed to drugs taken by the mother, either by transfer across the placenta before delivery, or via breast milk.

PHARMACOKINETICS

ROUTES OF ADMINISTRATION AND BIOAVAILABILITY

Oral

Liquid formulations of a variety of drugs can be administered to neonates. However, oral administration produces unpredictable variability in drug absorption, and hence in blood and tissue concentrations. Factors that affect absorption include milk, the higher neonatal gastric pH and slower rate of gastric emptying, differences in the neonatal gastrointestinal flora, pre- and postnatal maturity, and the presence of underlying illness.

Rectal

Solutions of drugs such as paraldehyde, paracetamol and diazepam are available for rectal administration. This route of administration is more reliable than oral dosing, and is occasionally useful, especially where intravenous access is not readily available. Calcium resonium may be administered as an enema to remove excess potassium in hyperkalaemia.

Respiratory

Drugs such as steroids, bronchodilators and the anti-respiratory syncytial virus drug ribavirin can be administered directly into the respiratory tract of ventilated babies using specific delivery devices. Theoretically, this can provide high concentrations of drug in the respiratory tract with less risk of systemic toxicity, but in practice the efficacy of drugs administered in this way is variable.

INTRAMUSCULAR (I.M.)

Lipid-soluble drugs can diffuse directly through capillary walls and are rapidly absorbed by this route. Drugs that are not lipid-soluble are absorbed much more slowly via the lymphatic system, provided that they are water soluble at physiological pH. The unreliability of the i.m. route is accentuated in neonates, because of the small amount of suitable skeletal muscle available and poor tissue perfusion, especially during illness. Occasionally, this slow absorption produces a depot effect that is clinically useful, for example with vitamin K, and with naloxone, where an i.m. dose administered to the baby at birth along with an i.v. dose can provide prolonged reversal of pethidine-induced respiratory depression.

INTRAVENOUS (I.V.)

This is the main route of drug administration in emergency situations and to babies in neonatal units. Intravenous administration gives rapid action and complete availability of the drug to the body without first-pass metabolism. Dosage is easily controlled, which is especially useful when titration of drug concentrations to within a therapeutic range is required.

ABSORPTION OF DRUGS APPLIED TOPICALLY

Significant systemic absorption of substances applied locally to the skin and the eye can occur. Systemic toxicity can occur from hexachlorophene powder (Ster-Zac®), which is commonly applied to the cord and other areas of staphylococcal carriage to prevent neonatal *Staphylococcus aureus* infections. Systemic atropine-like side effects have been seen after cyclopentolate eyedrop administration, and methyl alcohol poisoning has been reported in very immature babies following application of alcoholic cleansing solutions to the skin.

DISTRIBUTION

Neonates have a relatively larger total body water and lower body fat as compared with older children and adults. The proportion of total body water that is extracellular fluid is also higher in neonates, especially during the first 48 hours of life (*see p.10*). As a result, most drugs have a larger volume of distribution during infancy, and a larger dose related to weight is required. Extracellular fluid volume directly correlates with body surface area, therefore, theoretically, drug dosing based on surface area should be more precise. However, volume of distribution is only one variable influencing drug handling by neonates, and, for convenience, most drug doses continue to be based on body weight, together with gestational and postnatal ages. The lower total protein concentration in neonatal plasma, together with the lower drug-binding capacity of neonatal albumin, also contribute to a larger volume of distribution for drugs that are protein-bound.

Effect of bilirubin

Bilirubin can compete with some drugs for binding sites on albumin. Drugs such as indomethacin, aspirin, sulphonamides and some X-ray contrast media can displace bilirubin, leading to an increase in free bilirubin, and an increased risk of kernicterus.

METABOLISM

The most important site of drug metabolism is the liver. In general, enzymatic biotransformation of drugs is markedly slower in the newborn, especially if preterm. However, the various metabolic pathways differ in their maturity: glucuronidation, N-dealkylation and oxidation are important pathways that are especially immature in neonates. There is also considerable variation between individuals, which can be compounded by enzyme induction or inhibition by other drugs given to the neonate, or even to the mother before delivery. Drugs that can induce enzymes include phenobarbital, phenytoin and rifampicin. Inhibitors include chloramphenicol and cimetidine. Drug effects need to be considered when interpreting biochemistry and haematology results.

Drug metabolism can involve two phases. Phase I metabolism is a modification of the drug by oxidation, reduction or hydrolysis, usually catalysed by microsomal enzymes. Oxidation is the most common phase I reaction, and involves a group of haemoproteins called cytochrome P450 that act as the terminal oxygen carrier in the oxidation pathway. Phase II metabolism is a synthetic reaction that involves conjugation of the drug or its metabolites with another molecule, e.g. glucuronic acid, sulphate or acetate. Some drugs pass through only one phase, whereas others must undergo a phase I reaction before a phase II reaction can take place. Drugs that are eliminated by both phase I and II reactions (e.g. diazepam, chloramphenicol) have particularly unpredictable pharmacokinetics in neonates.

The following drugs exemplify the problems arising from slowed drug elimination in neonates.

- Pethidine is hydrolysed by an esterase that is present in low concentrations in neonates. The drug has an elimination half life of up to 22 hours, seven times that in adults. Pethidine used as an analgesic during labour can cross the placenta and cause prolonged respiratory depression in the newborn.

- The N-demethylation pathway for caffeine is deficient in neonates. A large proportion of the drug is excreted unchanged in the urine, and the half-life is four days, compared with around four hours in adults.

- Glucuronidation of chloramphenicol is an important elimination mechanism that is markedly impaired in the neonate. This leads to high circulating concentrations of chloramphenicol, which in turn can inhibit microsomal enzymes involved in phase I elimination. High circulating concentrations of chloramphenicol occur, which are toxic to mammalian cells. Without dose reduction and close monitoring of drug concentrations, this can lead to the fatal 'grey baby' syndrome with shock and circulatory collapse.

EXCRETION

Renal function is poor at birth, especially in the preterm or sick neonate. The glomerular filtration rate (GFR) can be as low as 2-3 mL/min in a baby of 28 weeks gestation, and increases only slowly in the first postnatal week. After the first week, the GFR increases more steeply and there is a sharp increase at the equivalent of 34-36 weeks gestation. Surface area adjusted adult levels are not reached until about two years of age. As a result, the half-life of drugs that are excreted unchanged in the urine can be greatly prolonged, e.g. digoxin ($t_{1/2}$ 100 hours, compared with 30 hours in adults) and gentamicin ($t_{1/2}$ 18 hours, compared with 2 hours). Drugs such as penicillin are mainly eliminated by active tubular secretion. Tubular function is poor, particularly in the preterm or sick neonate, resulting in diminished tubular secretion of such drugs. Frusemide is excreted unchanged by both filtration and secretion. The mean half-life in neonates is seven hours, compared with 1.5-3 hours in adults. This is associated with a sustained diuretic effect and increased risk of electrolyte disturbance and loss of minerals. Nephrocalcinosis has been reported in preterm neonates.

MONITORING FOR THE ADVERSE EFFECTS OF DRUGS

Adverse effects are usually concentration-dependent, resulting from an augmented pharmacological response to the drug. They are more common in neonates than in any other age group, both because drug pharmacokinetics are more unpredictable, and because of the immaturity of neonatal physiology. For example, increased sensitivity to opiates relates partly to markedly slower metabolism of the drug, but also to inefficiency of the immature blood-brain barrier.

Adverse effects rarely produce characteristic physical signs until they have become serious. The laboratory, therefore, has an important role in both reducing the risk of adverse effects by monitoring blood drug concentrations (see below), and in detecting biochemical and haematological changes that may either affect drug handling or be directly drug-induced (Figure 16.1).

Biochemical and haematological monitoring in neonates on drug therapy

Drug	Suggested monitoring	Minimum frequency of monitoring	Rationale for monitoring
Aminoglycosides*	Urea & electrolytes	2-3 times weekly	Potentially nephrotoxic Dosage adjustment required in renal impairment
Amphotericin B (systemic therapy)	Urea & electrolytes	2-3 times weekly	Biochemical disturbances predictable (especially raised urea and hypokalaemia). Less commonly, hypomagnesaemia
	Full blood count	1-2 times weekly	Haematological dyscrasias sometimes occur
β-lactam antibiotics (penicillins, cephalosporins, carbapenems)	Urea & electrolytes	Twice weekly	Electrolyte disturbances (hypokalaemia, hypernatraemia) may occur, especially with high doses
Diazepam	Urea & electrolytes	1-2 times weekly	Elimination is prolonged in renal failure
Digoxin*	Urea & electrolytes	Daily	Electrolyte disturbances (especially hypokalaemia and hypercalcaemia) may potentiate digoxin effect. Dosage adjustment required in renal impairment
Frusemide	Urea & electrolytes	Every 1-2 days	Biochemical disturbances common (especially hypokalaemia and hypocalcaemia)
Indomethacin	Urea & electrolytes	Daily	Biochemical disturbances may occur (especially raised urea and hyponatraemia)
Phenobarbital*	Full blood count	Weekly	Risk of anaemia with prolonged therapy
Phenytoin*	Blood glucose Full blood count	1-2 times weekly Weekly	Risk of hyperglycaemia Risk of anaemia with prolonged therapy
Ranitidine	Urea & electrolytes	Weekly	Elimination is prolonged in renal failure
Theophylline*	Urea & electrolytes	1-2 times weekly	Risk of hypokalaemia, especially with concomitant diuretic or steroid therapy

*Laboratory measurement of drug concentrations is usually also indicated (*see pp.282-3*)

Figure 16.1 Indications for biochemical and haematological monitoring in neonates receiving drug therapy

Idiosyncratic drug effects are comparatively rare events that are unpredictable and not dose-related. Allergic reactions are rarely seen in neonates. Genetic abnormalities may lead to abnormal and unpredictable responses to drugs. For example, infants with glucose 6-phosphate dehydrogenase (G6PD) deficiency or hereditary methaemoglobinaemia are susceptible to oxidant drugs, such as sulphonamides.

OBSTETRIC DRUGS AND THE NEONATE

Drugs administered to the mother late in pregnancy may cross to the fetus and produce direct drug effects in the baby. This particularly applies to drugs that are rapidly absorbed across membranes, that is, those with a low molecular weight, low ionisation and a high lipid:water partition ratio.

A neonate can be adversely affected by maternal drug therapy in a number of ways. Problems may be due to:

- a direct effect of *in utero* exposure to the drug
- the effects of abrupt withdrawal of supply after delivery
- an inability to eliminate the drug, leading to accumulation and toxicity
- accelerated development of some hepatic elimination pathways as a result of prolonged fetal exposure to enzyme-inducing drugs, e.g. phenobarbital
- idiosyncratic effects.

The effects of specific drugs that may adversely affect a neonate if taken by the mother late in pregnancy are shown in Figure 16.2. A more comprehensive list appears as an appendix in the British National Formulary.

DRUG WITHDRAWAL

This is the most commonly encountered problem in neonates relating to maternal drug exposure. Maternal drug addiction, particularly to narcotic agents, may lead to the development of a withdrawal syndrome in the neonate after delivery. Presentation is usually within four days of birth, but can be delayed until ten days and may last up to six months. Symptoms and signs are variable, and are predominantly those of autonomic overactivity: cerebral irritability, nasal congestion, sneezing, yawning, runny eyes, photophobia, poor suck, hiccups and diarrhoea have all been described. In more severe cases there is an abnormal, high-pitched cry, increased extensor tone, irritability, poor sleeping, tachypnoea, weight loss and convulsions. Treatment is with a reducing course of opiates, or with sedative drugs if the maternal drug was a benzodiazepine.

Drugs adversely affecting neonates if taken by the mother in pregnancy	
Drug	**Effect on neonate**
ACE inhibitors	Neonatal blood pressure control and renal function may be affected
Alcohol	Intrauterine growth retardation, fetal-alcohol syndrome
Amiodarone	Risk of neonatal goitre
Anaesthetics, general (high doses, or delivery prolonged by >20 minutes)	Neonatal respiratory depression
Anaesthetics, local	Neonatal respiratory depression Hypotonia and bradycardia after epidural block
Anticoagulants	Risk of neonatal bleeding
Antidepressants	Tachycardia, irritability, muscle spasms may occur
Anti-epileptics	Risk of bleeding
Antipsychotics	Extrapyramidal effects occasionally occur
Aspirin	Impaired platelet function Kernicterus in jaundiced newborn
Benzodiazepines	Risk of neonatal withdrawal symptoms
Beta-blockers	Risk of neonatal hypoglycaemia or bradycardia
Carbimazole	Risk of neonatal goitre and hypothyroidism
Iodine and iodides	Risk of neonatal goitre and hypothyroidism
Lithium	Risk of toxicity
Opioid analgesics	Depression of neonatal respiration Withdrawal effects in dependent mothers
Sulphonamides and related drugs	Risk of neonatal haemolysis and methaemo-globinaemia
Thiazide diuretics	Risk of neonatal thrombocytopenia

Figure 16.2 Drugs that may adversely affect the neonate if taken by the mother late in pregnancy

DRUGS AND BREAST MILK

Many drugs given to the mother postnatally will be excreted to some degree in the milk. Factors that affect the rate of excretion include maternal pharmacokinetics (blood flow to the breast, hormonal influence, etc.), the physiological composition of the milk and the properties of the drug. Drugs that are weak bases, highly lipophilic and/or have low protein binding, are excreted in the largest amounts. However, the amount of most drugs available in breast milk for absorption is small (usually less than 2% of the maternal dose). For drugs with low to moderate potential toxicity, an exposure of up to 10% of the weight-adjusted maternal dose is generally regarded as acceptable. Thus, there is only a small number of drugs where breast feeding is absolutely contraindicated (Figure 16.3). Laboratory tests are occasionally useful in monitoring the effects of maternal drug therapy on breast-fed infants, e.g. thyroid function tests when the mother is receiving anti-thyroid drugs. A comprehensive list of drugs that can be excreted in breast milk is provided as an appendix in the British National Formulary.

Maternal drugs for which breast feeding is contraindicated	
Lithium	Cytotoxic drugs
Immunosuppressants (excluding corticosteroids)	Radiopharmaceuticals
Phenindione	Ergot alkaloids

Figure 16.3 Maternal drugs for which breast feeding is contraindicated

THERAPEUTIC MONITORING

Monitoring drug concentrations is most valid when there is a direct relationship between the plasma concentration and the pharmacological and/or toxic effects. Sometimes there is no such relationship, e.g. when the drug has active metabolites, or where the drug action is irreversible and therefore unrelated to steady-state concentrations. Regular monitoring of blood concentrations in neonates is indicated for drugs with one or more of the following characteristics:

- unpredictable half-life
- toxic cumulative effects
- narrow therapeutic index (i.e. the difference between effective and toxic concentrations is small)
- where inadequate dosage leads to loss of efficacy.

A list of such drugs, and their therapeutic ranges at the appropriate sampling times, is given in Figure 16.4.

Therapeutic monitoring of drugs in neonates

Drug	Sampling time	Target range
Amikacin	Peak (30-60 min post-dose)	15-20 mg/L
	Trough (<60 min pre-dose)	<10 mg/L
Gentamicin	Peak (30-60 min post-dose)	6-10 mg/L
	Trough (<60 min pre-dose)	<2 mg/L
Vancomycin	Trough (<60 min pre-dose)	5-10 mg/L
Chloramphenicol	Peak (1-2 hours post-dose)	15-25 mg/L
Digoxin	>6h post-dose	1-2 μg/L
Caffeine	>6h post-dose	15-30 mg/L
Theophylline	Peak (60 min post-dose)	5-12 mg/L
Phenobarbital	>6h post-dose	15-30 mg/L
Phenytoin	>8h post-dose	10-20 mg/L

Figure 16.4 Therapeutic monitoring of drugs in neonates

FURTHER READING

British National Formulary. Published biannually by the British Medical Association and Royal Pharmaceutical Society of Great Britain, London. http://BNF.org

Comer AM, Perry CM, Figgitt DP. Caffeine citrate: a review of its use in apnoea of prematurity. Paediatr Drugs 2001; 3: 61-79.

Sato Y. Pharmacokinetics of antibiotics in neonates. Acta Paediatrica Jpn 1997; 39: 124-31.

Wagner CL, Katikaneni LD, Cox TH, Ryan RM. The impact of prenatal drug exposure on the neonate. Obstet Gynae Clin North Am 1998; 25: 169-94.

Appendix A

Routine specimen collection

BLOOD COLLECTION IN NEONATES

Blood can be obtained by capillary puncture, venepuncture or arterial sampling. The sampling site will depend on the quantity of blood required, the analytes requested and the clinical condition of the baby.

In general, small specimens sufficient for routine testing can be obtained from the heel by capillary puncture. For all capillary measurements, a free flowing sample, from a warmed heel, is required – this is particularly important for blood gas analysis (*see p.74*) and other analytes affected by haemolysis, e.g. potassium. Peripheral venepuncture should be used for larger quantities of blood for coagulation and bacterial culture (see below), or when capillary puncture is contraindicated. For repeated sampling (e.g. regular monitoring) an indwelling umbilical line or peripheral arterial cannula is preferred.

Veins in the hands and feet should be used in the first instance for venous sampling with more proximal veins being reserved for central venous access. Jugular and femoral veins must not be used for routine sampling. On no account should broken needles be used.

CAPILLARY BLOOD COLLECTION

GENERAL

Capillary collection from neonates is not without risk and should therefore be minimised and planned to coordinate collection for both haematology and clinical biochemistry. If specimens for both clinical biochemistry and haematology are to be collected, then the blood for haematology must be collected *first* (beware of possible contamination from potassium EDTA for the clinical biochemistry specimen – this will manifest as an artefactually low calcium). This arrangement should minimise the extent to which the platelet count falls in shed blood after skin injury and provide results similar to those from a venous specimen. Every attempt should be made to collect clinical biochemistry specimens without haemolysis and to avoid excessive pressure, as this will affect the results obtained for some analytes as well as producing discomfort.

Should a baby's condition be a cause for concern before, or during, a blood collection, it is essential to inform the doctor or nurse in charge, who will advise whether to proceed. The phlebotomist should discontinue the procedure if in any doubt. Similarly, if a baby's clinical condition appears to have changed after the procedure, the nurse or doctor in charge should be told. Staff performing capillary blood collection from neonates, whether doctors, nurses or laboratory-based phlebotomists, must be specifically trained.

SELECTION AND PREPARATION OF SITE FOR SKIN PUNCTURE

Before commencing, the parent(s) should be given an explanation of the procedure that is about to be performed and answers given to any questions they may have. Efforts should be made to allay any fears. If the parent is unhappy about the collection, a doctor or nurse should be consulted before proceeding.

The baby should be lying in a secure and comfortable position so that the heel is easily accessible. In children under one year of age, the thumb and fingers should not be used for capillary blood collection. An area of the heel, free from previous puncture sites and any skin problems, should be selected (Figure A.1). The ankle should be inspected to check that it has not been used for venous access, as there is a danger of re-opening wounds. Punctures should not be performed on the posterior curvature of the heel where the bone is closest to the skin. Before attempting any blood collection, the site should be warm and well perfused: this may be achieved by rubbing the site gently or wrapping it in a clean, warm nappy or towel (< 40°C). A dirty heel should be pre-washed with soapy water, rinsed and thoroughly dried.

Before performing the puncture, the following items must be close at hand and ready for use:

- swab
- cotton wool
- puncture device
- specimen tube(s).

The name and registration number of the baby must be checked immediately before starting the procedure.

The site must be cleaned with an antiseptic solution (isopropyl alcohol-impregnated pre-injection swabs) and wiped completely dry with clean cotton wool to prevent haemolysis. These swabs can be used in an incubator: the heel is given a quick wipe and the swab is then immediately removed from the incubator.

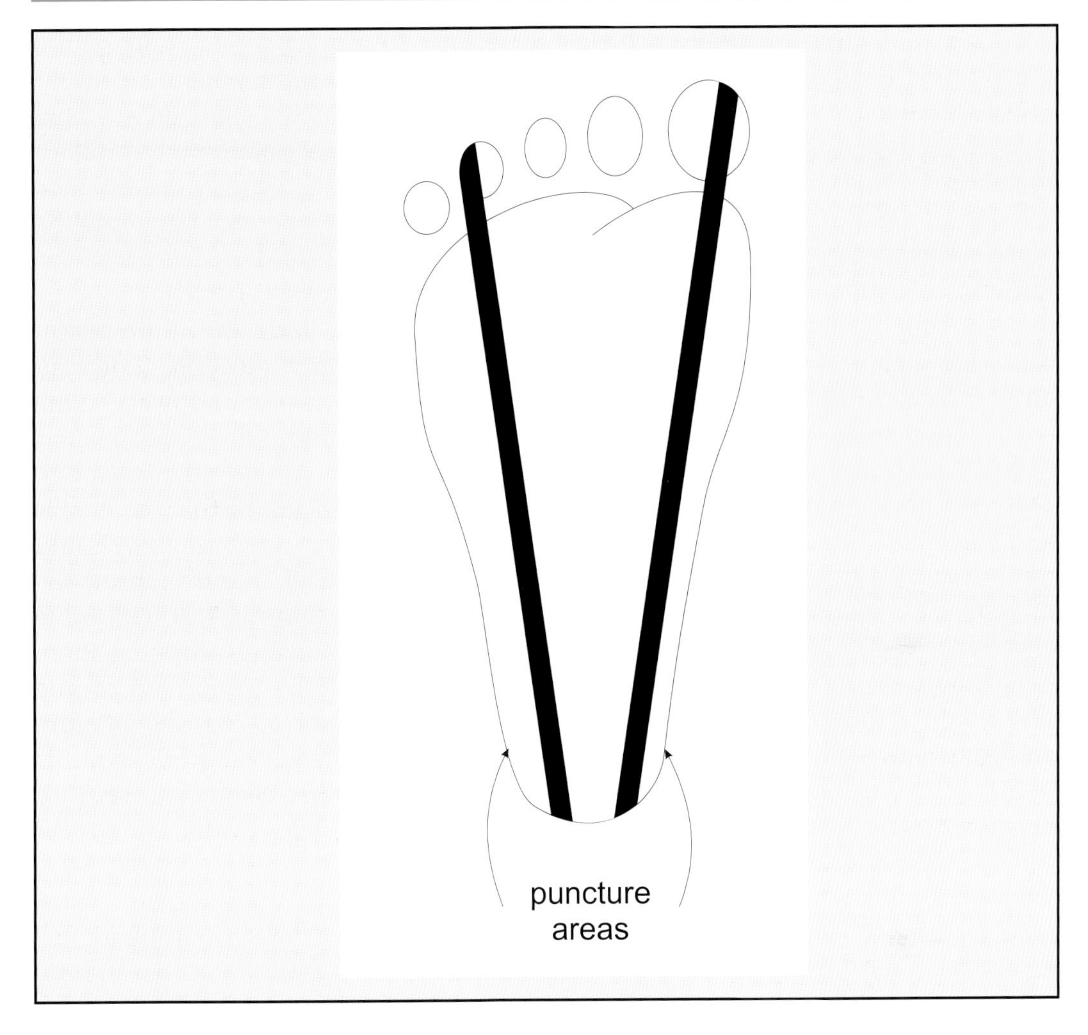

Figure A.1 Diagram of foot to show recommended sites on the heel for capillary skin puncture

Skin puncture

The phlebotomist should stand facing slightly away from the baby's head, holding the heel with the nearer hand. The baby's heel is gripped firmly by holding around the ankle with the index and middle fingers so that the sole of the foot is against the palm of the hand and the heel exposed. The thumb is placed around the heel and pressure is controlled with the thumb and index finger. Whilst maintaining tension on the heel, the puncture is made as one continuous deliberate motion in a direction slightly off perpendicular to the puncture site. Pressure is then released and the first drop of blood wiped off as it appears.

For a neonate, the puncture depth *must not exceed* 2.4 mm, and preferably be not greater than 1.6 mm, to avoid penetration of bone, and hence the potential complication of osteomyelitis. Several devices are available. The collection tube is held between thumb and forefinger. A hanging drop of blood is obtained; the side of this drop that faces away from the patient is touched against the inside of the tube which is furthest from the patient. The drop of blood is then knocked down to the bottom of the tube by giving the tube a sharp tap on a hard surface. Using a minimum of pressure, further drops of blood are obtained and touched against the same site inside the neck of the tube. They will follow the track of the initial drop. Pressure around the heel should be eased and then slowly and gently re-applied to allow more drops of blood to flow. Excessive 'milking' or massaging is not recommended as this may cause haemolysis. Should blood become smeared over the heel during the collection, it should not be scraped off into the collecting tube. The skin should be wiped with clean, dry cotton wool (*not* an alcohol swab) and the collection continued. Periodically, the tube should be gently flicked using the little or other free finger of the hand holding the tube. This is to ensure the mixing of the blood with anticoagulant. Blood will flow more easily if the heel is held low.

The blood volume required will obviously be dependent on which tests are required. This will vary for different laboratories depending on the methods in use; it should be possible to obtain the most commonly requested tests (i.e. full blood count, bilirubin (total and conjugated), sodium, potassium, creatinine, calcium and albumin) from a total blood volume of 1 mL, although this will depend on the PCV.

When the collection is finished, the cap is pushed onto the tube and the tube gently inverted several times to ensure mixing. A wad of dry, clean cotton wool is pressed firmly against the puncture site and the baby's heel held above the body for a few minutes to stop the flow of blood. Plasters may be applied to the puncture site but are best avoided if possible: neonates have sensitive skin and a plaster that becomes detached is at risk of being ingested. Also, later removal of the plaster may reopen the wound. If a plaster is used, the parents or nurse in charge must be informed.

The tube should be labelled either with a felt-tipped pen or a narrow adhesive label as a 'flag' (i.e. the label wrapped around the tube close to the top so that a portion overhangs at the side).

SPECIMENS FOR BLOOD CULTURE

There are two important considerations when collecting blood for culture: obtaining an adequate volume to be able to detect bacteraemia, and minimisation of the risk of contamination with skin bacteria.

Although neonates with bacteraemia tend to have a higher bacterial load than other age groups, it is not uncommon for there to be no more than 1-5 bacteria/mL of blood. Commercially available paediatric blood culture media are specially formulated for blood volumes as low as 0.5 mL. Nevertheless, the more blood that is sampled, the more likely it is that bacteraemia will be detected. Repeat blood cultures are always worthwhile where sepsis is suspected in the face of a negative initial culture.

Around 50% of blood culture isolates from adults and older children are caused by contaminants and are, therefore, not significant. The number of contaminants in blood cultures from neonates may be even higher because of the greater difficulty in obtaining samples cleanly. It is especially difficult to distinguish between contamination and infection in neonatal blood cultures, because coagulase-negative staphylococci are both the most common contaminants and true pathogens in neonatal units. Because of the high likelihood of contamination, capillary blood samples are not suitable for culture. Samples are best obtained by venepuncture after thorough skin disinfection. Iodine-based antiseptics are sometimes recommended for skin preparation, but there is a risk of systemic absorption through neonatal skin and there is no evidence that they are superior to isopropyl alcohol-impregnated swabs. Blood for culture can also be collected through intravascular devices, such as an umbilical catheter, either at the time of insertion or later. However, cultures taken at the time of insertion of the device may have an increased rate of contamination because of the extra manipulation that is usually required during insertion. Accessing indwelling intravenous long lines risks introducing infection. Therefore, whenever possible, collection of blood cultures via this route should be delayed until the device is being entered for another reason; this is especially important for lines that are, or may be, used for therapeutic purposes such as administration of parenteral nutrition.

URINE SAMPLES

Accurate monitoring of urine output is difficult in the neonatal period. When there are concerns about fluid balance, unmeasured insensible losses of water through skin and respiratory tract may be more relevant than polyuria, and water loss is best monitored by weighing the baby regularly, using electronic scales, and by monitoring plasma sodium concentrations.

A good estimate of urine volume can be obtained using weighed nappies (weighed pre- and post-use) and this is commonly done for babies requiring intensive care for the first 3 to 5 days. Urinary catheterisation is very rarely used in neonatal units unless there is a structural urinary tract problem.

Samples for microscopy and culture can be obtained by clean catch into a universal container (in a male), and by using a urinary collection bag (U-bag) or equivalent in a female. A convenient method of urine collection for biochemistry or culture, or to estimate volume of urinary output in a small baby in an incubator, is to use a transparent glove into which several sterile cotton wool balls have been placed, and to place this over the baby's nappy area. The sides of the glove may have to be cut open. When the cotton balls are observed to be wet, the glove is removed and a syringe used to aspirate the urine from the balls until they are dry. This method does not traumatise the baby's skin as a U-bag may, and can be used over long periods.

OTHER SPECIMENS FOR MICROBIOLOGICAL INVESTIGATION

Microbiological investigations may be undertaken on swabs and other samples from a wide variety of sites. Techniques for collection of these specimens should be determined locally, and will depend on the methodologies used by individual laboratories.

FURTHER READING

Blumenfeld TA, Tur GA, Blanc WA. Recommended site and depth of newborn heel skin punctures based on anatomical measurements and histopathology. Lancet 1979; **1:** 230-3.

Garvey K, Batki AD, Holder RL, Edwards C, Kenkre J, Thorpe G. Thirteen lancing devices. London: Medical Devices Agency evaluation report, 1998. MD/98/05.

Garvey K, Batki AD, Thomason HL, Thorpe G. Review of lancing systems. London: Medical Devices Agency evaluation report, 1999. MSA/99/08.

Lilien LD, Harris VJ, Ramamurphy RS, Pildes RS. Neonatal osteomyelitis of the calcaneous: complication of heel puncture. J Paeds 1976; **88:** 478-80.

Meites S, Levitt MJ, Blumenfeld TA, Hammond KB, Hicks JM, Hill GJ *et al*. Skin puncture and blood collecting techniques for infants. Clin Chem 1979; **25:** 183-9.

Meites S. Skin puncture and blood collecting techniques for infants. Update and problems. Clin Chem 1988; **34:** 1890-4.

Meites S, Hamblin CR, Hayes JR. A study of experimental lancets for blood collection to avoid bone infection of infants. Clin Chem 1992; **38:** 908-10.

Murray PR, Baron EJ, Pfaller MA, Tenover FC, Yolken RH (eds). Manual of Clinical Microbiology, 7th edn. Washington: American Society for Microbiology, 2001.

Slockbower JM, Jacoby H, Blumenfeld TA, Bruck E, Duffie ER, Mundschenk D. Approved standard procedures for the collection of diagnostic blood specimens by skin puncture. The National Committee for Clinical Laboratory Standards 1982; **2:** 132-46.

Verlio M, Siviero R, Trento M, Porta M. Finger-pricking devices; are they less painful than lancets? Diabetic Medicine 1996; **13:** 598.

Appendix B

Emergency specimen collection for the diagnosis of inherited metabolic disorders

In life-threatening situations where an inherited metabolic disorder is thought to be a likely cause (whether from family history, results of preliminary investigations or clinical presentation) the specimens detailed below should be taken. At the earliest opportunity, a specialist laboratory should be contacted to discuss appropriate investigations. If possible, urine and blood specimens should be taken before death. Appropriate policy and procedure for obtaining informed consent should be followed. Skin and tissue specimens are better taken as biopsy specimens when the baby is still alive. If this is not possible, then they should be taken as soon as possible after death.

If any of the specimens are taken after death, it is extremely important to record accurately both the time of death and the time when the specimens were taken. Appropriate storage as detailed below is *essential*.

URINE

Urine, *however little*, is extremely useful. Ideally, 5-10 mL of urine should be collected into a bottle with no preservative and stored deep frozen (- 20°C). If the sample is contaminated with blood, it should be centrifuged to remove cells before the supernatant is frozen.

BLOOD

Ideally, 5-10 mL blood should be collected in lithium heparin and 0.5 mL in fluoride oxalate; plasma samples should be separated as soon as possible and stored deep-frozen (-20°C). The packed red cells should be stored at 4°C (not frozen). If DNA analysis is likely to be required, a further 5-10 mL whole blood (EDTA) should be taken and kept at 4°C to be sent for analysis during the next working day.

SKIN (FOR FIBROBLAST CULTURE)

Skin taken up to 24 hours after death is likely to be viable provided it is not infected. A skin sample should be taken and placed in a suitable transport medium (obtainable from most virology or cytogenetic departments). In an emergency, sterile isotonic saline can be used; agar should not be used. If the specimen cannot be sent to the laboratory immediately, it should be stored at 4°C until despatch, and not frozen.

Sterility is of paramount importance when taking skin biopsy specimens, especially at necropsy.

TISSUE SAMPLES (LIVER, HEART MUSCLE, SKELETAL MUSCLE)

These should only be taken if there is a strong clinical suspicion of a primary defect in one of these tissues. It is very important that blood and urine specimens are also collected in addition to tissue specimens. Necropsy tissue samples are usually only suitable for biochemical analysis if taken within two hours of death. Tubes must be labelled clearly with the patient's details, the time taken *and* the type of tissue. This should be done before taking the biopsies.

Two or three needle biopsy samples of tissue should be taken, placed in a plastic tube and snap frozen in liquid nitrogen (or solid carbon dioxide). All specimens should be stored deep frozen, as cold as possible.

Note that these samples are required for biochemical analyses only. Appropriate fixed samples may also be required for histological investigation.

CEREBROSPINAL FLUID

Sometimes a cerebrospinal fluid sample may be useful. If the specimen is cloudy or blood stained, it should be centrifuged and the clear supernatant stored deep frozen.

Appendix C

Laboratory investigation of sudden unexpected death in infancy (SUDI)

(i.e. children under two years old who die suddenly and unexpectedly)

1. Break the news to the parents, explain about the urgency and nature of the investigations and the obligation to report to the Coroner.

2. Inform the Coroner and obtain permission to take specimens as part of the investigation of SUDI.

   Note: Coroners (or other appropriate officers) may vary in exactly what procedures they wish to follow and laboratories may differ in exact specimen requirements. Check your local arrangements. Once permission has been given, do not delay taking specimens for metabolic investigations.

3. Blood – perform a cardiac puncture within 30 minutes of death if possible, and preferably not more than four hours after. Drop some blood onto blood spot cards directly from the syringe (for acyl carnitines). Allow to dry at room temperature. Split the remainder into:

   - lithium heparin bottle for metabolic tests – centrifuge and store the plasma at -20°C; keep red cells at 4°C
   - plain bottle (clotted blood) for toxicology – centrifuge and store serum at -20°C
   - blood cultures – to incubate at 37°C
   - consider blood for chromosomes, especially if the baby was dysmorphic.

4. Urine – Suprapubic aspirate (SPA) from bladder. Divide the urine into three plain bottles for:

   - microbiology – store at 4 °C
   - toxicology – centrifuge and freeze supernatant at -20°C
   - biochemistry for metabolic tests (amino and organic acids) – centrifuge and freeze the supernatant at -20°C.

5. Nasopharyngeal swab, if less than eight hours post mortem – place into transport medium for virology. Any other body fluids, e.g. wound swabs, store at 4°C for microbiology.

6. Skin biopsy for metabolic investigations (see Appendix B) – place in culture or suitable transport media. Store at 4°C.

7. Muscle and liver biopsy – consider if there is a strong suspicion of an inherited metabolic disorder, e.g. family history. Contact specialist metabolic laboratory for advice.

Document in the clinical notes all the specimens taken (including a record of the site(s) from which specimens were taken, e.g. cardiac stab, SPA urine, etc.) Label tubes and complete request forms to include date and time taken. Ensure an unbroken chain of evidence for forensic specimens. All request forms and clinical notes must be signed, as they may become legal documents.

Appendix D

Investigation of neonatal hydrops

Hydrops is defined as the presence of excess subcutaneous fluid (oedema) with effusions in body cavities – pleural or pericardial effusions or ascites.

Hydrops that is suspected antenatally and confirmed by detailed ultrasound scanning can be investigated, and interventions may sometimes be undertaken, before birth (*see Chapter 1*).

The causes are broadly divided into immune (associated with blood group incompatibility, antiglobulin test positivity or fetal anaemia) and non-immune. The latter group includes numerous conditions variously affecting the heart, kidneys and urinary tract, gastrointestinal and respiratory systems, together with certain chromosomal abnormalities, e.g. trisomy 21, Turner's syndrome (45XO) and Noonan syndrome. Infective causes include viral infections (parvovirus B19, cytomegalovirus, Coxsackie viruses), *Treponema pallidum, Toxoplasma gondii, Listeria monocytogenes*. Non-immune haematological causes include haemoglobinopathies, haemolysis, fetal haemorrhage and erythrocyte underproduction.

Numerous inherited metabolic disorders (IMD) can present as hydrops. Many are lysosomal storage disorders. Details are given in Figure D.1.

It is estimated that, if full prenatal and postnatal assessments are performed, a precise diagnosis can be obtained in 85% of cases.

CLINICAL MANAGEMENT AND INVESTIGATION

Prenatally, interventions such as fetal blood transfusion, or aspiration of fluid-filled cavities, may be appropriate. Immediate interventions required at birth may include ventilation, aspiration of fluid and transfusion. Immediate investigations after delivery in suspected immune hydrops will include blood gases, blood glucose, blood group and direct antiglobulin test, full blood count and plasma bilirubin and albumin concentrations.

Inherited metabolic diseases that may present as hydrops	
Disorder	**Diagnostic test**
Sly's disease (mucopolysaccharidosis type 7)	Urine glycosaminoglycans Leucocyte or fibroblast β-glucuronidase
Sialic acid disorder	Urine oligosaccharides Fibroblast sialic acid
Mucolipidosis type 1 (sialidosis)	Urine oligosaccharides Leucocyte or fibroblast α-neuraminidase
G_{M1}Gangliosidase	Urine oligosaccharides
Galactosialidosis	Leucocyte or fibroblast β-galactosidase
Morquio disease type A	Urine mucopolysaccharides Leucocyte or fibroblast galactose 6-sulphatase
Niemann-Pick disease type C	Bone marrow biopsy Skin biopsy for cholesterol uptake studies and cholesterol staining
Gaucher's disease	Bone marrow biopsy Leucocyte or fibroblast β-glucosidase
Carbohydrate deficient glycoprotein syndromes (CDGS)	Plasma transferrin isoforms
Haemolytic anaemias e.g. pyruvate kinase, hexokinase, G6PD and glucose phosphate isomerase deficiency	Erythrocyte enzymes
I-cell disease	Plasma I-cell screen
Carnitine deficiency	Plasma carnitine
Cytochrome oxidase deficiency	Blood and CSF lactate Muscle biopsy ?Fibroblast cytochrome oxidase
Fumarase deficiency	Urine organic acids
Farber's disease	Fibroblast acid ceramidase
Neonatal haemochromatosis	Plasma iron, ferritin and TIBC Liver iron

Figure D.1 Inherited metabolic diseases that may present as hydrops

For non-immune hydrops, the following investigations should be performed (blood being taken before transfusion):

- plasma electrolytes, creatinine, ALT, AST, coagulation screen, total and conjugated bilirubin
- chromosomal analysis and sample for DNA to cytogenetics
- aspirated ascitic or pleural fluid for total protein concentration, microscopy (for lymphocytes, and fat globules in chylothorax), viral and microbial culture
- electrocardiogram with rhythm strip
- ultrasound examination of heart, kidneys and brain
- haemoglobin electrophoresis, blood film
- serological investigations (TORCH and parvovirus)
- urine for CMV PCR.

SPECIMENS TO BE COLLECTED FOR THE INVESTIGATION OF THE NEONATE FOR IMD

If an inherited metabolic disorder is suspected (i.e. no obvious other cause of the hydrops and features suggestive of IMD, e.g. family history of unexplained illness, sibling death) additional specimens should be collected as follows:

- 5 – 10 mL random urine for glycosaminoglycans, oligosaccharide and organic acid analysis
- 3 mL venous blood into lithium heparin for plasma carnitine and acyl carnitines, I-cell screen and transferrin isoforms, and 0.5 mL into fluoride oxalate for lactate
- 1 mL venous blood into a tube without anticoagulant for ferritin quantitation
- consider a bone marrow biopsy to look for foam cells
- blood for assay of red cell enzymes (if there is a haemolytic anaemia).

Should the infant with hydrops die before a diagnosis is made, the following specimens should be collected to allow a diagnosis to be established post mortem, to form a basis for genetic counselling:

- fetal skin for culture for chromosome analysis and biochemical tests (enzymes)

- fetal blood for investigation of haemoglobinopathies/haemolytic disorders

- placental tissue for histological analysis. Culture of this tissue is also possible; however such cell lines often show early senescence

- fetal urine if available

- liver and muscle for histology/histochemistry

- blood for leucocyte enzymes.

Specimens to be collected for the IMD investigation of a hydrops fetalis *in utero,* collect 10 ml amniotic fluid for culture and mucopolysaccharide electrophoresis (specific enzymes can be measured on cultured amniocytes).

FURTHER READING

Jones DC Non-immune fetal hydrops, diagnosis and obstetrical management. Seminars Perinatol 1995; **19:** 447-61

StephensonT, Zuccollo J, Mohajer M. Diagnosis and management of non-immune hydrops in the newborn. Arch Dis Child 1994; **70:** F151-4

Biochemical reference ranges

The values quoted below, and in the following section, are a guide to interpreting data for term neonates, from birth to the age of four weeks, and apply to laboratory methods currently in use at Birmingham Children's and Birmingham Women's Hospitals; they will not necessarily apply to methods in use at other hospitals. Ranges will differ significantly for some analytes for different methods; therefore, it is important you consult your local laboratory.

Blood/plasma	**Unit**	**Reference range**	**Comments**
Acid base status:			
Hydrogen ion	nmol/L	38-48	Arterial
pH		7.32-7.42	Arterial
*p*CO2	kPa	4.0-5.5	Arterial
Bicarbonate (derived)	mmol	17-25	
Base excess (derived)	mmol/L	-4-+4	
*p*O2	kPa	8.0-11.0	Arterial
Alanine aminotransferase (ALT)	IU/L	up to 40	May vary with method
Albumin	g/L	28-43 30-43 32-44	0-7 days 7-14 days 21-28 days Concentrations increase over first three weeks. Concentrations are lower in preterm babies and correlate with gestational age.
Alkaline phosphatase (ALP)	IU/L	150-700	Higher concentrations in first week due to placental ALP. Preterm concentrations higher and may be up to 1600 in the absence of active rickets. Range can vary widely with method.
α_1-antitrypsin	g/L	0.9-2.2	'Adult' concentrations at birth, with fall after two weeks. Gradual rise to adult concentration by one year. Genotype should be assessed if <1.6 g/L in infants with prolonged jaundice. Concentrations may be increased as part of an acute phase response.

Blood/plasma	Unit	Reference range	Comments
α-fetoprotein	kU/L	450-55,000 185-27,000 80-13,000	Birth 2 weeks 4 weeks After birth, concentrations fall ($t_{1/2}$ 5.5 days) in first 2 weeks. Concentrations are method dependent.
Ammonia	µmol/L	up to 100	Preterm and/or sick babies may have concentrations up to 200 µmol/L. Lower concentrations after one month (< 40 µmol/L).
Amylase	IU/L	up to 50	Reference range for children reached after one year.
Anion gap i.e. $([Na^+]+[K^+]) - ([Cl^-]+[HCO_3^-])$	mmol/L	less than 20	
Aspartate aminotransferase (AST)	IU/L	up to 100	May vary with method.
Bilirubin			
Total	µmol/L	up to 200	< 10 days of age (peak ~ 3-4 days).
Conjugated	µmol/L	less than 20	Total bilirubin > 50 after 14 days is
Direct reacting	µmol/L	less than 40	abnormal
Caeruloplasmin	g/L	0-4 months	Increases from birth throughout the first year.
Calcium	mmol/L	1.95-2.75 2.15-2.75	0-5 days After one week There is often a marked fall after birth with lowest concentration (1.8) at around 24-48 h of age.
Chloride	mmol/L	95-110	
Cholesterol (total)	mmol/L	1.5-4.0	Gradual increase from birth.
Copper	µmol/L	3-11	Rapid increase during first week.
Cortisol	nmol/L	180-550 at 09:00 <130 at 24:00	Cortisol is difficult to measure accurately at birth because of cross-reacting steroids. Concentrations are high at birth.There is a marked fall within 24 hours following delivery – partly due to a falling maternally-derived cortisol.

Blood/plasma	Unit	Reference range	Comments
Creatine kinase	IU/L	High levels up to 10 fold those in infancy/childhood	Range dependent on methodology. Marked fall during first week of life, following peak at 24-48 h.
Creatinine	µmol/L	15-55 20-80 15-55	0-7 days 7 days - 1 month 1 month - 2 years Method dependent. Sharp decline in concentration over first month. Also dependent on gestational age – see Figure 1

Plasma creatinine concentration (µmol/L)				
Postnatal age		**Gestational age (weeks)**		
	28	**32**	**36**	**40**
2 days	40-220	27-175	23-143	18-118
7 days	23-145	19-119	16-98	13-81
14 days	18-118	15-97	12-80	10-66
21 days	16-104	14-86	11-71	9-57
28 days	15-95	12-78	10-64	9-53

Figure 1 Plasma creatinine concentration (µmol/L) and gestational age

Blood/Plasma	Unit	Reference range	Comments
C-reactive protein (CRP)	mg/L	up to 10	Plasma half-life 5-7 h
Ferritin	µg/L	90-640	From two weeks (lower at birth). Falls to lower concentration by six months (upper limit 150).
Glucose (fasting)	mmol/L	2.0-5.5	For discussion of hypoglycaemia see p.108 15% lower in whole blood than plasma

Blood/Plasma	Unit	Reference range	Comments
17α-hydroxyprogesterone (17-OHP)	nmol/L	0.7-12.4	There is a rapid fall from the very high concentrations of 17-OHP (maternally derived) in the first 24-48 hours of life. This is therefore an inappropriate time to measure 17-OHP for diagnostic purposes. Premature and stressed neonates may have 2-3 fold higher concentrations of 17-OHP compared with values for full term infants.
Immunoglobulins			
IgG	g/L	5.2-18.0	Cord blood
	g/L	5.0-17.0	0-2 weeks
	g/L	3.9-13.0	2-6 weeks
IgA	g/L	<0.02	Cord blood
	g/L	0.01-0.08	0-2 weeks
	g/L	0.02-0.15	2-6 weeks
IgM	g/L	0.02-0.20	Cord blood
	g/L	0.05-0.20	0-2 weeks
	g/L	0.08-0.40	2-6 weeks
IgE	kU/L	<5	At birth
	kU/L	<11	At 3 months
Iron	μmol/L	10-30	May be much higher at birth (up to 60 μmol/L).
Lactate	mmol/L	0.5-2.0	
Magnesium	mmol/L	0.6-1.0	
Osmolality	mmol/kg	275-295	
Phosphate	mmol/L	1.3-3.0	Affected by type of milk feed.
Potassium	mmol/L	3.5-6.5	Capillary blood.
		3.5-5.5	Venous or arterial blood and not haemolysed.
Protein (total)	g/L	54-70	Term baby. Gradual increase from birth. Preterm babies have lower values.
Sodium	mmol/L	133-146	0-1 week
		134-144	1 week-1 month
Thyroid stimulating hormone (TSH)	mU/L	< 10 (whole blood) < 5 (plasma)	At 6-14 days; pre- and full term infants show a rapid increase in TSH during the first 24 h.

Blood/Plasma	Unit	Reference range	Comments
Thyroxine (total, tT4)	nmol/L	142-296 116-203	1-3 days 1-4 weeks Higher concentrations occur in first week of life.
Thyroxine (free, fT4)	pmol/L	14-28	Higher at 1-3 days.
Transferrin	g/L	1.05-2.65	
Triglycerides (fasting)	mmol/L	0.3-2.0	
Immunoreactive trypsin (IRT)	ng/mL	< 70 (dried blood spot) < 130 (plasma)	0-2 weeks
Urea	mmol/L	1.0-5.0	Infants fed on cows' milk formula may have higher concentrations than breast milk.
Urate	μmol/L	120-340	Values are higher at birth.
Zinc	μmol/L	9-22	0-5 days. Preterm infants have higher values

Urine	Unit	Reference range	Comments
Calcium	mmol/kg/24h	less than 0.4	
Calcium:creatinine ratio	mmol/mmol	up to 1.2	Term baby; first two weeks
Copper	μmol/24h	up to 1.0	
Phosphate	mmol/1.73m^2/24h	up to 2.0	Term baby; first two weeks. Higher in preterm babies.
Fractional phosphate excretion	%	1-6	Term baby; first two weeks. Higher in preterm babies.
Potassium	mmol/kg/24h	up to 2	Depends on potassium intake and gestational age.
Sodium	mmol/kg/24h	up to 1 (full term) up to 3 (preterm)	Depends on sodium intake and gestational age.
Fractional sodium excretion	%	< 0.3 term 2-5 preterm	During week 1
Urate:creatinine ratio	mmol/mmol	up to 2.0	

CSF	Unit	Reference range	Comments
Glucose	mmol/L	2.5-4.5	Normally 75% of blood glucose
Protein	g/L	0.4-1.2 0.2-0.8	Newborn Neonate

Haematological reference ranges

Normal haematological values

Value	Gestational age (weeks) 24	34	Full-term Cord blood	Day 1	Day 3	Day 7	Day 14
Hb (g/dL)	14.5	15.0	16.8	18.4	17.8	17.0	16.8
Haematocrit (%)	45	47	53	58	55	54	52
Red cells ($x10^9/L$)	4.0	4.4	5.25	5.8	5.6	5.2	5.1
MCV (fL)	120	118	107	108	99	98	96
MCH (pg)	40	38	34	35	33	32.5	31.5
MCHC (%)	31	32	31.7	32.5	33	33	33
Reticulocytes (%)	5-10	3-10	3-7	3-7	1-3	0-1	0-1
Platelets ($x10^9/L$)			290	192	213	248	252

MCV, mean corpuscular volume
MCH, mean corpuscular haemoglobin
MCHC, mean corpuscular haemoglobin concentration

Figure 1 Normal haematological values

Leucocyte values and neutrophil counts in neonates (10^9/L)

Age (h)	Total white cell count	Neutrophils	Bands/ metas	Lymphocytes	Monocytes	Eosinophils
Term infants						
0	10.0-26.0	5.0-13.0	0.4-1.8	3.5-8.5	0.7-1.5	0.2-2.0
12	13.5-31.0	9.0-18.0	0.4-2.0	3.0-7.0	1.0-2.0	0.2-2.0
72	5.0-14.5	2.0-7.0	0.2-0.4	2.0-5.0	0.5-1.0	0.2-1.0
144	6.0-14.5	2.0-6.0	0.2-0.5	3.0-6.0	0.7-1.2	0.2-0.8
Premature infants						
0	5.0-19.0	2.0-9.0	0.2-2.4	2.5-6.0	0.3-1.0	0.1-0.7
12	5.0-21.0	3.0-11.0	0.2-2.4	1.5-5.0	0.3-1.3	0.1-1.1
72	5.0-14.0	3.0-7.0	0.2-0.6	1.5-4.0	0.3-1.2	0.2-1.1
144	5.5-17.5	2.0-7.0	0.2-0.5	2.5-7.5	0.5-1.5	0.3-1.2

Figure 2 Leucocyte values and neutrophil counts in term and premature infants

Normal values for coagulation screening tests

Test	Older child	Full-term newborn	Healthy growing premature infant
Platelets (x10^9/L)	150-400	150-400	150-400
Prothrombin time (secs)	10-14	11-15	11-16
Partial thromboplastin time (secs)	25-35	30-40	35-80
Fibrinogen (g/L)	1.75-4.0	1.65-4.0	1.5-3.25
Fibrin degradation products (mg/L)	<10	<10	<10

Figure 3 Normal values for coagulation screening tests

Glossary

Agenesis	- Failure of development (of an organ or body part).
Amniocentesis	- Removal of specimen of amniotic fluid for analysis, usually at 16-18 weeks gestation.
Apgar score	- Widely used, rapid assessment system of baby's condition after birth, usually at 1 and 5 minutes. The maximum score is 10.
Apnoea	- Cessation of respiratory effort for a period longer than (usually) 20 seconds.
Biliary atresia	- Rare condition in which bile ducts are absent and there is progressive obstructive jaundice and liver disease.
Centile chart	- Chart derived from measurements (e.g. of weight) on large numbers of subjects. Lines on chart relate to centiles, i.e. number per hundred subjects whose measurement is below the line.
Cardiotocograph	- Derived signal representing fetal heart rate.
Cephalhaematoma	- Subperiosteal collection of blood over skull usually arising from trauma during delivery. Can be associated with underlying skull fracture.
Choledochal cyst	- Cystic malformation of major bile duct.
Chorionic villus	- Area of fetal tissue in early pregnancy that will develop into part of placenta.
Consanguinity	- Degree to which a father and mother are 'blood' relatives.
Cordocentesis	- Technique by which a blood sample is taken from the unborn baby, from umbilical cord vessels under ultrasound control.

Cryptorchidism - Undescended testes.

Dysplasia - Abnormal development (of a tissue, organ or part of the body).

Dystocia - Difficult or slow labour.

Erythroblastosis fetalis - Condition of the unborn baby secondary to severe (Rhesus) iso-immunisation.

Exomphalos - Failure of return of intestinal contents to the abdominal cavity during early fetal life. There is no normal umbilical cord.

Fontanelle - The soft spots on top of a baby's skull where the bones do not meet. They normally become undetectable between 12-18 months of age.

Gastroschisis - Malformation in which, in early fetal life, gut fails to relocate normally in the abdominal cavity and remains floating in the amniotic sac, the connection to the baby being to the right of a (normal) umbilicus.

Hydrops - Description of a baby or fetus with effusions in several body cavities, and subcutaneous oedema. This can be caused by fetomaternal blood group incompatibility ('immune') or by a wide range of external or intrinsic problems ('non-immune').

Hypospadias - Urethral opening is sited inferior to the normal position; this may give rise to problems in sexual differentiation.

Intrapartum - Occurring during labour or delivery.

Intraventricular haemorrhage - Blood clot within the ventricles of the brain (usually lateral ventricles) in a preterm baby. Bleeding originates from sinusoidal vessels just beneath the ventricle lining.

Kernicterus	- Clinical condition associated with bilirubin toxicity to the brain. Cerebral nuclei are stained yellow. Late complications include deafness and athetoid cerebral palsy.
Leucomalacia	- Softness and white discolouration of an area of brain due to infarction and death of tissue.
Meconium ileus	- Small intestinal partial obstruction due to abnormally sticky meconium; usually caused by cystic fibrosis.
Microcephaly	- A small head.
Multipara	- A woman who has had previous pregnancies.
Necrotising enterocolitis	- Inflammation of small or large intestine in neonate, sometimes leading to perforation or stricture.
Nullipara	- A woman who has had no previous pregnancies.
Oligohydramnios	- Abnormally decreased volume of amniotic fluid surrounding the unborn baby.
Opisthotonic	- Posture where the neck and back are extended.
Perinatal	- At or around the time of birth, e.g. perinatal mortality = death within 7 days of birth.
Pneumocytes	- Specific differentiated cells lining the small airways and air sacs of the lung. Some produce surfactants.
Polyhydramnios	- An excess in the amount of amniotic fluid.
Preterm	- Delivery before 37 completed weeks of gestation (timed from the last menstrual period).
Pyloric stenosis	- Condition presenting at 2-3 weeks of age with recurrent milk vomiting due to progressive narrowing of stomach outlet. Treated by surgery.

Reye's syndrome	- A rare disorder, usually presenting in infancy characterised by encephalopathy and hepatic dysfunction which may be due to an underlying inherited metabolic disorder.
Rhesus incompatibility	- Baby is affected when IgG antibodies cross the placenta from an immunised but unaffected rhesus negative mother. The antibodies destroy the baby's red blood cells if baby is rhesus positive.
SGA	- Small for gestational age (birth weight criterion).
Surfactant	- An agent reducing surface tension in the lung. A phospholipid with hydrophilic and hydrophobic poles forming a liquid surface lining to alveoli.
Symphyseal-fundal height	- Tape measurement of uterine size in a pregnant women from the pubic symphysis to the top (fundus) of the uterus.
Tocolytic	- A drug or substance given to delay or slow labour.
TORCH screen	- Antibody screen for congenital toxoplasma, rubella, cytomegalovirus and herpes infection.

Index

A

B

D

E

F

G

H